Zaleski   Integrating Device Data into
the Electronic Medical Record

The Author

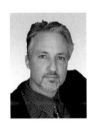

John Zaleski, Ph.D. is Principal Key Expert and Product Manager of the Critical Care product line at the Siemens Medical Solutions USA Health Services Division in Malvern, PA. He has been awarded Innovator of the Year by Siemens Health Services in three different years. He is responsible for coordinating research into leading edge technologies for the purpose of applying these to clinical information systems and medical devices.

Integrating Device Data into the Electronic Medical Record

A Developer's Guide to Design and a
Practitioner's Guide to Application

by John Zaleski, Ph.D.

Publicis Publishing

Bibliographic information published by the Deutsche Nationalbibliothek
The Deutsche Nationalbibliothek lists this publication in
the Deutsche Nationalbibliografie; detailed bibliographic data
are available in the Internet at http://dnb.d-nb.de.

www.publicis.de/books

Contact for authors and editors: gerhard.seitfudem@publicis.de

ISBN 978-3-89578-323-4

Editor: Siemens Aktiengesellschaft, Berlin and Munich
Publisher: Publicis Publishing, Erlangen
© 2009 by Publicis KommunikationsAgentur GmbH, GWA, Erlangen

Printed in Germany

Preface

The idea to write a book on the subject of device integration occurred to me rather suddenly about a year ago. I have been involved in the field of medical information technology and medical integration for well over a decade now. I first cut my teeth interfacing medical devices to computers back in the mid 1990s during my doctoral research days, when it was necessary to collect data automatically from mechanical ventilators as part of my clinical studies. My study of the weaning behavior of coronary artery bypass grafting patients necessitated a complete and accurate record of patient respiratory data and such a complete record was available only through direct connection to the mechanical ventilators in surgical intensive care. As the years passed I became heavily involved in the interactions between electronic medical records and medical device technology—a necessary by-product of the roles I held. I have developed and continue to develop and manage products that support clinical workflow at the point of care, and these require interaction with medical devices. In my current role as product manager for a critical care product line at Siemens, I spend a considerable amount of time and energy in the fielding of medical devices in conjunction with electronic medical records. Therefore, the by-products of physiological measurement and monitoring are keys to assessing patient state. A recent Frost & Sullivan Market Insight article observed that the "most common problem with patient monitoring systems has always been their interoperability."[1]

In writing this text I struggled with the fact that there simply is too much to say on the topic in the limits of a single text to express all points of view, methods, testimonials from the field, and approaches.

As I complete this text efforts continue and evolve in the areas of medical device networking standardization. The proposed IEC 80001 standard, "Risk management of networks incorporating medical devices," is under development. This standard focuses on patient safety and connectivity within the healthcare enterprise networking infrastruc-

---

[1] Gideon V. Praveen Kumar, "Lack of Medical Device Interoperability – Is there a way out?," Frost & Sullivan Market Insight: 15 September 2008.

ture. Connectivity specialists, such as Tim Gee of Medical Connectivity Consulting, describe activities surrounding this standard and the implications for the healthcare enterprise.[2]

No doubt, critical review by those practitioners in the field will find areas requiring greater coverage or different approaches to similar topics based upon diverse experiences. To those critics let me simply say that any omissions were not intentional based on my belief that they were not important, but rather simply that space being limited, this represents in my judgment a first extensive treatment on the subject. I also struggled with single authorship. I imagine that some may suggest a broader array of authors may have provided for a more distilled, wider ranging treatment of the topic. I acknowledge this and humbly submit that I am not suggesting that I have "cornered the market" on intelligence in the area—simply that I believe a single point of view would make for a more homogeneous treatment—all the while recognizing that to the standard practitioner "your mileage may vary." I welcome differing viewpoints and hope to engage in a broader dialogue in the field. Improving our capabilities in this area as an industry will ultimately help every patient and every medical practitioner. Therefore, I see pursuit as a noble goal.

John R. Zaleski, Ph.D.
October 2008

---

[2] Tim Gee, Medical Device Connectivity Consulting, Inc.
http://medicalconnectivity.com/2008/05/26/iec-80001-an-introduction/

Contents

1 The Medical Device Integration Landscape

1.1 Introduction

Data inundate us.

More and more data are presented to us to review, analyze, and digest. We, in turn, generate data from those data in order to produce even more data that others must review, analyze, and digest. In short, we are a data-rich society made more so by ubiquitous computer and software programs. The benefits of data accessibility become obvious as insights drawn from its rapid access make plain in our everyday lives. Gone are the days of paper memoranda, paper facsimile, and even standard telephone calling. Today we have Internet-based communication, Web logs, remote meeting capabilities, and email. The need to be present at a vast majority of business meetings is mitigated by technology—a benefit that impacts other aspects of life and society, to include the ability to reside just about anywhere, thereby minimizing the need to commute to and from specific locations in our workaday lives.

Increasing healthcare costs are a factor in motivating this need. In the United States, national healthcare expenditures are anticipated to grow from just shy of 16.5% to approximately 19.5% (as a percentage of US Gross Domestic Product) in the 10 years from 2007 to 2017[1]. Clearly, providing greater automation and integration of healthcare data is consistent with the need to manage and mitigate these rising costs.

Patient data retrieved from medical devices at the point of care are an important subset of healthcare data. Automating medical device data collection is a logical extension for allied health professionals in that it can be brought to bear to assist in clinical decision making and assist in clinical workflow. However, the need to collect data is also

---

[1] Cinda Becker, "Slow: Budget Danger Ahead." Modern Healthcare. March 3rd, 2008. Pages 6-7.

consistent with the general direction the healthcare industry is taking towards globalizing the use of electronic medical records (EMRs).

What is an EMR? The National Alliance for Health Information Technology developed definitions for various terms, chronicled in its report titled "Defining Key Health Information Technology Terms." Healthcare IT News reported the definitions on several of these, including the EMR. As quoted from this source[2], here is the definition of the Electronic Medical Record as offered by The National Alliance for Health Information Technology:

"Electronic Health Record: An electronic record of health-related information on an individual that conforms to nationally recognized interoperability standards and that can be created, managed, and consulted by authorized clinicians and staff across more than one healthcare organization."

To be clear, in this book I address a specific class of medical devices and communicating their data to the EMR: those associated with vital signs, measurement, respiration, glucose, and general physiological function. Medical image data standards are well documented and are described elsewhere[3]. Data (or, perhaps more accurately, metadata) descriptive of medical imagery can be transmitted to EMRs using a Health Level Seven (HL7) Standard. Patient identification and admission, transfer, and discharge (ADT) messages can be associated with image metadata to enable linking to existing medical imagery. High-resolution medical imagery normally created using magnetic resonance imaging (MRI), X-Ray, or Computed Tomography (CT) equipment typically has very large data storage requirements (Gigabytes to Terabytes) and therefore cannot be practically stored within EMRs. Data about these images (i.e., *metadata*) can be stored but are normally text-based data that identify an image pointer together with patient identifying information.

The ability to access and make use of medical device data begets other uses that were not so obvious when the interest in and ability to retrieve it first became available more than 20 years ago. Such is the creativity, facility, and ingeniousness of the human mind. While aspects of society such as financial institutions, manufacturing, and service sectors have embraced the use of data, it is somewhat surprising that medicine is still in the early stages of implementation. This is

---

[2] Bernie Monegain, "Healthcare IT definitions are in." Healthcare IT News. 05/21/08. http://www.healthcareitnews.com/story.cms?id=9274&page=2

[3] Example: the DICOM Image Standard, available from http://medical.nema.org.

not to say that sophisticated software offerings do not take advantage of the ability to draw upon medical device data to better clinical care. Lags typically exist in the adoption of techniques by healthcare providers (hospital enterprises, physician offices, clinics, etc.) in the use of medical device data. Difficulties with data collection and the knowledge of how to do it is partly to blame. However, there are providers who have embraced and rolled out enterprise-wide software and computing solutions that take full advantage of medical device data collected from patients in the enterprise from the perspective of electronic medical record integration, computerized physician order entry (CPOE), laboratory information systems (LIS), and pharmacy (Rx) systems (to name a few). These individual subsystems, taken together in their collective whole, become what has been commonly referred to as a health information system (HIS) or computerized health record (CHR) that incorporates the sum total of all information available on any given patient within a health enterprise.

While critically important to patient care, these subsystems are not the primary focus of this book. Rather, my focus is to discuss medical device data, their measurement, and how their collection can be accomplished and used to assist in forming the basic understanding of patient state—i.e., the condition of the patient. Findings and measurements—how they are collected, displayed, used, and assessed—are key pieces of evidence for guiding the treatment of disease.

Before proceeding, definitions are necessary. The term electronic medical record, or EMR, is defined as a computerized repository of medical data consisting of patient findings, physiological information, identifying and demographic information, medications, diagnoses, orders, etc.

Definitions of EMR abound[4,5] which further qualify this definition based upon content and purpose. While these are recognized, the definition provided above will establish the basis for the analysis to follow and can be mapped into other definitions as need be. A drilldown into the details of the electronic medical record is the subject of Chapter 5.

In essence, the focus of this book is the mechanics of data acquisition, review, analysis, and presentation to the physician, nurse, and other

---

[4] Thomas J. Handler, M.D.,"Magic Quadrant for U.S. Enterprise CPRs, 2007," Gartner Industry Research ID Number G00152518; 31 October 2007.

[5] Wes Rishel, Thomas J. Handler, M.D., Jonathan Edwards, "A Clear Definition of the Electronic Health Record," Gartner Industry Research, ID Number G00130927, 4 October 2005.

allied health professionals (respiratory therapists, technicians, home health aides, etc.) who make up the team of care providers for any given patient. When I speak of medical device data I am referring primarily to that used in normal physiological measurement or assessments, such as blood pressure, temperature, pulse, etc., and on the periodic measurement and analysis of physiological parameters used in guiding patient care.

Gartner Industry Research[6] advises that medical device management & standardization currently reside (2007) at the peak of the industry hype cycle, and growth will occur in the field of medical device interface development and use in medicine as an important adjunct and enabler of clinical workflow and patient care management. Gartner further recognizes that the path ahead in the area of device integration is still not entirely clear in terms of the evolutionary roadmap. As a result, one of their key recommendations is to focus on interoperability as industry standards continue to evolve. This is an important point, because the lack of universal adoption of concise and clear standards is a key reason why medical device data collection is still not the norm in many, if not most, healthcare enterprises.

The use of medical device data for patient care is expanding as a result of the call to improve workflow in the clinical environment. Faster response to patient complaints, improved delivery of care, and reducing errors during treatment are but a few reasons why this value is recognized. The value proposition in medical device integration to the EMR is that it enables complex clinical workflow implementations, enhances patient care management, ensures data accuracy, and reduces the latency in recording data from devices when patients are in highly technologically dependent states, such as the case in intensive care units (ICUs).

Gartner also acknowledges the use of proprietary interface protocols between individual medical devices and the EMR. They suggest that medical device integration systems[7]:

"1) Provide physical or Internet Protocol-based connectivity to the instrument;

---

[6] Barry Runyon et al., "Hype Cycle for Healthcare Provider Technologies and Standards, 2007." Gartner Industry Research. ID Number: G00148328. Publication Date: 11 July 2007. Page 16.

[7] Barry Runyon et al., "Hype Cycle for Healthcare Provider Technologies and Standards, 2007." Gartner Industry Research. ID Number: G00148328. Publication Date: 11 July 2007. Page 36.

2) Map between the instrument proprietary data format and a format that works for the CPR [e.g. Health Level 7];

3) Provide a means to select representative data for charting;

4) Provide buffering to continue the data capture when the CPR is unavailable; and

5) Provide at least some support for adding patient ID information to the stream coming from the instrument."

The need for seamless and straightforward medical device data integration will grow as the population ages. Patients with chronic illnesses will of necessity require devices to assist in managing diabetes, chronic obstructive pulmonary disease (COPD), heart disease, cancer, and others. The aging population will require and benefit more fully from the ability to monitor and manage chronic health problems from the comfort of home. Indeed, devices that measure basic physiological parameters necessary for diagnostics and therapeutics provide invaluable data for management, prevention, and monitoring of disease. Specific measurement instruments that are often used for home health monitoring include flow meters, glucometers, blood pressure and pulse oximetry monitors, medication tracking meters, and cholesterol monitors[8].

In addition, medical device integration into the EMR provides other benefits, including simplifying analysis and clinical decision support assessments, automated charting, and, as we will see later on in Chapter 10, establishing the basic foundation for automatic control of medical equipment at the bedside and simplifying clinical documentation and charting. Some of these functions, and strategic as well as tactical benefits, have been described in the literature of the American College of Clinical Engineering[9]. Medical device integration is receiving much more attention within senior management in healthcare enterprises. Indeed, Gartner[10] suggests that

> *"...the CIO will take on more responsibility for medical device oversight and ultimately will bring the associated biomedical engineering staff under the office of the CIO."*

---

[8] Shekar Rao, "Prognosis for Medical Electronics—Growth and Technology Convergence," 9th Texas Instruments Developer Conference India, 30 Nov – 1 Dec 2006, Bangalore.

[9] Stephen L. Grimes, "Convergence of Clinical Engineering and Information Technology," College of Healthcare Information Management Executives, August 24th, 2006. Pages 9, 35.

[10] Barry Runyon, et al. "Hype Cycle for Healthcare Provider Applications and Systems, 2007." Gartner Industry Research. ID Number: G00148329. 11 July 2007. Page 25.

Furthermore, technological advances in networking, improvements in positive patient identification, and the uses of barcodes and radio frequency identification (RFID) will further enhance automated data collection as they will enable near error-free association of patient data with patient identity, thereby facilitating automatic data capture.

Positive patient identification is a subject that will be addressed more fully in Chapter 8, where methods and technologies will be discussed.

The Joint Commission Perspectives on Patient Safety reported that "incorrect patient identification was involved in 13% of surgical errors and 67% of transfusion errors."[11] Gartner reported a study at a single Florida hospital in which an error rate of 4.4% was associated with transcribing vitals parameters data into the EMR[12].

1.2 Medical Device Integration Landscape

Medical devices for vitals measurement span the range from single value to multi-measurement, network-enabled machines. Figure 1-1, influenced by the work of Norgall[13], illustrates medical device technology dimensions along three axes each representing the evolving states of connectivity, access to data, and device complexity. The simplest of devices and interfaces are those shown closest to the origin, with increasing complexity further out along the axes.

Three key features of any medical device are

- the type of device and the complexity of the measurements it produces, and
- the data it measures and transmits externally,
- the method by which it communicates to external systems.

These are reflected in the three axes of Figure 1-1: Data, Device, and Connectivity Technology.

Beginning with the Data axis, the simplest of measurement devices, such as home-care meters including glucometers, stethoscopes, or

---

[11] "Technology in Patient Safety: Using Identification Bands to Reduce Patient Identification Errors." Joint Commission Perspectives on Patient Safety, April 2005, Volume 5, Issue 4. Page 1.

[12] Wes Rishel, "The Evolving Market for Universal Medical Device Busses." Gartner Industry Research. ID Number: G00149688. 26 June 2007. Page 2.

[13] Thomas Norgall, "Interoperability and Medical Device Communication Standardization," Fraunhofer-Institut fuer Integrierte Schaltungen—Angewandte Elektronik; Erlangen, Germany; 10-12 October 2002; Slide 3.

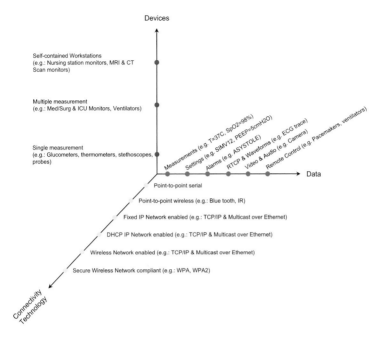

Figure 1-1 Medical device domain with ever increasing complexity

simple non-invasive blood pressure measurement cuffs, all measure one or two parameters discretely. The parameters typically will not contain personal identifying information and some of the data that are measured may not even have time or date stamps. These are the most basic of measurement devices.

Moving further along the axis we arrive at devices that accept specific settings, including thresholds. Some of the more sophisticated glucometers and multi-parameter measurement devices (cholesterol meters, blood pressure cuffs) fall into this category.

Next, devices that sound and transmit alarms are indicated. These devices typically produce an alert when a specific user-defined threshold is exceeded. Devices residing within this class of medical device can include ad hoc point of care monitors. The measurements obtained from these devices may be queried continuously.

Moving further out we arrive at devices that support real-time streaming protocol (RTSP) transactions. ICU monitors, mechanical ventilators, and infusion pumps are in this category. Continuous waveforms are produced and transmitted using a proprietary protocol along a high-speed network to a nursing station or other end-user

15

device that displays results, waveforms, and alarms that can indicate life-threatening problems.

Live video and audio communication can be included within the realm of real-time communication, together with the real-time control of medical devices from a remote location. Although automatic control system theory is used internally to medical devices in the management of systems vital to patients, generally available forms of external automatic control, whereby medical devices are controlled remotely and automatically in response to user input, are still a long way away. For example, automatically controlled weaning algorithms that can be adjusted by allied health professionals from afar (possibly through a Web portal over a hospital enterprise network). The use of such methodologies are beginning to be considered for the monitoring and maintenance of patients in a controlled environment, such as ventilated patients being weaned according to a specific protocol. Such functionality would reside within the realm of expert systems. In the future, routine or redundant activities may be automated as the level of acceptability and confidence in such systems grows through continued use, validated through extensive clinical trials.

Certain implantable pacemakers allow for bi-directional communication in which pacemaker settings can be adjusted using an external device that communicates transdermally. Data can also be downloaded from these devices.

Proceeding along the Device axis we evolve from discrete single measurements through multiple measurements and to self-contained workstations. Single measurement devices are those that are designed for a specific, single task (temperature, glucose, etc.) Multiple measurement devices provide a collection, or vector, of measurements that describe many aspects of the patient state. Critical care telemetry monitors, mechanical ventilators, and infusion pumps typically fall into this category. Surgical monitors can also be considered as a multi-measurement device.

Beyond this realm lies the region of self-contained workstations: devices that can collect measurements and also perform on-line analysis of measurement data. Nursing workstations, MRI and CT Scan systems populate this region. However, telemetry monitors are moving into this area as their level of sophistication advances.

In terms of the level of sophistication associated with connectivity technology, these have evolved, as well.

Looking at the Connectivity axis of Figure 1-1 we see the evolution from simple point-to-point communication using a physical serial interface up through network-enabled technology. Whether wired or wireless technology is used for point-to-point communication, such as infrared (IR) communication devices or Bluetooth, these communication technologies are differentiated from large-scale networking protocols in that they support communication of (primarily) one device to one computing client and checks on data integrity are performed to ensure data integrity.

True data redundancy and delivery checking occurs once we enter the domain of Ethernet via Transmission Control Protocol / Internet Protocol (TCP/IP) communication. Here, TCP/IP is the preferred protocol due to its verified delivery mechanism. Many medical monitors communicate patient critical information to nursing stations using TCP/IP but use a less reliable mechanism, such as User Datagram Protocol (UDP), which I refer to as "fire and forget." This form of transmission does not verify packet delivery. Oftentimes multicast transmission is used as a broadcast mechanism within a networking subnet to enable devices to communicate with each other.

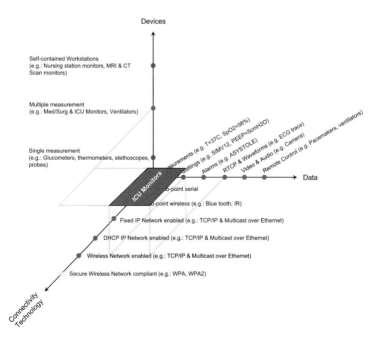

Figure 1-2 Range of technologies and measurements represented by typical ICU monitors

Most of the sophisticated telemetry monitors today communicate via wired or wireless TCP/IP over Ethernet. They do so using fixed or static Internet Protocol (IP) addressing.

Figure 1-2 illustrates the span or range of technologies typically associated with critical care telemetry monitors.

Critical care telemetry monitors collect a wide range of measurements (i.e., multi-measurement devices) and provide the capability to set thresholds which establish acceptable range limits corresponding to alarm triggers. The range of communication technologies span fixed IP wired to fixed IP wireless communication. By contrast, we can compare a typical single-parameter measurement device, such as a glucometer, with the ICU monitor. This is illustrated in Figure 1-3.

A limitation of these simple devices is their native inability to be networked within a large enterprise—this severely limits widespread and standardized data integration with the EMR. The scalability of devices having only point-to-point connectivity can be extended by bringing in third-party network extenders. One such example is the Moxa Tech-

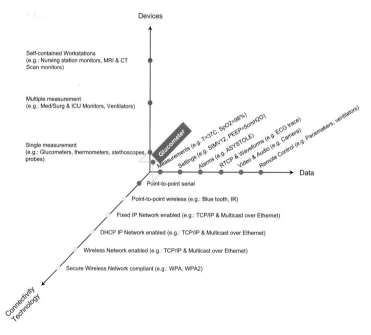

Figure 1-3 Single parameter measurement device using point-to-point communication

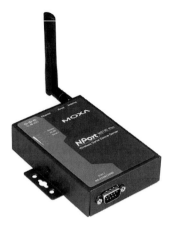

Figure 1-4
Moxa Technologies NPort W2150
Wireless 802.11g to Serial adapter
(Courtesy Moxa Technologies,
used with permission)

nologies *Airworks* device illustrated in Figure 1-4. I will cover devices such as these in Chapters 2 and 3.

In the case of point-to-point devices that employ serial communication interfaces, these can be extended to attach to existing (standard) Ethernet networks using a device like the one shown in Figure 1-4. The state of this technology is such that communications can be supported in an 802.11 wireless environment and serial devices—those normally isolated to lab or small networks—can now be accessed throughout the enterprise remotely.

In reviewing the current and future needs of medical device measurement technologies, Figure 1-5 (via the arrows) provides a high-level assessment of where the industry should focus. The arrows in the diagram identify the gaps in current technology but also show areas of needed future focus.

The use of single, multiple, and workstation data collection and measurement devices will and must continue in order to meet future patient care management needs. Advances in the complexity and sophistication of data analysis, clinical decision support, and workflow methods will also require seamless, automated, and continuous data integration to the EMR, thus motivating more rapid integration solutions.

The ability to both receive data and to control medical devices will continue. This will occur both organically and out of business need: medical hardware and software manufacturers recognize this today and collaboration between hardware manufacturers and software developers will increase as the solution will involve both—the soft-

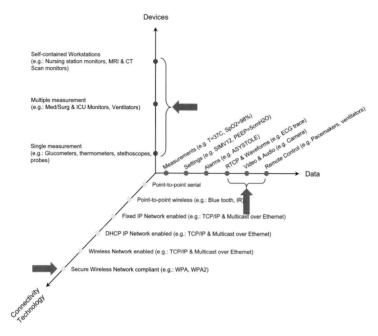

Figure 1-5 Areas of future technology capability and growth for measurement devices

ware will become integrated and fully coupled with the medical device. Stethoscopes, glucometers, ventilators, and similar devices are already migrating in this direction.

To ensure data integrity and security, medical device manufacturers will need to evolve their physical communication standards to align more with those of the communication & networking industry. The FDA[14] has already weighed in on this subject with a draft guideline focusing specifically on wireless technology and the need for standardization requirements that must be met as part of the regulatory evaluation and certification process of medical devices that rely on this technology.

Finally, standards-based application-level communication such as HL7 will continue to grow and become the common "language" by which medical device manufacturers enable transaction exchange between device level "gateways" and existing clinical repositories.

---

[14] "Draft Guidance for Industry and FDA Staff—Radio-Frequency Wireless Technology in Medical Devices," http://www.fda.gov/cdrh/osel/guidance/1618.html

Future areas of monitoring can include noninvasive ischemic stroke monitoring, prosthetic monitoring, monitoring for congestive heart failure, bed monitoring for patient movement, weight, and fowler angle, infusion pumps, intra-arterial balloon pumps, and beyond[15]. A discussion, along with examples of the details of device communication, is the subject of Chapter 2.

1.3 Evolving Standards in Medical Device Communication (IEEE/ISO & MD PnP™)

Standards and working groups focusing on medical device interface standardization have been in existence for years and have endeavored to establish a common architectural, data, application, and communication framework for device connectivity with computer-based information systems and with each other.

The challenge remains to enable common interfaces to secure information while protecting it from unauthorized or hostile access. The Workgroup on Electronic Data Interchange (WEDI) and other standards-setting organizations such as X12, Health Level 7 (HL7), the American Society for Testing and Materials (ASTM), the National Institute for Standards and Technology (NIST), the Computer-based Patient Record Institute (CPRI); and various associations such as Healthcare Financial Management Association (HFMA) and the Association for Electronic Health Care Transactions (AFEHCT) are involved in establishing standards both for data interchange between and among different systems and also the security policies associated with protecting those data. Independent researchers and academic institutions are also engaged in research to align on common standards[16,17,18]. While manufacturers of medical hardware and software are engaged in the production of next-generation technologies to support and enhance clinical diagnosis and treatment, they must also dedicate time and effort to enabling their systems to communicate according to these new standards.

---

[15] Shekar Rao, "Prognosis for Medical Electronics—Growth and Technology Convergence," 9th Texas Instruments Developer Conference India, 30 Nov – 1 Dec 2006, Bangalore.

[16] Richard Schrenker and Todd Cooper, "Building the Foundation for Medical Device Plug-and-Play Interoperability." Medical Electronics Manufacturing. April 2001.

[17] http://mdpnp.org

[18] Richard A. Schrenker, "Software Engineering for Future Healthcare and Clinical Systems." Computer, Published by the IEEE Computer Society. April 2006.

The Institute of Electrical and Electronics Engineers (IEEE) along with the International Standards Organization (ISO) have proffered standards and working groups that are investigating and evolving the area of universal interoperability. The IEEE 1073 standard which has essentially been supplanted by the IEEE/ISO 11073/20601 standards have made important strides towards achieving this standardization. The Medical Device "Plug-and-Play" Interoperability Program is pursuing open standards leading to seamless, universal connectivity among medical devices and systems[19]. MD PnP™ was initiated by Massachusetts General Hospital and the Center for Integration of Medicine & Innovative Technology (CIMIT)[20]. This is an interdisciplinary program focusing on medical device interoperability to improve patient safety and workflow-related efficiency. In short, the MD PnP™ program is championing standards adoption, positing the regulatory path to facilitate adoption by the larger manufacturing community, among others, and working towards providing a proof-of-principle laboratory for demonstrating and eliciting requirements related to medical device connectivity.

In the area of Connectivity Technology, I have combined two concepts together: that of physical connectivity and data integrity. At its most basic, data are collected typically via serial connection according to specific standards ("Standard for Medical Device Communications—Transport Profile—IrDA Based—Cable Connected", IEEE 1073.3.2, for example). These are point-to-point connections with no verification of transmission beyond the basic hardware layer and no validation of role or data integrity.

The IEEE 11073 standards provide for an evolving framework around the enablement of medical device communication with computer-based health information systems. The goals, as enunciated in the standards, are[21]:

1) Provide real-time plug-and-play interoperability for patient-connected medical devices; and,

2) Facilitate the efficient exchange of vital signs and medical device data, acquired at the point-of-care, in all health care environments.

Versions of these standards in draft form are in review and date as recently as February 2008. These standards describe recommended

---

[19] Information available at http://mdpnp.org/Home_Page.html

[20] Information available at http://www.cimit.org

[21] International Standard ISO/IEEE 11073, Health Informatics—Point-of-care medical device communication—parts 10101, 10201, 20101, 30200, 30300; First Edition 2004-12-15

communication mechanisms associated with cable-connected devices, infrared (IrDA) devices, and interconnectivity speeds (e.g.: baud rates, stop bits, link disconnect timing, etc.)

The primary collection of these standards is described briefly below:

- ISO/IEEE 11073-10101 standard describes common nomenclature, syntax, and terminology for identifying findings and vitals parameters. This standard describes the nomenclature architecture for medical device communication at-point-of-care (APOC);[22]

- ISO/IEEE 11073-10201 standard proposes a domain information model describing medical device data attributes and their structure for communicating with external systems[23];

- ISO/IEEE 11073-20101 standard proposes application-level communication profiles including medical device encoding rules (MDER), allocation of object identifiers, time synchronization protocols, state transition, and some sample code segments for implementing these[24];

- ISO/IEEE 11073-30200 standard describes suggested connectivity for cable connected communication, including RS-232, RJ45, and others[25]. This standard discusses details such as medical information bus (MIB) cable lengths using CAT-5 cable[26]. Signaling speeds are suggested relating to serial transport, both through cables and via infrared; for example, signaling speeds of 9600 bits per second, data size in any received frame of 64 octets, and link disconnect times of 3 seconds[27]; and finally

- ISO/IEEE 11073-30300 focuses on infrared wireless connectivity. The IrDA physical communication and architecture are described here[28].

---

[22] International Standard ISO/IEEE 11073-10101; Health Informatics—Point-of-care medical device communication—Part 10101: Nomenclature. First Edition 2004-12-15

[23] International Standard ISO/IEEE 11073-10201; Health Informatics—Point-of-care medical device communication—Part 10201: Domain Information Model. First Edition 2004-12-15

[24] International Standard ISO/IEEE 11073-20101; Health informatics—Point-of-care medical device communication—Part 20101: Application profiles—Base standard. First edition 2004-12-15

[25] International Standard ISO/IEEE 11073-30200; Health informatics—Point-of-care medical device communication—Part 30200: Transport profile—Cable connected. First edition 2004-12-15

[26] Ibid.

[27] Ibid.

[28] International Standard ISO/IEEE 11073-30300; Health informatics—Point-of-care medical device communication—Part 30300: Transport profile—Infrared wireless

Since the medical device plug-and-play initiative was launched, the focus of MD PnP™ has been on integrating these devices into a clinical environment in the context of use cases that are specific to application at the point-of-care. An important extension of this vision is that of enabling individual medical devices to seamlessly communicate with one another[29].

The work in the standards arena is extremely important and must continue. Enabling seamless communication among medical devices is a noble goal. Pragmatically, though, the state of the situation as it exists today is far from being standardized. This is one reason I decided to write this book. The fact today is that the standards related to electrical connectivity, networking, suggested data modeling, and nomenclature are necessary components relating to the overall goal of achieving universal medical device communication. But adoption aside, the details of the data content, and the query-response mechanisms of the health information systems that retrieve the data and validate for the purposes of storage within the EMR, have practical business implications in terms of costs to implement. The adoption, recognition, and creation of common data communications software and models will require extensive development efforts; the modification of medical hardware and firmware to conform to these standards must occur; and alignment between industry and healthcare enterprises on the specific needs and content of the interface specifications must occur. All of these can happen, and will happen eventually. But in the meantime, the problem of medical device data integration into an EMR remains. Participation in the standards organizations and working towards an accepted and sufficiently-detailed standard must occur in parallel with pragmatic device integration. For the present, the 'sub-optimal' methods for data integration using third-party software and hardware must still be used to achieve the end result in the operational environment. This work cannot stop while a standard is being developed, balloted, approved, and adopted.

While standards are necessary for assuring continuity and consistency, the use of common data models by manufacturers for extracting data from medical devices must also evolve towards consistency. As I will show in Chapter 2, devices performing the same functions may even have different data definitions and some medical devices may not even produce the same results (that is, may produce variants of the same data or additional data that are not produced by medical

---

[29] "'Plug and Play' Connectivity Initiative Launched." AAMI News. Vol. 40, No. 1 January 2005.

devices even supporting similar functions). For instance, two mechanical ventilators may be queried for values related to respiratory rate. One ventilator may provide an inspiratory and expiratory value while another may only provide an average between the two values. The aforementioned standards describe recommended communications mechanisms and data models for medical devices. Yet, currently, devices specify differing syntax, communication rate, and even physical access mechanisms.

1.4 Data Integration: A First Look

Figure 1-6 illustrates the process flow involved in the basic storage of medical device data as they are collected manually by a clinician. This process flow is oftentimes referred to as a scenario—a descriptive sequence of events that capture the steps involved in achieving the goals of a use case, which can be described as an overall model of system and user interaction to achieve a specific goal.[30,31] While greatly simplified, the essence of the process is as follows.

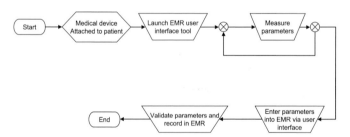

Figure 1-6 A simple functional representation of the manual data entry and EMR storage processes

In the example provided, an EMR tool—such as a system involving a user interface that allows on-line, manual interaction—provides the means for an allied health professional (typically, a physician, nurse, respiratory therapist, or technician) to enter data measurements obtained from a patient. For example, a user interface as part of a

[30] Allen Holub, "OO design process: Use cases, an introduction," IBM on-line article, 01 Dec 2000, http://www.ibm.com/developerworks/java/library/co-design5.html.

[31] http://en.wikipedia.org/wiki/Use_case.

medical application operating on a laptop computer would provide data entry fields for blood pressure, temperature, and pulse. The user "attaches" a medical device to a patient (such as a blood pressure cuff), launches an EMR user interface tool into which data can be manually entered, measures and reads the parameter using the medical device, enters the parameter into the user interface, validates the parameter to affirm that it is a true recording of the measurement from the medical device, and then transmits the newly measured value to the EMR for storage and later retrieval and review.

Within Figure 1-6, the summing junction is added to indicate that more than one parameter can be measured. Once all parameters are collected they are transmitted together as a finding to the EMR. In our simple example of blood pressure, pulse, and temperature, these three values, taken together, comprise the finding. They become part of the patient medical record once validated by a health professional. They define specific, quantitative physiological measurements of patient state at the time of measurement.

The finding establishes what I will refer to as a data "vector" of patient physiological findings, otherwise termed "vitals" measured on a particular date and at a particular time, t:

$$FindingsVector(t) = \{BP, HR, T, \cdots, t\}$$

where BP is patient blood pressure typically represented as the ratio of systolic and diastolic components (usually measured in millimeters of mercury—mmHg), HR is pulse or heart rate (measured in beats per minute), T is temperature (measured in either Celsius or Fahrenheit), and t is the date/time stamp of the measurements. Each value can be compared with normally accepted ranges to determine their compliance.

The process of measuring and reviewing these findings is part of findings validation—the process by which measurements are determined to be accurate, true, and representative of the patient physiological state at the time of measurement. The validation process is critical as it affirms the confidence in the validity of the measurements. Thus, while physiological measurement data are necessary, bad data are useless: a blood pressure measurement taken while a patient is moving about or agitated is not indicative of a resting value and is not a valid indicator of true resting blood pressure. This also applies to pulse measurement (unless a patient is undergoing a stress test). Hence, the patient's environment and status is important as it establishes the context in which the finding was measured. The user interface to the EMR is illustrated in the notional diagram of Figure 1-7.

The notional diagram depicts several user interface "tabs" located vertically on the left side of the user interface. This serves to illustrate that different forms of data may be stored in the EMR. Those shown are examples and include laboratory data (e.g., complete blood count or blood gas information) and patient medications.

The user interface is the entry point for findings. The clinician, via this point of entry, validates the findings. Once the clinician enters parameter values a method of entry and transmission is then provided ("Enter" button) to cause the results to be written to the EMR. Because the finding is entered manually, the health professional is afforded the opportunity to correct parameters as necessary in the event of error or changes to physiological state should invalidate a particular measurement.

Once the "Enter" button is pressed the process of storing the finding occurs when the data are transmitted to the EMR for storage and later retrieval and review. This completes the simple process of storage within the electronic medical record. Although greatly simplified,

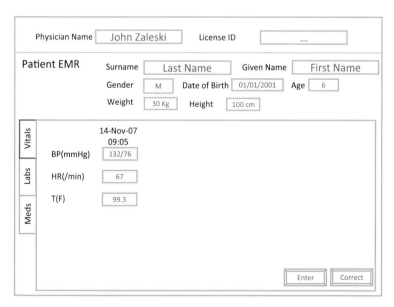

Figure 1-7 A notional depiction of a generic EMR user interface display into which parameters are entered manually by a health professional

this process serves to illustrate the essentials of data retrieval. Most electronic medical records and health information systems provide for much more complicated functionality.[32]

Various developers of electronic medical records and health information systems today provide the essential features described in the example here.[33] Accurate and timely medical record data recording is essential to clinical decision making. Hence, mechanisms for medical device data measurement and storage within the electronic medical record enable a better longitudinal understanding of a patient's state.

The process for viewing already-existing information within the clinical record in much simplified form is illustrated in Figure 1-8.

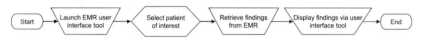

Figure 1-8 A simple functional diagram representing the process for retrieving patient findings from the EMR

A user interface tool provides the health professional with the ability to select a patient of interest from those within the EMR. The patient is selected and the findings are retrieved and displayed. Details have been left out of this process flow, including user authentication, which are necessary but outside the scope of this current discussion. Rather, this process is taken up at the point where the user has "logged" into the EMR system. Authentication and role-based access are assumed.

Once authenticated, the user may be provided with a census list of patients for whom the health professional is authorized to review. The user then selects one particular patient from within the census list. This triggers the retrieval of that particular patient's EMR. The medical record might depict the information in Figure 1-9 together with older results that can be reviewed in comparison, just as in the case of legacy paper charting of medical records. Figure 1-9 shows the comparison with a previously measured finding. The health professional can view the data historically and comparatively so as to obtain a view

---

[32] For example: Siemens Soarian® Clinicals Health Information System.

[33] Examples of developers of health information systems that feature robust electronic medical records include Cerner, Epic, GE, McKesson, Meditech and Siemens.

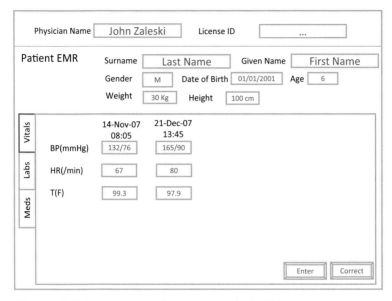

Figure 1-9 Update showing prior data stored in the EMR

of patient "state" change over time. In the instance shown here this patient's blood pressure rose over a period of approximately 5 weeks.

The purpose in showing this example is to establish a common basis for understanding the underlying processes and work flows inherent in measurement and recording of findings. The primary differences between paper chart recording and electronic recording has been reduced to the medium used for the task—that is, paper versus a virtual user interface and computer database access application. While paper charting has worked for decades as the standard for clinical charting, in the age of electronic media the process of automating the collection of medical device data is a natural extension.

In the case of simple medical charting in which discrete findings are recorded during the course of a patient visit, the data comprise only a small portion of the patient EMR. Recording such values manually becomes a trivial undertaking. In non-emergent environments in which patient findings need be recorded only on an ad-hoc basis and in limited quantity, entering measurements into an EMR for later retrieval and analysis is straightforward and demands very little time or effort on the part of the clinician either to enter parameter values initially or to retrieve and review them. The benefits of automating the process of findings collection become apparent when the scale is increased in terms of quantities of measurements and number of parameters in a finding. Improved data security and accuracy are also realized by automating the medical device data collection process.

Consider the sampling of patient findings in Table 1-1. While not a complete list, these parameters make up a subset of those patient

Table 1-1 Sample patient findings recorded by health professional during a typical stay in an ICU

Finding Name	Symbol	Description	Typical Values (adults)
Systolic Pressure	SP	Arterial pressure measured during contraction	120-140 mmHg
Diastolic Pressure	DP	Arterial pressure measured at the end of the cardiac cycle	80-95 mmHg
Mean Arterial Pressure	MAP	Mean component of blood pressure, estimated as DP + 0.333 x (SP - DP)	90-110 mmHg
Stroke Volume	SV	Volume of blood pumped by heart in one contraction	40-70 ml/m^2
Cardiac Output	Q	Volume of blood pumped by heart in one minute	2.4-4 liters/minute
Respiratory Rate	Resp	Quantity of inhalations and exhalations per minute	12-20 /min
Pulse	HR	Quantity of left ventricular contractions per minute	60-100 /min
Arterial pH	pH	Blood acidity / alkalinity index	7.33-7.49
Temperature	T	Body Temperature	36-38C
Inspired O2 Fraction	FiO2	Fraction of O2 contained in inspired gas (ventilated or masked patients)	21-100%
Tidal Volume	Vt	Volume of gas inspired in a single breath	5-7 ml/Kg
Minute Volume	Ve	Volume of gas inspired in a single minute	5-7 liters/minute
O2 Saturation	SpO2, SaO2	Percentage of oxygenated hemoglobin, measured via pulse oximetry or blood gas	>95%
Positive End-Expiratory Pressure	PEEP	Residual pressure maintained in lungs at the end of spontaneous expiration, typically employed as a technique to maintain gas in lungs at end of expiration	5-10 cmH2O
End Tidal CO2	etCo2	Measure of carbon dioxide determined on the expiratory side of intubated and non-intubated patients (for instance) correlated to changes in cardiac output and used to estimate low cardiac output or to establish a measure of respiratory viability in mechanically ventilated patients.	35-45 mmHg

parameters monitored during a stay in an intensive care unit (ICU). These represent only the key cardiovascular and respiratory findings that are typically available from in-room patient monitors.[34]

Other findings include laboratory data, infusion pump data, patient intake and output fluid data (intake being partially comprised of infusion data), and notes recorded by allied health professionals (e.g.: physicians, nurses, respiratory therapists). In the past, findings were recorded in a paper flow sheet in the ICU. The process of recording patient vitals consumes a large quantity of nursing time as they are updated many times per hour. Standard nursing care involves monitoring devices for the purpose of collection, identification, assessment, and treatment of the patient. This can be a daunting task. A seemingly obvious answer to capturing the readily available data is to automate its collection by providing a means to transmit it directly into the electronic medical record. The quantity of data recorded becomes obvious especially as data collection frequency increases. This is apparent from Figure 1-10 in which the quantity of findings is shown parametrically against the data collection frequency, assuming the simple list of 15 findings shown in Table 1-1 is the base set of those to be recorded over a 24 hour period.

The amount of data that must be recorded becomes time consuming, requiring the complete attention of the health professional, even to the point of possibly impacting patient care. The frequency of data collection causes the nurse to focus on the role of a scribe for informa-

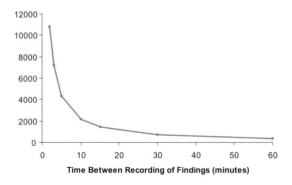

Figure 1-10 Quantity of findings recorded in the medical record over a 24 hour period as a function of collection frequency

---

[34] Paul L. Marino, The ICU Book, 2nd Edition, Williams & Wilkins, 1998; Pages 4, 271, 367, 470, 876.

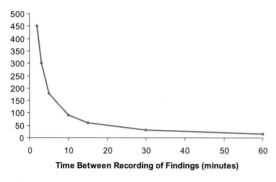

Figure 1-11 Data recorded on a typical patient over one hour
(with 15 findings per entry)

tion readily available from bedside telemetry monitors, laboratory data, and ancillary equipment. Because this places a burden on the health professional, a balance must be achieved in the frequency with which data are recorded without dominating the valuable time which must be devoted to patient care. Typical data recording intervals are approximately once every 15 minutes, or 4 findings entries per hour. The quantity of data recorded in a single hour is shown in Figure 1-11.

Concerns also exist with recording accuracy. Erroneous recording of data, while unfortunate, does occur.

In a typical ICU, the process of recording findings occurs around the clock. Because of the manual interaction and the intensity of the ICU environment it becomes inevitable that errors can and do occur, especially in the process of transcribing findings from bedside monitors to paper records or an EMR. A hypothetical assessment of the number of errors in the recording of findings during a 24 hour stay in the ICU is illustrated by Figure 1-12. Given a 1% likelihood of recording a finding in error (i.e., a nurse records findings correctly and accurately 99% of the time) the number of errors expected to be recorded within the medical record is approximately 15. If, instead, a 5% likelihood of recording an error is the norm (i.e., a nurse records findings correctly and accurately 95% of the time) the number of errors expected to be recorded within the medical record is approximately 72. Mathematically, these may be expressed as:

$$E\{error = 1\% \,|\, 24hours\} = 14.4$$

$$E\{error = 5\% \,|\, 24hours\} = 72$$

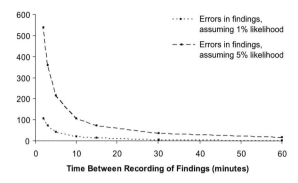

Figure 1-12 Expected error rate over a 24 hour period associated with the recording of findings versus recording interval

Neither of these expected values is necessarily an indication of what will absolutely occur, but rather what may occur in a typical encounter within the ICU with a patient over a normal 24 hour period. Of course, this is an estimate of error rate based only on the recording of findings. This does not take into account medication errors and other errors that may be independent of the analysis above—but which also have some correlation to errors in recording of medical device parameter data. The accurate recording of information is recognized in the industry and has been codified. Items 9 and 14 of the 30 safe practices[35] for improved healthcare identify explicitly under the subsection for Facilitating Information Transfer and Clear Communication state that:

> "...care information, especially changes in orders and new diagnostic information, [must be] transmitted in a timely and clearly understandable form to all of the patient's current health care providers who need that information to provide care..." and

> "...standardized protocols to prevent the occurrence of wrong-site or wrong-patient procedures [should be implemented]."

Errors can cost lives and money. The Institute of Medicine (IOM) report estimated the total cost of preventable adverse events to be approximately $17 billion[36]. These represented between 2% and 4%

---

[35] Agency for Healthcare Research and Quality, "30 Safe Practices for Better Health Care." AHRQ Publication No. 05-P007. Current as of March 2005.

[36] Linda T. Kohn, Janet M. Corrigan, Molla S. Donaldson, editors, "To Err Is Human: Building a Safer Health System (2000)," Institute of Medicine & National Academy Press. Page 41.

of U.S. national health expenditures in 1996[37]. The report refers to a study of 1,047 patients admitted to two intensive care units at large teaching hospitals where 45.8% were "identified as having an adverse event" related to or defined as "situations in which an inappropriate decision was made when, at the time, [an] appropriate alternative could have been chosen."[38]

While the bulk of these errors are related to artifacts surrounding medication error administration, a subcategory within these was identified as inadequate monitoring and documenting patient information, such as findings and responses[39]. The point must be underscored that the root cause of errors being projected here is not only because of incorrect recording of data, but rather the entire process, or system, for monitoring the patient in general. Health professionals can be notified more rapidly when clinical information is available for analysis within the EMR. More timely, complete, and accurate information can translate into notifications to clinicians of adverse events whereby multiple care providers can review and be made cognizant of patient status. Such information has historically remained within the "data island" of the monitoring device or the subsystem responsible for directly interacting with the patient (e.g.: infusion pumps, bedside vitals monitors and mechanical ventilators, etc.).

Once data from these devices can be made available within the EMR, then care providers have a means of accessing this information from anywhere within the health enterprise, thereby enabling more thorough and complete review by individuals spanning the spectrum of care for any given patient (i.e., therapists, nurses, physicians). The need for device-level data integration becomes obvious especially in large healthcare enterprises wherein health professionals may be widely distributed and unable to be present at the bedside of a patient for extended periods of time. Intensive care units, medical/surgical wards, post-operative acute care units, operating theatres, emergency departments, and in certain situations, home-health environments all can benefit from medical device integration for these reasons.

The challenge remains taking information at the point of care and developing a universal mechanism for migrating it into the EMR, as illustrated in Figure 1-13. Many devices provide information (data)

---

[37] Ibid. Page 27.

[38] Ibid., page 31.

[39] Ibid., pages 36, 38.

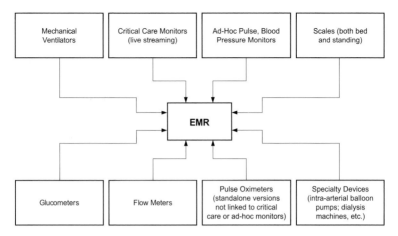

Figure 1-13 Examples of medical device findings transmitted to the electronic medical record

communication mechanisms. These will be discussed later on. The device data must be downloaded and communicated to a processor that can format them for standardized transmission and storage within the EMR. Central collection points, or devices hubs, can provide a single point of connectivity to the EMR.

The purpose of the device hub is to perform query-response communication to the medical instrumentation. This mechanism involves requesting data asynchronously from each device using its own proprietary "language." To date, most devices communicate using their own peculiar formatting and data translation schema. As pointed out earlier, efforts are underway to recommend standards and focus the medical and health information technology communities at large on developing common interface and communication mechanisms[40]. Key among organizations focused on driving standards in medical device connectivity include the Integrating the Health Enterprise (IHE) initiative, the Institute for Electronic and Electrical Engineers (IEEE) 1073 workgroup, the American College of Clinical Engineers (ACCE), the Association for the Advancement of Medical Instrumentation (AAMI), et al. Device standardization initiatives within these and other standards development organizations (SDOs), such as the American National Standards Institute (ANSI) work to achieve com-

---

[40] Tim Gee, "Plug and pray?" Medical Device Connectivity, November 2006, 24x7 e-magazine; www.24x7mag.com/issues/articles/2006-11_04.asp

mon data representation and communication mechanisms for the healthcare sector. Chief among these data representation mechanisms is the HL7 communications model. Examples of the application of HL7 communications will be described in Chapter 2. The IHE initiative has drafted and codified a patient care device technical framework[41,42] to provide guidance in the application of existing standards for medical device integration and interoperability (e.g.: HL7, IEEE, DICOM, etc.). The IHE further fosters device connectivity efforts through many initiatives, including its *Connectathons*—one-week events organized annually by IHE to invite EMR developers, medical device vendors, consultants, and academics to participate in interoperability testing of software and hardware for proof-of-principle evaluations. As advertised on the IHE *Connectathon* Web site, the *Connectathons* provide "a detailed implementation and testing process to promote the adoption of standards-based interoperability by vendors and users of healthcare information systems."[43]

The IHE has through its member partners (e.g.: ACCE, HIMSS, RSNA) proffered an integration and interoperability framework involving actor interaction and behavior and specific scenarios (e.g.: subscribe to point-of-care data at a specific interval) to assist in developing specific implementations of established standards (e.g.: HL7) to achieve integration goals supportive of optimal patient care[44]. As stated above, the IHE initiative promotes the use of existing standards. The HL7 standards for communicating data are well described and are available through that organization[45].

While more widespread implementation and acceptance of the HL7 standards motivates medical device manufacturers to embrace further standardization, healthcare enterprises are still required to develop proprietary communication device interface mechanisms to those devices that still do not. Many devices do not. This impacts scalability and ease of data collection. My experience in this area reveals that peculiarities in interfacing and query-response mechanisms demonstrate the broad challenges that still exist in device communi-

---

[41] IHE Patient Care Device Technical Framework Year 1: 2005-2006. Volume 1: Integration Profiles. 15-Aug-1006. Version 10 (trial implementation) Copyright ACC, ACCE, HIMSS, RSNA

[42] IHE Patient Care Device Technical Framework Year 1: 2005-2006. Volume 2: Transactions. Version 6.0 (trial implementation). Copyright ACC, ACCE, HIMSS, RSNA

[43] http://www.ihe.net/Connectathon/index.cfm

[44] IHE Patient Care Device Technical Framework Year 1: 2005-2006. Volume 1: Integration Profiles. 15-Aug-1006. Version 10 (trial implementation) Copyright ACC, ACCE, HIMSS, RSNA. Page 2

[45] http://www.hl7.org

cation[46]. Over the course of the past decade many companies have sprung forth that provide data translation and communication mechanisms from medical devices to EMR[47] systems. Yet, regardless of the current recognition with which device interfacing standardization has been given by standards organizations, the reality is that the corporate business cases of device manufacturers must align with the larger community needs. This is a prerequisite for seamless data communication between medical devices and EMRs—a systematic versus individualistic and proprietary approach. There are many sound business reasons why data communications mechanisms have not aligned towards a standard more quickly. Device manufacturers need to evaluate all of the implications of changing device technologies that can have impacts on manufacturing practices, which in turn can impact intended use. Medical devices are, of course, regulated products and, as such, changes in design, manufacturing, etc. carry a large burden associated with respect to validating and verifying that these changes do not impact patient safety or otherwise create hazards for both patients and health professionals. Therefore, it is understandable that migration towards device standardization has been slow or has not resulted in the adoption of one single model, especially when that one model does not yet exist. Even the HL7 data model can be tailored to the point at which no two findings transactions are precisely alike. Changes in medical device hardware, firmware, and even medical software carry concomitant design, development, and manufacturing burdens which must pass the muster of Good Manufacturing Practice (GMP) and Quality System Regulations (QSR) standards and procedures. Changes can be costly and time consuming affairs.

Hence, for now and the foreseeable future, medical device data communication into the EMR will remain more of an art form rather than a proven and standards-based process. The intent here is to evaluate, compare, educate, illustrate, and inform the "student" of medical device interfacing and integration as to the types of interface mechanisms that can be applied regardless of medical device manufacturer; current and proposed methods for communicating these data effectively to the EMR; ways of ensuring that patients and data are positively identified; and ways to validate, verify, and display these data.

---

[46] John R. Zaleski, "Modeling post-operative respiratory state in coronary artery by-pass graft patients: a methodology for weaning patients from mechanical ventilation," Ph.D. Dissertation; The University of Pennsylvania, 1996; page 53.

[47] DataCaptor by Capsule Technologie; CareTrends by Sensitron; IDM-MG Appliance by Nuvon; Enterprise Service Bus by Emergin; CMSense by Cain Medical; Soarian Device Connect by Siemens Medical; iSirona SmartAdapter & DeviceConX

The student is also prompted to ask specific questions of manufacturers of hardware and developers of medical device integration and interfacing software to ensure that correct enterprise decisions are made to save time, costs, and above all, to promote patient safety.

1.5 Discussion

In the chapters that follow I will focus not only on the rather dry topics of data acquisition and communication to the EMR, but also on what to do with those data once they are there. Chapter 2 discusses device networking and communication. Chapter 3 delves into medical device communication methods. Chapter 4 discusses real-time data collection challenges. Chapter 5 focuses on the computer-based patient record, its content, design, how it can be structured, how data arrive, their clinical implication, and management. This leads into Chapter 6 which discusses positive patient identification techniques and their importance in reducing risks to the patient. Chapter 7 describes some statistical techniques for analyzing and reducing data, especially when large quantities are present. Chapter 8 branches out into how these data should be displayed within an EMR flow sheet: visualization and presentation. Chapter 9 takes a look at patient safety, security, and regulatory issues and implications of medical devices interfacing. Chapter 10 looks to the future: methods for automatically controlling or enabling closed-loop feedback control for medical devices. My own thoughts as well as my research into this area, its challenges, and the approaches for overcoming these will be presented. Finally, Chapter 11 lists a number of methods I have developed over the years for communicating with medical devices. These include Java code samples a student may use as building blocks upon which to develop his or her own methods for communicating with medical devices and for analyzing and displaying their data.

2 Device Networking and Communication

2.1 Medical Device Interfaces

Software methods for communicating with medical devices vary by device manufacturer, type of medical device, and their physical attributes. This wide ranging variability, together with the lack of formalized standardization in this area, is a reason why no one approach is best for medical device communication, although commercial software does exist that can make the task much easier. Not only are the logical mechanisms important to consider, but the approach that meets the needs of the healthcare enterprise in terms of optimizing and simplifying workflow considerations must be taken into account. For example, any method that requires clinical staff to operate sophisticated and esoteric software is not advised simply because this takes attention away from their primary task of caring for the patient.

Let's consider a typical situation in which a mechanical ventilator is located within a patient room in an intensive care unit. The collection of ventilatory data is desired for patient care management; that is, mandatory support parameters as specified by the minimum respiratory requirements for the patient should he or she not be able to sustain spontaneous breathing. If a patient is breathing spontaneously then those parameters associated with actual breaths will be recorded. These parameters will be collected and validated by healthcare professionals for inclusion within the EMR. Measured parameters that are collected automatically via software from the mechanical ventilator can also be used for clinical decision support applications to assist clinicians in predicting and guiding future outcomes or to assess the patient's state in comparison with other patients.

Although the precise physical approach for connecting a medical device, such as a mechanical ventilator, to an existing information network can vary, many employ the standard for communicating via an RS232, or a EIA232, serial adapter[48]. For instance, Figure 2-1 illustrates a 9-pin serial adapter attached to the serial communications port on a Servo[i] mechanical ventilator. The mechanical ventilator in question is illustrated in Figure 2-2.

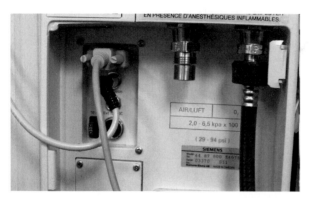

Figure 2-1 Serial adapter (9-pin) attached to the serial communications port of a Servo^i mechanical ventilator (Photo by author)

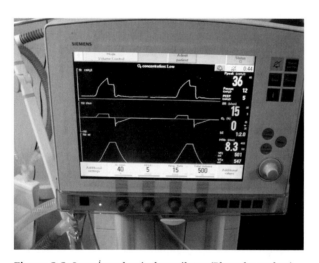

Figure 2-2 Servo^i mechanical ventilator (Photo by author)

Both inbound and outbound communication use a translation mechanism to re-cast the data into a form that can be communicated to the EMR. That is, communication to the ventilator operates in a query-response format. Software requests information and the medical device responds based on the information requested. This form of communication is frequently referred to as asynchronous.

---

[48] RS232 was renamed to EIA232 (Electronic Industries Association) upon introduction of the EIA232F standard in 1997.

From the perspective of physical connectivity, serial connections are usually hard-wired, implying that the mechanical ventilator (in this case) must have a physical connection to a computer, and that the computer must have some type of connectivity to a hospital information system. Depending on the specific approach employed by the information technology and biomedical engineering organizations within the enterprise, there are several approaches—at varying levels of cost and investment—that can be pursued. One approach is to provide a fixed, hard-wired computer connection between the mechanical ventilator and the network. This could be done by simply affixing a laptop computer to the mechanical ventilator via an RS232 cable and then communicating from the laptop over a wired or wireless Ethernet connection to the EMR.

This approach has its benefits in that the laptop can communicate over a high-speed communication interface that is becoming more commonplace throughout any healthcare enterprise.

Wireless connectivity provides the added flexibility to communicate anywhere within the enterprise that already supports wireless coverage. The one challenge would still be the hard-wired connection between the laptop computer and the medical device. It is preferable to make a permanent connection between the mechanical ventilator and the computer as it is clumsy to have a healthcare professional continually make and tear down such connections.

However, there are approaches to solving even this problem. Many portable notebook or tablet computers (such as those manufactured by Motion Computing, Inc.[49]) can sit in docking stations. These docking stations can remain affixed to the medical device or remain permanently in a patient room and the computer may be docked and removed to another patient room as required. Several regrets associated with this approach, though, are when the tablet PC is not docked, there is no way to communicate data. Hence, data can only be collected when the tablet is present in the room. Furthermore, additional hardware in the form of a docking station is required per medical device to provide the mechanism for communicating with the tablet PC.

A dedicated computer, laptop or otherwise, enables continuous collection of medical device data. There are some drawbacks to this approach. Specifically, a single computer (laptop or otherwise) must

---

[49] http://www.motioncomputing.com/products/

be dedicated to each device, which will require both software and physical security and maintenance measures to ensure that (1) the laptop is not removed without authorization, (2) the laptop is maintained with the latest application and operating system software to ensure accurate usage throughout the enterprise, and (3) the laptop cannot be compromised to reveal private patient data to unauthorized individuals. The cost of dedicating a laptop for use with each mechanical ventilator is prohibitive and not very efficient. Furthermore, other medical devices would require their own dedicated computing hardware thus compounding the cost and logistics challenges.

In addition, permanently attaching a medical device such as a mechanical ventilator to a computer is not practical: devices such as mechanical ventilators require servicing and cleaning and must be mobile. Certain models can remain dedicated to patient rooms. But, the ability to do so depends on the requirements of the healthcare enterprise and cannot simply be the assumed solution in the general case. Hardwiring a device such as a mechanical ventilator to an existing room is also impractical from the perspective of movement. It is unrealistic to expect healthcare professionals (nursing, respiratory therapy, even physicians) to possess the knowledge or the time to disconnect or reconnect to a hardwired environment within another patient's room. The ancillary issues of ensuring that data are being correctly communicated from the medical device once reconnection occurs can cause delays while connections are retested, further consuming the time required for patient care—the primary task of a healthcare professional. This is inherently unsafe. Thus, this is altogether an impractical approach.

Networking equipment does exist that enables medical devices to communicate over an existing enterprise network to a central server or directly to an EMR. However, this can be problematic in the case of medical devices which provide no direct networking capability and, thus, are not readily scalable. Fortunately, methods for enabling such devices for direct network communication are available. An example of a networking device like this is shown in Figure 2-3, a serial-to-Ethernet converter. They are available today, are highly reliable, and are very useful for enabling a proprietary RS232 serial interface to communicate remotely over a standard Ethernet network via TCP/IP.

These devices are also available to support wireless ("Wi-Fi") communication via a standard 802.11a/b/g network. A rather elaborate example of a wirelessly-enabled medical device—in this case, a simple glucometer—is shown in Figure 2-4. It should be noted that the rather elaborate measures taken to wirelessly enabled serial devices can bor-

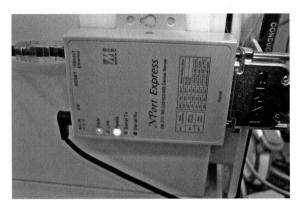

Figure 2-3 Example of a commercially available serial-to-Ethernet adapter (Moxa NPort model DE-211; Photo by author)

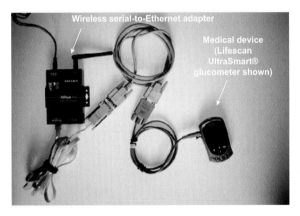

Figure 2-4 Example of Serial-to-Ethernet connection using a wireless communication adapter (Moxa NPort Wireless-G adapter shown; Photo by author)

der on the amazing in terms of complexity. This is one such example I have constructed to illustrate that case.

Although complex, this is indeed a viable approach. Again, care must be taken to ensure that the wireless adapter remains associated with the wireless network. Data security mechanisms must be employed to ensure that both patient identifying information as well as patient findings cannot be intercepted over the wireless network by a rogue individual possessing an unauthorized access point. One approach to mitigating this problem is by using a form of data encryption as well as wireless equivalency protocol (WEP) keys in addition to the encrypted SSIDs[50]. Data should be encrypted prior to transmission to the hospital enterprise and the EMR.

The price for using wireless data connectivity is the need for robust security. This applies to both 802.11 and 802.15 (Bluetooth) networks. Wireless 802.11a/b/g connectivity to the hospital network is more acceptable today as many enterprises support homogeneous access to the Internet over wireless broadband connections. Thus, the infrastructure is usually in place to begin with, especially in large and modern equipped hospitals. In situations where this is not the case, an alternative may be to use Bluetooth. Bluetooth operates according to 802.15 IEEE standards. While not as robust in terms of connectivity, range, and enterprise-wide access as 802.11 Wi-Fi, it offers radio frequency connectivity that is reliable and can be made secure via the application of methods that impose media access control (MAC) layer networking access protocols to restrict access to data and can be used to ensure that medical devices correctly communicate data on the right patient.

Medical devices that only contain serial communications ports can also be served by serial-to-Bluetooth adapters that communicate wirelessly with a laptop or a computer-based Bluetooth device over a standard serial port. An example of such a device is shown in Figure 2-5. These devices can be paired with Bluetooth receivers on remote computers or laptops as healthcare professionals make rounds. Again, the

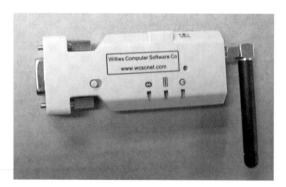

Figure 2-5 Example of a commercially available serial-to-Bluetooth adapter (Photo by author)

---

[50] A Service Set Identifier: character string contained in networking communication packets transmitted over a wireless local area network (WLAN) required to authenticate the receipt and communication of these packets over such networks.

specific workflow requirements of the enterprise will dictate the best and most efficient approach for accomplishing this. In certain cases where devices remain at the patient bedside throughout the course of a patient's stay, a healthcare professional may be wheeling a computer from room to room in the process of collecting data (such as vitals within a medical/surgical ward). For example, when a clinician enters a patient room the pairing between the device and the laptop on the mobile cart can be made and medical device data can be downloaded directly and transmitted to the EMR.

Consider the physical connectivity of devices to a laptop or desktop computer running the Microsoft Windows XP operating system. It should be noted that while I use the example of Microsoft Windows XP, the configurations described below also apply to Microsoft Windows 2000, and even to Microsoft Windows 2003 Server. However, in the case of Windows 2003 Server, there may be driver compatibility issues.[51]

One approach I've found to be useful is mapping device ports (i.e., serial ports) from the computer to the communication device (e.g.: Bluetooth adapter). Many Bluetooth-to-Serial devices support these virtual mappings. Some virtual port adapters provide drivers to ease this process.

Bluetooth adapters can also be used in situations in which laptops or medical devices come equipped with universal serial bus (USB) ports rather than RS232 communication ports. Hard-wired adapters are also available to translate serial port communication cables to virtual serial ports via Serial-to-USB adapters. Before addressing the Bluetooth example, let's consider the hard-wired connection.

An example of this type of attachment modification is illustrated in Figure 2-6. One such type of adapter which I have used and have found to be reliable is the Belkin F5U109 Serial-to-USB adapter. These devices are sold with an installation Compact Disk (CD) which contains the drivers to recognize and map the USB device to a serial port, as if the adapter plug were an actual standard serial connector.

The settings on these devices are manipulated using the normal settings under device manager within the operating system of a Microsoft Windows XP or 2000 laptop operating system. These devices are identified within the Device Manager setting of the Hardware Tab under the System Properties Menu.

---

[51] The author has not evaluated Windows Vista.

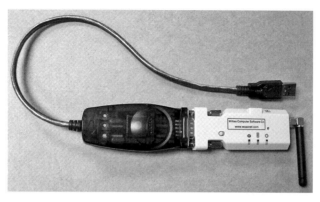

Figure 2-6 Serial-to-USB adapter configuration attached to a Bluetooth
adapter (Belkin F5U109 Serial-to-USB adapter; Photo by author)

Once drivers are installed the device is normally plugged into a USB port on the laptop. Detailed installation instructions accompany these adapters. If all goes well, the operating system will locate the drivers and install the device. Once installed properly, the user will receive a message so indicating. Now a virtual serial port is established. The port can be treated precisely as a standard serial port (i.e., an active physical serial attachment—usually a 9-pin serial adapter) resident on the laptop itself.

Setting the physical configuration of this virtual serial port is a simple matter, described below. It is important to ascertain the required serial connector settings of the medical device to be attached. Some off-the-shelf configuration and connectivity software will automatically detect such settings, so it is unnecessary even to configure the virtual serial port on the laptop. It is possible for the user to develop a serial communication method that will also enable automatic discovery of active serial ports.

The virtual serial communications port is accessed through the System Properties menu, found by right-clicking on the My Computer icon on the Microsoft Windows desktop. Selecting Properties at the bottom of the System Properties menu will reveal the System Properties sheet itself, which will normally contain 7 tabs. To configure the virtual serial adapter the user clicks on the Hardware tab, revealing the Device Manager pages shown in Figure 2-7.

Right-clicking on the port displays the serial communications port properties page, as shown in Figure 2-8.

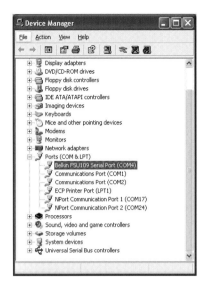

Figure 2-7
Device Manager tab showing serial port mapping for USB-Serial adapter port

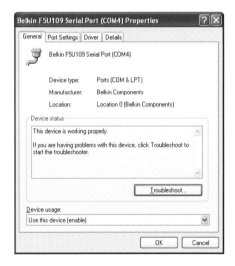

Figure 2-8
Communication properties page for selected virtual serial port

Settings for the virtual serial port are shown in the Port Settings tab, an example of which is shown in Figure 2-9.

Once configured, communication with the medical device may begin. It should be noted that even when using commercially available medical device communication software, it is necessary to manually configure port settings.

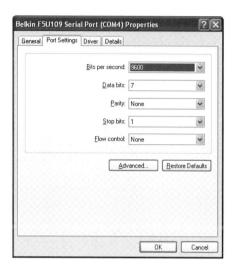

Figure 2-9
Virtual serial port
settings

Software is available for download with which serial port communication methods may be derived. The Java Communications Applications Programming Interface is an example. More information can be found at the Sun Microsystems Website http://www.java.sun.com/download.

2.2 Communication Methods

Hard-wired data communication is perhaps the most inexpensive means of establishing physical and logical connectivity between devices and the EMR. However, it is also the most problematic in terms of scalability within the healthcare enterprise. The most obvious reason for this is the potential for interference with clinical workflow. Device configuration is both time-consuming and inconvenient unless equipment is permanently installed in hospital rooms. Unless a well-staffed and knowledgeable biomedical or clinical engineering department is available to assist healthcare professionals, it is disruptive to the clinical workflow process and unrealistic to expect clinical staff (nursing, respiratory therapy, and physicians) to make these connections. I recall my own experience a number of years ago in a related manner where a recall of an arrhythmia trace was requested by a cardiac surgeon on a patient in ICU: clinical engineering responded and had to search the databases for data on a specific telemetry monitor, requiring almost an hour of hunt-and-peck searching within the arrhythmia database of a single telemetry monitor. While there certainly are exceptions to this rule, to expect that clinical staff—already taxed by the burdens of patient care—to expend time and energy in software or hardware configuration is unreasonable.

Thus, hard-wired connectivity should only be used in patient rooms dedicated to technologically-dependent patients. Most intensive care units and some emergency departments as well as operating theatres fall into this category with vital signs monitoring equipment. Other ancillary yet important devices, such as mechanical ventilators, must be mobile as they are required for different patients on an as-needed basis and must be disinfected between uses. This normally requires moving them to locations where they can be configured with new disposable components (intubation and extubation tubing, filters, etc.) and then moved back to patient rooms. Infusion pumps usually fall into this category, as well.

A substitute for hard-wired connectivity that supports the aforementioned scenarios is wireless connectivity to either an existing hospital or dedicated device network. Both of these fall into the category of local area networks (LANs). Enabling the device to communicate over Wi-Fi (i.e., un-tethering the device) is the key to its usability in the clinical environment.

There are several methods for communicating wirelessly. All three have their benefits. These are:

1) Communication using infrared data association (IrDA),
2) Radio frequency communication (e.g.: Bluetooth or Communication over TCP/IP via 802.11a/b/g through wireless access points), and
3) Sound or audio-based communication.

Infrared communication involves transmitting and receiving data through line-of-sight connections between the computing hardware and the medical device. Some medical devices can be configured with manufacturer supplied IrDA receiver hardware that attach directly to serial ports on the devices themselves. These receivers handle the mechanics of translating and communicating the infrared signal to an EIA232-compliant format and hardware handshake that acts as the physical interface mechanism to the device itself. A communicating laptop then transmits queries for data and receives responses (i.e., asynchronously) via the line-of-sight linkage. One benefit of this approach is that positive identification is established between the device and the computing device which receives the data, thereby virtually guaranteeing the likelihood that data collected from the device is indeed associated with the correct patient. This communication mechanism supports various baud rates, is simple, and requires little in the way of knowledge to configure for biomedical hospital information technology staff. However, the simplicity of this communication mechanism (i.e., line-of-sight) is also one of its key drawbacks. Firstly, clinical staff collecting these data at the bedside must establish this link between the laptop and the bedside device.

To ensure proper connectivity, the clinical user must confirm both the transmitters and receivers are properly aligned. Anyone who has worked with these connections even between adjacent laptops knows that they can be finicky: connections can drop in the middle of transmission, establishing the connection in the first place can require movement of the device around the line-of-sight, and for handheld devices in which the clinician (frequently, the nurse) is holding the receiving laptop or personal digital assistant (PDA), this process can be quite tedious, especially if the nurse is otherwise distracted.

Secondly, the laptop and the on-board device IrDA receiver must be in close proximity to one another: typically, within 1 to 2 feet. This may be difficult to achieve if the laptop is located on a mobile cart which has a limited range of motion and the medical device has limited accessibility or cannot be moved easily due to tubing, proximity to other equipment, or location with respect to the patient. Thus, drawbacks to using IrDA exist that can limit its use with highly mobile (and light) devices, such as glucometers or some medical/surgical monitors that are easily manipulated by staff.

For these reasons, radio frequency communication is preferable. Radio frequency communication via Wi-Fi or Bluetooth requires no line-of-sight connectivity. Furthermore, unique identification can be established between a querying device (that is, a laptop configured with either a Bluetooth adapter or a Wi-Fi networking card) via a unique media access control (MAC) address that positively differentiates the device from those around it. If these devices are to be attached to the hospital network, their signals must be sufficiently strong to enable communication with an existing hospital network, or with a laptop in proximity to the patient. With wireless communication, the potential for device identification confusion can result if any two (or more) adjacent devices are radiating in a sufficiently large radius so as to overlap with neighboring devices. This poses a rather obvious patient safety problem from the perspective that the user may attempt to retrieve data on the wrong patient.

The actual communication between the medical device and laptop itself requires establishing an open port to the device and then querying for results. I prefer the Java programming language, because a very mature library for serial device communication is available using the Java communications application programming interface (API). This library enables developing communication methods for the Win32 and Sun/Solaris operating system platforms that comply with the EIA232 standard for RS232 serial port communication, as discussed several pages ago. While the documentation associated with this communication library is extensive, and examples are provided, I'll briefly discuss the essence of serial communication with a typical medical device. In Java, the following import command is required in the header in order to make use of these libraries:

```
Import javax.comm.*;
```

Let's begin by defining some variables that we will use throughout the process of opening and communicating through a serial port. These parameters are defined in Table 2-1. Then, Table 2-2 defines a basic try-catch block that outlines the opening of a serial communication port, establishing an inbound and outbound communication stream, and transmitting and receiving data through the established serial communication port.

Table 2-1 Serial port communication private parameter definitions

```
Private CommPortIdentifier    portId = null;
Private SerialPort            serialPort = null;
private String               commPort = "COM5";
private int                  baudRate = 9600;
InputStream                  inputStream = null;
OutputStream                 outputStream = null;
```

In Table 2-2, I open a serial port and assign it a timeout setting of 2 seconds (2000 milliseconds). This must be placed in a try-catch block. The actual name of the COM port (e.g.: comPort variable) is that mapped to the physical port itself. This can be an RS232 port on the laptop from which you are working or even a virtual COM port, as was discussed previously when using a Serial-to-USB adapter. Regardless, this must reflect the actual port through which communication will take place.

Table 2-2 An example of a simple try-catch block method for opening
a serial port

```
try {
portId = CommPortIdentifier.getPortIdentifier(comport);
serialPort =
(SerialPort)portId.open("name_of_method_connection",
2000);
} catch (PortInUseException piue) {
System.out.println(" Exception thrown in " +
 "Communicate opening serial port: " + piue + "\n");
}
```

The next step involves opening the connection to the port for read and write access. I illustrate this in Table 2-3. First, set the serial port parameters. Specifically, the baud rate, data bits, stop bits and parity—the usual parameters required for serial communication. I then open an input and output stream. We are now prepared to read and write data. Note that this code segment is captured within the bounds of a try-catch block. I will be completing the remainder of the block in a few moments. Also make note of it so that the reader does not lose sight of the fact that we shall capture the input and output stream read and write process in such a block.

Table 2-3 Opening serial port input and output streams

```
try {
  serialPort.setSerialPortParams( baudRate,
              SerialPort.DATABITS_8,
              SerialPort.STOPBITS_1,
              SerialPort.PARITY_NONE);
  serialPort.enableReceiveTimeout(500);
  inputStream = serialPort.getInputStream();
  outputStream = serialPort.getOutputStream();
```

The next part of the communication process becomes specific to the particular medical device. Here are the details of precisely how to communicate with the device.

In order to provide an informative example, I use a code segment that may be used in communicating with the GE Dinamap ProCare 400 monitor. In this particular instance I query the monitor for an O_2 saturation measurement. The query command for the O_2 saturation measurement for this particular monitor is "<sp>OA!3<cr>" where

<sp> stands for space.[52] This command has a checksum (!3) and carriage return <cr> appended to it prior to transmission to the monitor. It is important to note that devices oftentimes require checksum commands that are used to verify the correct transmission of data to and from the medical device. Calculation of and selection of appropriate types of checksums is outside the scope of this book. Nevertheless, I include several methods as examples which are illustrative of the point made above. While the specifics of the following code segment will, indeed, vary by device, it is a useful experience to understand to what extent the details must be represented so that there is no loss of understanding by the reader in the process. Then, in Table 2-4, I transmit a command to and receive a finding from the medical device.

Table 2-4 Serial port transmission O2 saturation command

```
Int        nChars = 0;
String     O2SatCmd = " OA";
String     O2SatCmd_chksm = "";
char       O2SatCmd_chksm_cmd[] = new char[10];
O2SatCmd_ chksm = checksum( O2SatCmd );
nChars = convertToCharArray (O2SatCmd_chksm_cmd,
               O2SatCmd_chksm );

for (int i = 0; i < nChars; i++ )
{
   outputStream.write( O2SatCmd_chksm_cmd [i] );
}
```

Several items will be noted. A checksum variable and a character array are created to hold, respectively, the communication command and the character array containing the individual characters comprising that command. This character array also contains the character representation of the checksum. The character representation is necessary in order to write to the serial communications (COM) port—this cannot be done as a command string, but instead requires copying the command string to individual characters in a character array. Once the string command is copied to the character array, the characters are written individually through the serial communication port to the device. Note that both the input and output streams can remain open during the write and read processes.

---

[52] GE Medical Systems: Dinamap Host Communications Manual, Document Reference 20/0566D Page 29, June 5th 2003

Once the command is written through the serial communications port, the application attempts to read a response. Sun, through its communications API examples, describes and implements a novel approach based on a serial event listener that awaits data arrival at the communications port. In lieu of this, the code segment included in Table 2-5 may be substituted, which simply attempts to retrieve data from the serial communications port immediately following the write command.

Table 2-5 Serial port retrieval of O2 saturation data

```
StringBuffer readBuffer = new StringBuffer();
int c;

while ((c=inputStream.read()) != 13)
{
  if(c!=13) readBuffer.append((char) c);
}
String scannedInput = readBuffer.toString();
```

Characters are read in integer "decimal" format. If data are not read, then an exception will be thrown. Data are read as integers corresponding to the decimal values and are re-cast as characters and appended to a string buffer which "assembles" the individual characters into a new string containing the resulting data. The end of the line associated with the received finding is detected using a check for decimal 13: this is used to determine when a carriage return character is read. Once read this terminates further read attempts.

The readBuffer variable is then copied to a string (scannedInput). The value contained in the string may be further parsed or printed as desired. Once this process is complete, the remaining "cleanup" activity required is to close the streams. This is depicted in Table 2-6.

Table 2-6 Finalizing and closing file streams

```
}
   catch (Exception e) {
   System.out.println( "Error: " + e + "\n");
}
closeStreams();
```

Now look at several of the complementary functions that enable this communication. I'll begin with the checksum function. In short, checksums are used to verify data integrity and validate pedigree. In the context presented here, they serve as a means of verifying whether data are transmitted accurately. Checksums can follow standard conventions or may be customized depending on the complexity desired. I have found the Java Checksum utility available from SourceForge[53] to be a fairly reliable and flexible utility for experimenting with checksum calculation. This checksum utility, referred to as JACKSUM (JAva cheCKSUM), supports 58 hashing algorithms and is easy to use. This utility is distributed under GNU public license and is, therefore, typically not available for resale. So, individuals requiring checksum calculation for use in a saleable product must obtain commercially available utilities or write their own. However, the JACKSUM utility can be very educational and can assist users in developing their own proprietary methods for computing checksums. I will illustrate a simple method below.

As pointed out, checksums can be used to ascertain data integrity. One use is to verify whether data have been correctly transmitted over a network from a client to a server application. A string or other data being prepared for transmission to a server could have a checksum calculation that would be transmitted together with the original data. The checksum would be recalculated on the server side. If the transmitted and newly computed checksums match, then data integrity are likely to have been preserved. A simple example method to illustrate whether two strings (one transmitted, one received) are the same employs the exclusive OR (XOR) operator. Consider the following two strings:

```
String s1 = "This iS a test";

String s2 = "this is a tAst";
```

Upon inspection it is obvious that several characters differ between strings s1 and s2: the 'T' versus 't'; the 'S' versus 's'; and the 'e' versus 'A'.

An XOR calculation performed character for character between the two strings results in the following values, illustrated in Table 2-7.

---

[53] http://sourceforge.net/projects/jacksum/

Table 2-7 Exclusive OR calculation between two strings

Character Number	Character in s1	Hexadecimal Value	Character in s2	Hexadecimal Value	XOR
1	T	0x54	t	0x74	20
2	h	0x48	h	0x48	0
3	i	0x69	i	0x69	0
4	s	0x73	s	0x73	0
5		0x20		0x20	0
6	i	0x69	i	0x69	0
7	S	0x53	s	0x73	20
8		0x20		0x20	0
9	a	0x61	a	0x61	0
10		0x20		0x20	0
11	t	0x74	t	0x74	0
12	e	0x65	A	0x41	24
13	s	0x73	s	0x73	0
14	t	0x74	t	0x74	0

The highlighted rows show the characters that differ between the two strings. The XOR column shows the result of the XOR calculation carried out character by character (e.g.: XOR 'e' versus 'A' is 24, from 0x65 compared with 0x41). A Java program used to compute these elements is provided in Table 2-8.

Given this understanding it is then possible to suggest a mechanism for computing a checksum of a string that can be used to verify data integrity. Let's consider a new string:

```
String s = "jG7zChyk";
```

Compute the XOR between adjacent characters in this string. Note, the Java XOR operator is the symbol '^'. The checksum computes to be 0x59. Hence, the string with checksum added would include the hexadecimal string '59'. Table 2-9 lists a simple program for computing the checksum using XOR. Figure 2-10 shows the program output for this particular string and shows how this checksum is determined.

One of the most used methods for computing checksums is the cyclic redundancy check (CRC)[54]. The CRC operates in general as above in that it can be used to detect changes in data (e.g.: data transmitted

Table 2-8 Listing of XOR.java

```java
import java.awt.*;

public class XOR
{
        String s1 = "This iS a test";
        String s2 = "this is a tAst";

   public XOR()
   {
     computeXOR( s1, s2 );
   }

   public static void main(String[] args)
   {
     XOR xr = new XOR();
   }

   public void computeXOR(String cmd1, String cmd2 )
   {
     int xorDiff[] = new int [20];
     int xor1 = 0;
     int xor2 = 0;

     if ( cmd1.length() == cmd2.length() )
     {
       for (int i = 0; i < cmd1.length(); i++)
       {
       xorDiff[i] = cmd1.getBytes()[i] ^ cmd2.getBytes()[i];
          System.out.println( " xor diff ["+i+"] = " +
Integer.toHexString(xorDiff[i]).toUpperCase() );
             }
           else {
               System.out.println( " Error: two strings are
not of equal length " );
             }
   }
}
```

from source to destination) and, thus serves to verify data integrity. The JACKSUM library contains a number of methods for computing checksums using cyclic redundancy checks.

---

[54] Created by W.W. Peterson and D.T. Brown. Referenced here: Peterson, W.W.; Brown, D.T. "Cyclic Codes for Error Detection." Proceedings of the IRE. Volume 49, Issue 1, January 1961. Pages: 228-235.

Table 2-9 Listing of checksum.java

```java
import java.awt.*;

public class checksum
{
  String s = "jG7zChyk";

  public checksum()
  {
    computeChecksum( s );
  }

  public static void main(String[] args)
  {
    checksum cs = new checksum();
  }

  public void computeChecksum(String cmd )
  {
    int chksum = 0;

    for (int i = 0; i < cmd.length(); i++)
    {
      chksum ^= cmd.getBytes()[i];
      System.out.println( " i = " +
        i +
        "; intermediate chksum: " +

        Integer.toHexString(chksum).toUpperCase() );
    }
    System.out.println( "\n Final checksum: " +
      Integer.toHexString(chksum).toUpperCase() );
  }
}
```

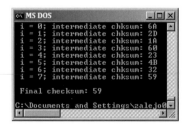

Figure 2-10
Output from checksum.java

In order to operate on individual elements within a string it is necessary to access individual characters. This can be facilitated by transforming a string to a character array. When converting a string variable to a character array, it is necessary to pay attention to the makeup of the string as well as the terminator. In the example included in Table 2-10, a string, *stringVal*, is passed to the function. The size of the string is determined. Then, a character array, *charArray*, is created element by element using the *charAt* function—a standard Java character and string function.

Table 2-10 Sample Java code segment for converting a string variable to a character array

```
public int convertToCharArray( char charArray[],
                String stringVal )
{
  int m = stringVal.length();
  for ( int k = 0; k < m; k++ )
  {
    charArray [k] = stringVal.charAt(k);
  }
  array[m] = 0x0D;
  return m;
} // end convertToCharArray
```

A hexadecimal carriage return is appended at the end of the string—this is necessary so as to notify the device that the end of the command has been reached. Finally, we close the input and serial streams. This function is shown in Table 2-11.

Table 2-11 Method for closing serial communication streams

```
public void closeStreams()
{
  try
  {
    inputStream.close();
    outputStream.close();
    serialPort.close();
  } catch ( Exception e ) {}
}
```

Using this standard serial approach it is possible to build custom interface applications to medical devices.

2.3 Interface Standardization

The IEEE 1073 and 11073 standards on medical information buses (MIBs) took important steps in defining the various communication layers as well as requirements on networking and robustness. These are specifically delineated as[55]:

1) Must withstand frequent reconfiguration due to patient and equipment movement;

2) Must support a simple plug-and-play capability; and,

3) Must provide for positive, unambiguous association between patients and devices.

MIB follows the ISO Open Systems Interconnection 7-layer Reference Model (OSI) 7-layer model which includes lower level physical device connectivity while the upper layers incorporate data encoding including the Medical Device Data Language (MDDL)[56]. A frequent misunderstanding is that devices can be seamlessly integrated with any information technology system. Historically, this has not been the case[57,58,59]:

"The core of the so-called plug-and-play interoperability problem is this: In the absence of a communications standard that extends from the physical device connection through the application-language level, every interface between a medical device and any device or system with which it is to communicate must, at a minimum, be examined to determine what physical and logical interfaces must be developed to effect communication."

In 2002, the IEEE announced plans to create three Health Infomatics standards[60]:

---

[55] Robert J. Kennelly, "Improving Acute Care Through Use of Medical Device Data," Chair, IEEE 1073 "Standard for Medical Device Communications" Committee; Eden Shores Consulting; 42 Loch Eden Shores Road; Meredith, NH 03253.

[56] Mike Gass, "ANSI/IEEE 1073: Medical Information Bus," Health Informatics Journal, Vol. 4, No. 2, 72-83 (1998).

[57] Jan Wittenbar, M. Michael Shabot, "The medical device data language for the P1073 medical information bus standard," Journal of Clinical Monitoring and Computing; Springer Netherlands. Vol. 7, Number 2 / April 1990. PP 91-98.

[58] Richard A. Schrenker, "Software Engineering for Future Healthcare and Clinical Systems," IEEE Computer Society; April 2006. MD PnP Sidebar.

[59] Richard Schrenker and Todd Cooper, "Building the Foundation for Medical Device Plug-and-Play Interoperability," Medical Electronics Manufacturing (MEM) April 2001.

[60] Karen McCabe, "IEEE Starts Work on Three Health Informatics Standards." http://standards. ieee.org/announcements/hisstds.html. April 2nd, 2002.

- IEEE P1073.1.3.16: "Health Informatics-Point-of-Care Medical Device Communication-Device Specialization-Dialysis Device," focusing on standardizing dialysis device communication with information technology.
- IEEE P1073.2.1.2: "Health Informatics-Point-of-Care Medical Device Communication-Device Specialization-Application Profiles-MIB Elements," focusing on definitions for non-transport-specific MIB objects targeting network management and communication.
- IEEE P1073.2.3.2: Health Informatics-Point-of-Care Medical Device Communication-Device Specialization-Application Profiles-Optional Package, Symmetric Communication," focusing on standardization of the communications interface for receiving, as clients, information from health information systems.

All three of these standards were sponsored by the IEEE Engineering in Medicine and Biology Society. Furthermore, the National Institute for Standards and Technology (NIST) has announced a collaborative effort with the IEEE 1073 Working Group to develop conformance tests and software tools to assist the medical device industry to ensure medical device communications standards are followed[61]. It is understood that the IEEE MIB standards extend from critical care monitors, infusion devices, and mechanical ventilators to glucometers, flow meters, pulse oximeters, etc. The target objective is simplified plug-and-play mechanical, logistical, and information interoperability from the bedside.

Apart from device-level communication, many manufacturers of networked devices, to include telemetry or vitals monitors (such as those used in ICUs) and some infusion pumps, employ internal networks that provide isolated conduits for communication among devices and a central service point, typically known as Gateways. An instance of such a network is illustrated in Figure 2-11.

These Gateways typically operate on sub networks ("subnets") that are separated physically or logically from an enterprise network as they enable the devices contained within the proprietary network to communicate unmolested. These networks support communication not only among monitors and the Gateway, but also to central nursing stations that enable alarms, notifications, and raw waveforms to be delivered rapidly. These medical subnets are, in effect, a system of medical devices within one larger medical device—the network itself.

---

[61] NIST request for participation, November 16, 2005. Point of contact: Lynne Rosenthal (lynne.rosenthal@nist.gov).

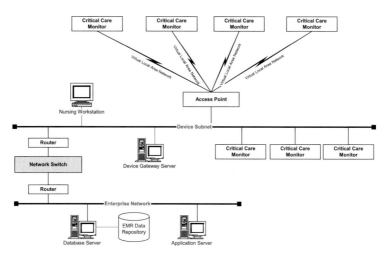

Figure 2-11 Example of a Medical Device Gateway network topology

Device communication within the subnet is of a proprietary nature, specific to the design of the manufacturer. The manufacturer provides a mechanism for communicating with the enterprise through the Gateway. This communication is more standardized—often supporting a traditional HL7 communication interface. This interface usually provides for outbound transactions or findings in the form of either solicited or unsolicited observations and an inbound transaction containing patient identifying information, usually termed an admission, discharge and transfer, or ADT, transaction. The purpose of the inbound transaction is to associate specific patient identifying information with particular monitors. Once patient identifying data are applied to particular monitors, all outbound results and waveforms will then be electronically identified with them, thereby ensuring positive identification of results with patients—which mitigates the risk of misassociating a patient with his or her vitals data. To illustrate this point, the proprietary communication within the subnet is transmitted to the Gateway and, from there, a more standardized feed of vitals transactions are sent to the enterprise network.

2.4 Medical Device Gateways

The Medical Device Gateway (MDG) is a model that provides the capability to retrieve data directly from the medical devices using a network that is dedicated to their communication using a standards-based messaging model.

Proprietary versus standardized communication is illustrated via the two separate outbound communication feeds shown in Figure 2-12. These outbound results from the medical devices are formatted as specified per manufacturer design requirements for communication among the devices and the Gateway.

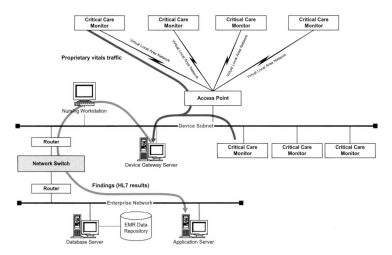

Figure 2-12 Outbound vitals transactions from Gateway

This controlled Gateway environment ensures that no ancillary or uncontrolled traffic will affect the performance, delivery, or integrity of the data retrieved directly from monitors or other devices. As will be discussed in Chapter 9, there is an important regulatory requirement satisfied by this architectural consideration.

One immediate benefit of this communication approach is that the communication mechanism within the system incorporating the devices and the Gateway can be manufacturer-defined and proscribed. On the outbound side of the Gateway, a more universal interface can be supported—through what is identified as a Device Bus Software & Hardware interface mechanism. This device bus could be, for example, a solution such as Capsule Technologie's DataCaptor product that communicates directly with the device Gateway. The outbound side of this interface can be a standard such as HL7. Many device Gateways already communicate using an HL7 standard, obviating the need for this intermediary interface. However, should the gateway interface use a proprietary format, then the intermediary can be used to translate data into a more standard format for communicating with a messaging or interface engine. The messaging engine provides the capability to tailor the HL7 message from the device Gateway to a format required by a specific instance of EMR. As we discussed, the HL7 interface provides a more universal mechanism for communicating. However, because components and segments within the standard messaging framework can vary, it will be necessary to alter this interface as required to meet specific needs.

The outbound traffic of this interface is representative of the results (HL7 R01) findings transaction. These gateway interfaces also support inbound admission, transfer, and discharge messaging so that patient demographic identifying data may be posted back to the devices through the device Gateway. This is very important from the perspective of positively identifying the findings from a particular patient.

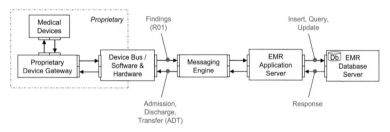

Figure 2-13 Example of gateway-based device interfacing

Figure 2-13 illustrates the communication mechanism typical of MDGs, in which proprietary medical device networks communicate outbound results to an EMR using a standard interface such as HL7, and can receive inbound identifying information from the EMR.

2.5 Medical Device Gateway Networking

The communication traffic within this proprietary network includes multicast, UDP, and TCP/IP. Because of the highly dynamic and real-time aspect of this communication traffic, the volume can be quite high, especially where many medical device monitors are present (>10). Thus, it is important to firewall this traffic from the enterprise so as not to flood that network with these data. Furthermore, the subnets on which the devices, their Gateway, and real-time workstations exist are typically "flat": that is, they are not decomposed into further subnets. One mechanism whereby some Gateways associate monitors with specific rooms and beds is via network IP addressing. Although the details of communications networking are outside the scope of this book, there are significant overlaps across fields so a rudimentary understanding is necessary to facilitate the basic understanding of the medical device communication area itself.

Standard network communications via TCP/IP, UDP, or multicast over Ethernet adhere to the IEEE 802.1x standards. Local and Wide Area Networks (LANs & WANs) employ a standardized network addressing mechanism for identifying computing and networking hardware. All computing hardware on LANs and WANs possess internet protocol addresses (IP). These addresses conform to specific standards in terms of ranges and values that are dictated both by the standards themselves as well as the specifics of the enterprise networks within which the devices and computing hardware are resident. The revised definition of the Internet Protocol was chronicled by the Defense Advanced Research Projects Agency (DARPA) in 1981[62]. This standard defines the Internet Protocol (IP) ranges for specific classes of networks, as shown in Figure 2-14.

Table 2-12 shows the IP ranges for the various classes of subnets for a local area network.

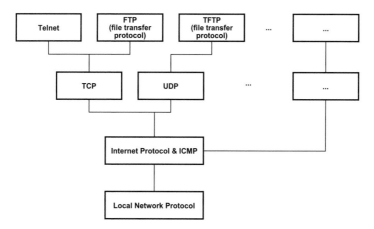

Figure 2-14 Internet Protocol hierarchy as codified by DARPA

---

[62] Internet Protocol: DARPA Internet Program Protocol Specification. September, 1981. Prepared for the Defense Advanced Research Projects Agency, Information Processing Techniques Office; 1400 Wilson Boulevard; Arlington, VA 22209. Prepared by Information Sciences Institute; University of Southern California; 4676 Admiralty Way; Marina del Rey, California 90291.

Table 2-12 IP and subnet ranges for various networking classes
(IPv4 Networking Standard)

Class	Start IP range	End IP range	Subnet Mask
A	0.0.0.0	127.255.255.255	255.0.0.0
B	128.0.0.0	191.255.255.255	255.255.0.0
C	192.0.0.0	223.255.255.255	255.255.255.0
D	224.0.0.0	239.255.255.255	undefined

For instance, a Gateway may be designed in the Class B range in which the subnet mask third and fourth octets (that is, "0.0") would define the care or monitoring unit and the bed number, respectively. In such situations, as medical device monitors are affixed within a patient's room in critical care, this establishes a method for assigning a bed to a specific monitor, which in turn is associated with a specific patient. This establishes the positive identity and association of the medical device with a patient.

The importance of this assignment process becomes evident when considering the assignment of patients to device monitors from an enterprise health information system through the Medical Device Gateway. Having examined the outbound communication, let's consider the inbound communication. Such an example is illustrated in Figure 2-15.

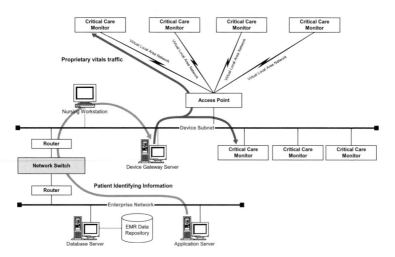

Figure 2-15 Patient identifying information transmitted to the medical device network

A sample workflow for transmitting patient information to the medical monitors might consist of the following scenario:

1) A patient arrives at the emergency department, or is admitted through standard registration.

2) This patient is assigned a medical record number (MRN) and a visit identifier or patient number (PTN). This information may be captured in text, barcode, or even through a radio frequency identification tag on a wrist bracelet.

3) The patient is admitted for a reason that mandates the clinical need to be placed on telemetry in an intensive care unit or other high-acuity ward.

4) The patient identifying information (i.e., MRN & PTN) is then transferred from the enterprise information system to the ward and nursing unit to which the patient will arrive.

5) The patient identifying information is assigned via an in-unit departmental information system to the medical device monitors, using the logic and methods intrinsic to the Medical Device Gateway subnet to assign this information to that device associated with an inpatient room.

Suppose an ICU were identified with a specific unit number (say, unit number 1). Then, suppose the unit contained 10 beds. Further suppose that this patient will be assigned to bed number 4. The Class B subnet capturing the range of IP addresses associated with the rooms and beds could be assigned to patients on the basis of MRN, PTN, or some combination therein, is 255.255.0.0. Thus, in this case, an example association might be as follows, illustrated in Table 2-13.

Here we have positively associated the patient with a monitor. I will be discussing positive patient identification and its need in monitoring and communicating data to the EMR in Chapter 5. However, frequently overlapping concepts require repeated exposure in order to foster better understanding of the primary idea being discussed: medical device communication.

Table 2-13 Example of patient assigned to ICU bed and suggested IP address mapping

First Name	Last Name	MRN	PTN	IP Address	Subnet Mask
John	Doe	123456	987654321	172.50.1.4	255.255.0.0

The assignment of patient identifying information to the medical devices within the proprietary network is thus accomplished through this closed-loop association. All outbound vitals data from these monitors will then be coupled to a specific patient.

This provides for closure of the round-trip loop between patient identification and the raw findings from the medical devices. The clear benefit offered by using Medical Device Gateways is that of the blending of the proprietary communications environment with that of the standard, more universal communication mechanism such as HL7. By maintaining the proprietary network, this alleviates the need for major modifications to the medical devices which will have the strong potential for impacting not only the design of the devices but will have regulatory impacts and their concomitant costs.

The Gateway concept isolates the medically proprietary network from the enterprise network and enables communicating with enterprise networks using an interface model which is standardized. Furthermore, the Gateway model enables receiving patient identifying information by which the proprietary network can associate from the enterprise with individual medical devices. This obviates the need to establish complex workflows between the enterprise information system and these medical devices, including the de-confliction of the associated patient data with these devices. This will save costs, custom software development, and the need for evaluating the individual hazard and risk mitigation processes with their obvious and inevitable regulatory implications. In short, this is the way to go. Other smaller devices (that is, ad-hoc monitors, pulse oximeters, glucometers, etc.) would also benefit from this model in the healthcare enterprise—to include the home healthcare market, physician office, and distributed clinical network.

2.6 Summary

The balance between proprietary and standardized medical device communication is achieved, at least in the near term, by the use of Medical Device Gateways (MDGs). This is an important reason why they should be implemented in healthcare enterprises as a preferred mechanism for communicating with EMRs. While the internal proprietary communication among medical devices, be they telemetry monitors or infusion pumps, can be defined in a manner preferred by the manufacturer, the interfacing communication mechanism is typically via a standardized interface such as HL7. Both inbound admission, discharge, and transfer information are normally able to be received by these MDGs, and observations (findings) can be transmitted by them to the EMR. This makes the task of communicating between EMRs and medical devices developed by different companies much easier than establishing custom interfaces that may require contractual relationships and expensive development timelines to achieve.

3 Mechanisms for Interfacing and Integrating Device Data

3.1 Medical Device Interfaces

Device communication between computing hardware and a medical instrument or device is represented in its most basic design in Figure 3-1. Methods to retrieve data from medical instrumentation have existed since the time devices contained microprocessors that enabled extraction from their firmware. Perhaps the most simple and straightforward of these is the terminal emulator program[63]. Even today, however, many systems only provide the capability for retrieving and archiving data in ASCII[64] format[65].

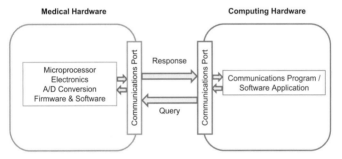

Figure 3-1 Simplified communications mechanism between computing hardware and medical device

In this chapter I will focus on several medical devices and their data communication mechanisms. I will then generalize these data communications mechanisms to include a broader spectrum of medical devices. The chapter concludes with a description of the HL7 standard segments for importing these data into the EMR.

---

[63] Examples include (a) the Columbia-University-developed Kermit (versions available as of this writing include Kermit 95 2.1.3 for MS Windows and Kermit 3.15 for MS-DOS); (b) Microsoft HyperTerminal; (c) PCommLite by Moxa Technologies.

[64] American Standard Code of Information Interchange

[65] Examples include the Siemens Servo[i] and Puritan Bennett mechanical ventilators.

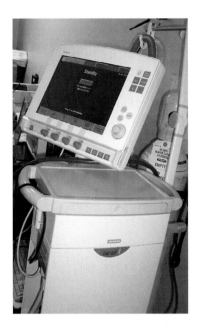

Figure 3-2
Siemens Servo*i* ventilator
(Photo by author)

Data-rich medical devices that are of utmost importance within acute care units include mechanical ventilators and critical care telemetry monitors. Two examples of mechanical ventilators that capture a large market in both the U.S. and Europe include the Siemens Servo*i* and the Puritan-Bennett 7200ae brands, although many others may be considered. Photographs of these two ventilators are included in Figure 3-2 and Figure 3-3, respectively. These two brands of mechanical ventilators provide data in accord with the communication mechanism of Figure 3-1 in that each must be queried prior to data being transmitted from them to the requesting information system. Data are retrieved via serial communication ports: the 9-pin serial communications port on the Siemens Servo*i* is shown in Figure 3-4.

Data are queried using proprietary communication protocol language. The syntax of this protocol language is provided in documentation published by the manufacturers. Specific examples associated with these two ventilators will be discussed to illustrate the rather proprietary nature of these data communication protocols. Examples of transmitted and received data from the Servo*i* ventilator are shown in Table 3-1. Data query response proceeds according to a process by which the specific data items being requested of the Servo*i* are defined for, requested of, and received from the ventilator[66]. Command definitions are preceded by the two-character acronym "DB,"

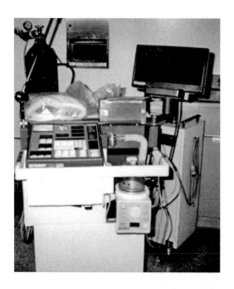

Figure 3-3
Puritan-Bennett 7200ae
mechanical ventilator
(Photo by author)

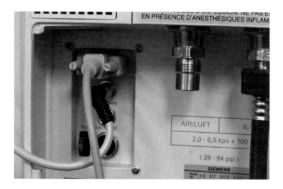

Figure 3-4 Serial communications port on Siemens Servoⁱ ventilator—
9-pin male RS232 cable attached (Photo by author)

for Define Breath. Then, two-digit integers follow, corresponding to the codes of specific parameters for which values are to be retrieved. Each code is concatenated: the more commands, the more data to be retrieved. For example, in column 1, row 1 the following command is displayed:

DB 01 03 08 10 11

---

[66] Command reference manual: Servoⁱ Computer Interface Reference Manual, reference number E382 E407E 119 01 01 02

Table 3-1 Servo^i commands transmitted and corresponding data retrieved

Command Transmitted	Command Received	Command Transmitted	Command Received	Time the command was transmitted
DB01 03 08 10 11	*	RB	2558 2554 2161 2271 2145	03 1218 112855

This command establishes specific parameter values to be retrieved from the mechanical ventilator in accordance with a mapping of these coded entries to a known table of available parameter channels. These known channel entries are listed in Table 3-2.

I will illustrate one data retrieval example here. The complete list of commands are available from the manufacturer in their Computer Interface Emulator reference manual.

The breath entries "01" "03" "08" "10" and "11" correspond to the parameter names "inspiratory tidal volume," "expiratory tidal volume," "respiratory rate," "expiratory minute volume," and "mean airway pressure," respectively.

When the command "DB0103081011" is transmitted, the acknowledgement "*" is received, indicating that the Servo^i successfully received and processed the command. Next, when the command "RB" (Read Breath) is transmitted, the response will contain the data associated with the DB command parameters, in the form of a vector of integers in coded format. In this instance, "DB0103081011" results in "25582554216122712145".

Considering the coded value response for the breath value "01" (inspiratory tidal volume), we see the corresponding "RB" entry is "2558." To translate this coded value response (CVR) into the actual finding value (FV) involves the following transformation equation:

$$FV = \frac{(CVR - 2048) \times 4.883}{ScaleFactor} \qquad (3.1)$$

The scale factor for this parameter from the Servo^i Computer Interface Emulator Reference Manual, is 5000.

$$FV = \frac{(2558 - 2048) \times 4.883}{5000} \qquad (3.2)$$

$FV = 0.50$ liters

Table 3-2 Resulting findings values for Servo[i]

Channel Number	Channel Value	Channel Scale Factor	Finding Value	Finding Name	Finding Units	Finding Date/Time
01	2558	5000	0.50	Inspiratory Tidal Volume	liters	2003 December 18 11:28:55
03	2554	5000	0.49	Expiratory Tidal Volume	liters	2003 December 18 11:28:55
08	2161	50	11.04	Respiratory Rate	breaths/ minute	2003 December 18 11:28:55
10	2271	200	5.44	Expiratory Minute Volume	liters/ minute	2003 December 18 11:28:55
11	2145	50	9.47	Mean Airway Pressure	cm H2O	2003 December 18 11:28:55

This process is repeated for all parameters in the "RB" finding vector. Upon completion, the values in Table 3-2 result. When paired with their corresponding units, the values for inspiratory tidal volume, expiratory tidal volume, respiratory rate, expiratory minute volume, and mean airway pressure are revealed together with their snapshots in date and time.

The query-response mechanism for the Puritan-Bennett (PB) 7200ae ventilator, by comparison, is much different. Of course, there is no expectation that they would be the same, but the point is to illustrate that the same information can be retrieved from two different kinds of medical hardware in differing formats. The data communications

Table 3-3 Summary of 7200ae SPD Command Structure

Ventilator Command	Definition/Description
SPD<sp><CR>	Send Patient Data:
	1. Ventilator time
	2. Respiratory rate – patient value
	3. Minute volume – patient value
	4. Mean airway pressure – patient value
	5. I:E ratio – patient value (inspiratory : expiratory ratio expressed as expiratory component)
	6. Tidal volume – patient value
	7. Spontaneous minute volume – patient value
	8. Peak airway pressure – patient value
	9. Plateau pressure – patient value

Table 3-4 SPD Query and Response

Query: SPD Response: PD,12:54 ,12 ,11.1 ,10.4 ,1.9 ,0.92 ,0.00 ,23.0 ,	
Ventilator Time	12:54 (pm implied)
Respiratory Rate (patient value)	12 (/minute)
Minute Volume (patient value)	11.1 (liters/minute)
Mean airway pressure (patient value)	10.4 (cm H2O)
I:E Ratio	1/9 (expiratory component)
Tidal volume	0.92 (liters)
Spontaneous minute volume (patient value)	(liters/minute)
Peak airway pressure (patient value)	23.0 (cm H2O)
Plateau pressure (patient value)	N/A (none present)

query-response format is available in models of the 7200ae and 7200spe ventilators configured with the Digital Communications Interface (DCI) 2.0 option[67]. PB 7200ae commands are structured in 4-character, fixed-length words—all uppercase—followed by a carriage return.

Table 3-3 summarizes the "Send Patient Data" command for the PB 7200ae ventilator. Complete listings of all commands and their definitions are provided in the PB 7200ae operator's manual.

Table 3-4 shows the response received to one SPD command transmission.

3.2 Communication Interface Architectures

These two examples serve to illustrate the point that medical devices and device manufacturers tend to employ their own proprietary mechanisms at the device level for data communication which mandates the need for an independent—third party—interfacing mechanism (software device) to translate the data into the correct format and to ensure that data are interpreted correctly. For instance, in com-

---

[67] "Puritan Bennett 7200 series ventilator system Ventilator, Options and Accessories Operator's Manual," Part Number 22300 A, September 1990. Includes Supplemental DCI 2.0 Option Part Number 22427 A (December 1993) & Option 20 Digital Communication Interface (DCI) Part Number 20521 B (January 1990).

paring Table 3-2 with Table 3-4, it can be seen that there is no precise translation between inspiratory & expiratory tidal volume identified in the former, and the simple tidal volume defined in the latter. A reasonable inference can be made that the inspiratory and expiratory tidal volumes are approximately the same, or that the average between the two might be considered as an approximation for the definition of the tidal volume represented in Table 3-4. However, there is no automated mechanism for performing this translation: a human must make the interpretation and instruct the computer in this interpretive methodology prior to making use of the data. Hence, if an enterprise contained mechanical ventilators of both types and the objective was to be able to interchange ventilators seamlessly within the environment, then in order to make their use transparent to the EMR, the data items comprising the data dictionaries associated with each of these ventilator devices must be taken into account and somehow sorted out so that similar data items can be represented as existing fields within the EMR database. Despite the fact that the syntax is different, the methodology is the same.

To further an understanding of the device interface illustrated in Figure 3-1, it is extended to include the processes described in Figure 3-5, which provides an overview of the methodological process flow.

At the initiating request of a user, a "Command Manager" receives and parses the request for specific content (i.e., retrieve parameter X) or as a general request for data (i.e., retrieve all) from a specific device. The "Command Manager" is meant as a generalized process for what could be a simple piece of software that interacts via a user interface or command prompt to receive a request to perform some task, to include communicating with a medical device. In its simplest form, this "Command Manager" could even be a terminal program.

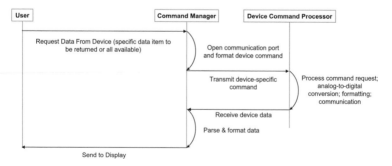

Figure 3-5 Device data query response functional flow

The "Command Manager" establishes a communication link with the medical device in order to transmit this command to the "Device Command Processor." The "Device Command Processor" is a generic name for the processing hardware, firmware, and software responsible for receiving the request, processing the request through the hardware and firmware logic, performing the analog-to-digital conversions necessary to translate analog signals into digital data, and then the communication logic to transmit the response back to the "Command Manager." Once device data are received at the "Command Manager," the next step can vary depending on the intended use case: data may be parsed and displayed to the user; they may be parsed and stored in a data repository for future review; they may be used in clinical decision making as part of a clinical decision support (CDS) system, etc.

The key to the use of this methodology for medical devices, as previously explained, lies in the generation of device queries that are specific to the device under investigation as well as to the parsing and interpretation of their data. From the preceding example it is now clear that how data items are intended or defined by the device manufacturer is essential to their incorporation into the EMR. This can be illustrated with the aid of Figure 3-6.

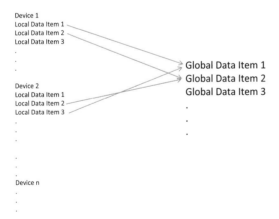

Figure 3-6 Local device data item mapping to global definitions

To ensure proper interpretation of device-specific data, clear definitions of those data elements must be provided and, in some instance, caveats for their use based upon the device. For instance, inspiratory and expiratory tidal volumes are approximately equal to the average tidal volume. However, the fact that these parameters are available from the Servo^j and not from the PB 7200ae is an important fact and to assert the tidal volume measurement from the 7200ae as being either an inspiratory or an expiratory value is to add information about the data that are interpreted. Rather, it is more reasonable to state that the average inspiratory and expiratory tidal volume measurements from the Servo^j approximate a mean, or average, tidal volume measurement, and this tidal volume measurement is what is measured by the PB 7200ae.

Figure 3-7 shows the location of each of the software components associated with the data query-response process model. In the proprietary communication language of a specific device, the "Command Manager" assumes all responsibility for properly formatting and transmitting the commands to the medical hardware and for retrieving and parsing the responses from that hardware. In this model, the "Command Manager" architecture is designed to communicate in the proprietary format of the specific medical device.

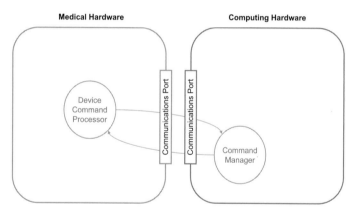

Figure 3-7 Compute and medical hardware connectivity augmented with functionality

The architecture of Figure 3-8 alleviates some of the need for coding proprietary commands within the "Command Manager" as now those commands can be retrieved from a data repository in preparation for transmission to the medical device. The "Command Manager" parses the data request per the above and transmits a query to a "Database Manager" to provide the specific and syntactically correct command structure associated with the requested data item back to the "Command Manager." The "Database Manager" could have a simple tabular-formatted structure that retrieves the syntax for a specific device

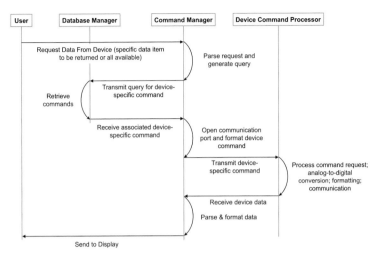

Figure 3-8 Device data query response functional flow with a database query feature for command selection

whereby the device identity is automatically detected at the communication interface to the computing hardware upon which the "Command Manager" is resident, or it could even be human logic to send a specific command (in the case of a terminal program). Regardless, the idea here is that of associating a device-specific command with the data item being requested.

Figure 3-9 augments Figure 3-7 by incorporating the command database functionality. The communication mechanism now involves retrieving device-specific commands from the database and then transmitting these through the communication channel to the medical hardware. The medical hardware responds, in turn, by transmitting data back to the "Command Manager". The process is more flexible and less proprietary because the command sequences that are transmitted to the medical hardware can now be stored in a data repository that segregates different device commands from one another.

The selection of the appropriate commands to be transmitted could be further augmented using either a manual or an automated mechanism for testing the type of device attached to the computing hardware and then selecting the commands to transmit based on that test (e.g.: a device identifier), or via a simple user selection mechanism, whereby a user identifies the device prior to transmitting the commands to the medical device.

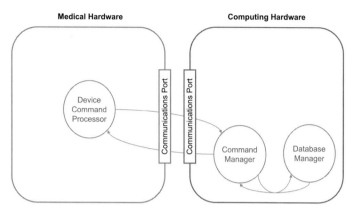

Figure 3-9 Compute and medical hardware connectivity with device database functionality added to support simple message command query-response

However, other aspects of the communication and query-response methodology are still rather proprietary; specifically, the selection of the device interface itself—this includes the physical connectivity, such as RS232 serial communications port, universal serial bus (USB), Ethernet, Bluetooth, or other. Processing of the retrieved data must occur, and the parsing of these data items that are transmitted from the medical device back to the computing hardware is dependent on the type of medical device. Thus, a data post-processing function that can be tied or linked to the device commands transmitted to the medical device (that is, the type of device commands sent translates into the types of parsing functions required) must be taken into account. This is done by adding the capability to determine the mechanics of the device interface (i.e., port settings, communications type, etc.) automatically in functionality, separate from the selection and transmission of commands. This is illustrated in Figure 3-10.

The "Comm Manager" or "Communications Manager" now handles interface selection. That is, if the attached device requires specific serial port connectivity settings, then this would be captured here. For instance, if the Servo[i] required serial device communication settings using 9600 baud, 8 bits, 1 stop bit, and even parity, and the 7200ae required serial port device communication settings using 9600 baud, 8 bits, 1 stop bit, and no parity, then the "Comm Manager" would ensure that these were selected automatically. Note also that the database can become the repository for this information: the message transmitted from the "Database Manager" to the "Comm Man-

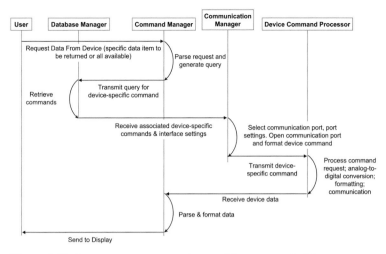

Figure 3-10 Query response processing model augmented with Communications Manager

ager" now includes interface settings. Figure 3-11 updates the hardware connectivity illustration showing the "Comm Manager."

The final component to add to this model is the "DP" or "Data Processing Manager." This function receives the data parsing structure from the "Database Manager" associated with the specific device under query and parses the output from the device so that individual data items can be separated into individual attributes that may then be dis-

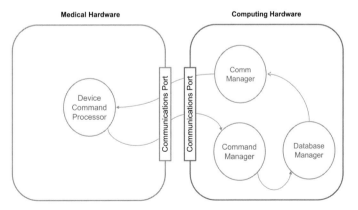

Figure 3-11 Compute and medical hardware connectivity with Comm Manager added

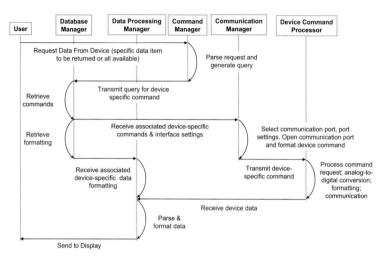

Figure 3-12 Query response processing model augmented with
Data Processing Manager

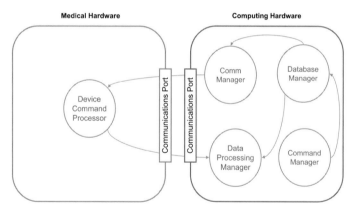

Figure 3-13 Compute and medical hardware connectivity with
Data Processing Manager added

played to the user, stored in an EMR, or transmitted to other applications. Figure 3-12 depicts this query-response processing model. Figure 3-13 is the hardware connectivity view of this functional implementation.

The device query-response process has now evolved to the point at which device query commands can be retrieved from a database. By knowing the identity of the device, the command manager can request device-specific commands from the database which can also supply information to the communications manager on how to actually communicate with the device physically. At the same time, device-specific information is passed to the data processing manager which uses this identifying information from the database to "understand" how to parse the output data, when received. This model provides for an extensible architecture for general device communication.

The communication mechanism between device and computing hardware is now scalable and flexible because the device commands can be selected from a database, obviating the need for hard-coding. However, the commands used to retrieve and parse data from the medical device are only valid so long as the medical device manufacturer provides for the continuing maintenance of those device commands and then regularly publishes updates. Up to now the assumption has been that the medical hardware all responds in accord with published message-type interfaces in which query-response commands in the form of simple syntactical transactions are the norm. Moreover, some device manufacturers only publish their device interfaces as part of proprietary software development kits or under contractual partnerships. In such cases, the communication mechanisms are not message-based at all. Hence, the query-response model for medical hardware interaction is only one form of data communication model that is used. The model works quite well when the interfaces are publicized by the medical hardware manufacturers; otherwise, a different model is required. For cases when a medical hardware manufacturer employs a proprietary messaging architecture that relies on developing or coding interfaces to exposed application programming inter-

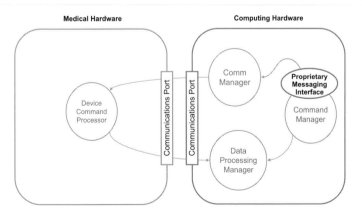

Figure 3-14 Medical hardware device connectivity when proprietary messaging interfaces are embedded into the processing functionality in the computing hardware

faces (APIs), then the functional model for communication remains essentially the same. However, the concept of using a database to retrieve individual commands is no longer applicable. In this case, conceptually, the connectivity diagram can be modified to reflect the new embedded interface, such as shown in Figure 3-14.

The "Command Manager" responsible for issuing commands now must employ the proprietary messaging interface mechanism that is built into it through vendor-supplied software development kits, or SDKs, to communicate with the medical devices. The "Comm Manager" can still be used to establish the physical communication between the computing and medical hardware. However, there is no command selection based upon device type. The mechanism for communicating still involves a query-response model, and they are proprietary in that they can only be made through the software interfaces established using the SDKs. A more concrete example of this is requiring the use of specific functions to retrieve data from medical hardware in which these functions are defined as dynamic link libraries (.dll) that must be compiled into the source code of the "Command Manager". These functions must be called with specific arguments in order to retrieve the requested data from the medical hardware. In such cases, the "Command Manager" now becomes a proprietary piece of software that is specific to this one type of medical device. It may be possible to provide this capability within the "Command Manager" as part of a larger overall device communication system, and to only use the proprietary components as required. But, the code will now have the proprietary components embedded, and this can limit its redistribution within an enterprise, especially if there are contractual restrictions as to the quantity of computing platforms on which the medical device manufacturer's Software Development Kit (SDK) may be deployed.

This point can be further illustrated. Let's consider two examples of Medical/Surgical monitors. Medical/Surgical monitors are typically those patient monitors that accompany nursing technicians throughout a ward on rounds during the process of vitals collection. This process typically occurs at least three times daily, notably at nursing/technician shift changes. These monitors measure basic patient vitals parameters, including non-invasive blood pressure (NIBP), temperature (T), pulse or heart rate (HR), and hemoglobin oxygenation, usually determined using a pulse oximetry finger cuff (SpO2).

Figure 3-15 and Figure 3-16 illustrate the user interface screens on two popular monitors: The GE Procare 400 Auscultatory Monitor and the WelchAllyn Spot Vitals LXI Monitor, respectively.

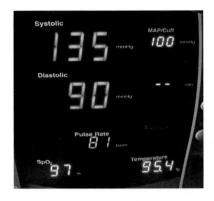

Figure 3-15
GE Dinamap Procare 400
user interface screen
(Photo by author)

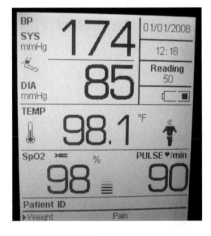

Figure 3-16
WelchAllyn Spot Vitals LXI
user interface screen

Communication with these monitors is rather easy using serial and USB cables, respectively. Figure 3-17 shows hard-wired cabling involved in a typical communication configuration from the Dinamap monitor. All cabling is standard off-the-shelf hardware available from the manufacturer, save the author's selection of a serial-to-USB adapter that facilitates connecting to a laptop computer.

The WelchAllyn Spot Vitals LXI monitor can receive either 9-pin RS232 cables or can be communicated with using a standard USB cable with miniature jack on the monitor side of the connection, as shown in Figure 3-18.

The detailed communication between the monitors and a querying application can be studied quite readily using a serial or USB port monitor. I have used several of these types of port monitors but have found two to be superior. These include the Advanced Serial Port

Monitor and the Advanced USB Port Monitor by AggSoft[68]. These monitors can be purchased today (October 2008) at a cost of about USD 60 for each tool. With these monitors it is possible to view the detailed interaction (both queries and responses) between the monitors and the querying application.

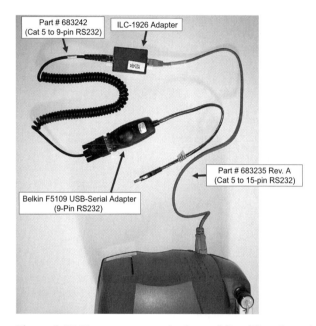

Figure 3-17 Dinamap communications cabling (Photo by author)

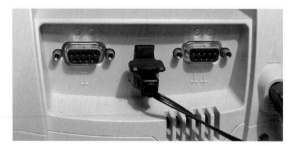

Figure 3-18 WelchAllyn Spot Vitals LXI communications cabling (Photo by author)

---

[68] Available for download for free trial with purchase required for continuing use at http://www.aggsoft.com.

For instance, Table 3-5 displays an example of the detailed serial port communication between the GE Dinamap and the querying application for blood pressure. As discussed in the preceding chapter, commands for the GE Dinamap are published by manufacturer[69]. Many manufacturers supply these communication manuals to enable customers to retrieve information directly from the medical devices.

Table 3-5 Advanced Serial Port Monitor trace between the querying
application and the GE Dinamap

```
NA!2<CR>
NA1100658141084109&3<CR>
TA!8<CR>
TA20957#$<CR>
OA!3<CR>
OA1099402#C<CR>
RA!6<CR>
RA2069"K<CR>
```

In this table we see responses to a series of queries for blood pressure (NA), temperature (TA), oxygen saturation (OA), and pulse (RA), respectively. The characters immediately following each command represent checksums.

I have underlined the output to make it more visible. In the case of blood pressure, the systolic, diastolic, and mean components here are 141, 84, and 109 mmHg, respectively.

Similar translations occur for temperature, oxygen saturation (SpO2), and pulse. For the sake of brevity these are 95.7F, 99%, and 69/minute, respectively.

The amount of data transferred both to and from the device is very small. Figure 3-19 plots the outgoing and incoming transaction throughput rates for communicating between the WelchAllyn Spot Vitals LXI Monitor and the querying application. These values will vary depending on the type and quantity of data retrieved from the monitor. The plot serves to illustrate the throughput scale of a typical transaction containing all four vitals components.

---

[69] "Host Communications Reference Manual," GE Dinamap, GE Medical Systems Information Technologies. Part Number 2010566 D. June 5th, 2003.

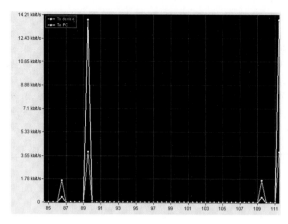

Figure 3-19 Transaction throughput rate between a querying
application and the WelchAllyn monitor
(plot created using the Advanced USB Port Monitor)

As shown, the outgoing query required a throughput of only 3.5 Kbits/
second. The data-carrying response throughput rate was approximately 14 Kbits/second.

I have referred to a "querying application" to describe the software
that requests data from a medical device. As pointed out earlier, this
can be a terminal program. I have created my own querying application whose user interfaces are shown in Figure 3-20 and Figure 3-21,
illustrating results taken from the Dinamap and WelchAllyn monitors, respectively.

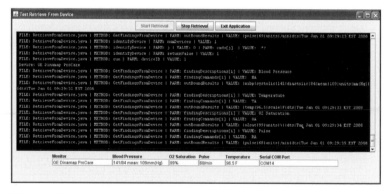

Figure 3-20 Querying application developed by author showing
Dinamap monitor data

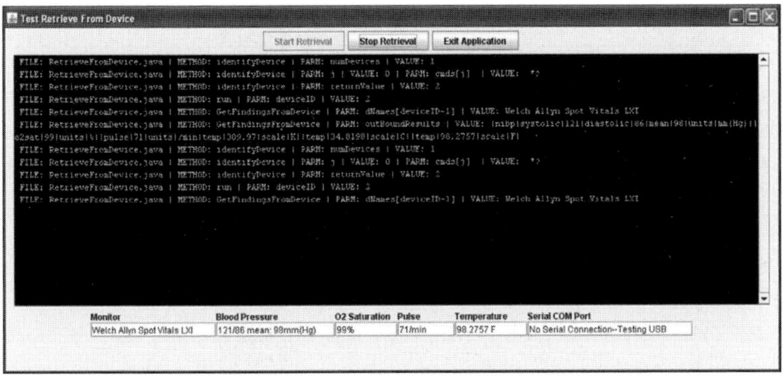

Figure 3-21 Querying application developed by author showing WelchAllyn monitor data

3.3 Standardized Data Interfacing Formats

Existing device integration solutions in the market place[70] provide the necessary device-level interfacing to include the communication and data processing components described above. These can be licensed and provide a clean mechanism for device interfacing. The data can be retrieved and stored in flat files on the computing hardware platform for tertiary processing and transmission to the EMR. It is important to understand the mechanics behind the interactions between the software and the medical devices themselves so that information technology and biomedical engineering departments can gain an understanding of what is involved in the data query and post-processing, in order to remove the sense of mystery from the device interface software.

The data themselves can be stored locally on the computing hardware. They can also be transformed directly into a more standardized message, such as HL7 Observation Report—Unsolicited (ORU) transactions (also referred to as an HL7 ORU^R01 message). The HL7[71] is one of the ANSI standards developing organizations focusing on the interoperability in the healthcare sector. The HL7 provides messaging templates to support communication of observations, orders, laboratory data, pharmaceutical information, demographics, etc. While a

---

[70] Examples: DataCaptor by Capsule Technologie; Sensitron Wireless Healthcare Innovations, Inc., et al.

[71] Health Level Seven information and models available from their Web site at http://www.hl7.org.

complete treatment of the HL7 history and structure are beyond the scope here, an overview is appropriate to aid in understanding.

The HL7 standard has evolved to an approved, industry-wide messaging template—versions 2.x, with the latest approved release of Application Protocol for Electronic Data Exchange in Healthcare Environments, version 2.5[72]. The newest versions of the HL7 standard provides for a more fully descriptive object model: a Reference Information Model (RIM). This is reflected in Version 3.0 of the HL7 Standard. This model adds rigor to message definition based on an object-oriented methodology and implementation. In particular, the versions of the HL7 Standard prior to the Reference Information Model provide great flexibility in terms of defining HL7 messages. While the specific format of the message is defined, the use of various component segments can vary greatly, requiring end users and developers to adapt interfaces in existing health information systems to meet the specific needs of these HL7 messages. The goal of Version 3.0 and the Reference Information Model is to promote uniform conformance by individual health information system vendors.

However, widespread HL7 message formatting today typically conforms to version 2 of that standard. In the discussion that follows I will reference message formats with respect to Versions 2.5 and the newly available (as of this writing) version 2.6 of the Health Level Seven Standard for electronic data exchange[73].

The messaging format for reporting of vitals parameters is described in Chapter 7—"Observation Reporting" of the HL7 Standard Version 2.6. Details of the contents of the messages are described thoroughly by this source. Therefore, I will focus on explicit implementations and on key elements of a typical Observation Result—Unsolicited (ORU).

The ORU[74] has traditionally been used for communicating results and findings using a standard messaging format. The explicit message content will be described below and can be referenced in detail from its source document[75]. The ORU Message is one of many message structures that are delivered in response to events. The ORU is termed an R01 Event, to coincide with its use for transmitting laboratory

---

[72] http://www.hl7.org, version 2.5 approved as ANSI standard as of June 26th, 2003.

[73] Health Level Seven (HL7) Standard for Electronic Data Exchange specification (SEDES), Version 2.6 © 2004.

[74] Ibid. Chapter 7, Section 7.3.1

[75] Health Level Seven (HL7) Standard for Electronic Data Exchange Specification, June 2003. Section 7.3: General Trigger Events & Message Definitions.

results to tertiary systems. While the object is laboratory results, the R01 event is oftentimes used as the primary message for communicating vitals transactions from a source system (in this case, a medical device) to an EMR.

Clinical messages are constructed using a hierarchy of segments, called observation records, or OBX segments. Multiple observation records can be transmitted in the body of a single message. The following format represents the complete R01 event for an ORU. Each observation record comprises a series of segments which define the content of the observation, its value, units, text qualifiers or descriptors, and time & date stamps. I tailor out components of the message associated with this event for specific sets of findings to illustrate how such a message would be created from flat file data or a data record returned from a medical device. Refer to Table 3-6.

Table 3-6 Tailored R01 Event—ORU

Event—R01 message segment identifier	Description
MSH	Message header
PID	Patient identification
PV1	Patient visit
OBR	Observation order
OBX	Observation result

Each of the message segments are compiled together to create the event R01. The message header, MSH segment, contains the fields defined in Table 3-7. Field separators are always vertical "pipe" characters: '|'.

An example transaction that represents the construct shown is:

```
MSH|^~\&|<source_app>|<source_care_unit>|
<destination_app>|<enterprise>|<date/time>|
|ORU^R01|<date/time>|P|2.5
```

Here, the date/time stamp is used both to stamp the message as well as be a unique message identifier. Fields 13 & 14 can be omitted for standalone R01 events as they are optional. Many receiving systems do not mandate a number of these fields. Usually, MSH fields 1, 2, 3, 5, 7, 10-12 are those necessary for communicating simple observation results with receiving systems.

Table 3-7 MSH segment content and definition

Field Number	Definition
0	Segment identifier
1	The escape character sequence. ^ separates adjacent components of data fields; ~ separates multiple occurrences of fields; \ escape character & separates adjacent subcomponents of data fields. Required content: ^~\\&
2	Source or sending application (from where data originate)
3	Sending facility or organizational unit
4	Receiving application (function or application to which message is being transmitted)
5	Receiving facility or organizational unit
6	Date and time stamp of the ORU
7	Not used
8	Message type
9	Message control identifier
10	Processing ID
11	Version ID
12	Sequence number
13	Continuation pointer

We can substitute fields in the MSH segment to further illustrate content:

```
MSH|^~\&|Medical_Device_Application|EMR|Hospital|
20071229071502||ORU^R01|20071229071502|P|2.5
```

The patient identification (PID) segment establishes the identity of the patient and associates information such as medical record number, patient number, name, and other associating information. The segment comprises many fields, many of which are optional, depending on the requirements of the receiving system. An example of a typical PID segment is as follows. Two identifiers are prescribed with a field separator to separate the identifiers and numbers from each component:

```
PID|1||[ID1_number]^ID1_Check_Digit^Check_Digit_
Scheme^Assigning_Authority^[ID1_Type_Code]~
```

```
[ID2_number]^ID2_Check_Digit^Check_Digit-Scheme^
Assigning_Authority^[ID2_Type_Code]||[last_name]^
[first_name]|||||||||||||
```

By substituting example values we can further clarify the specific content of the PID segment, using fabricated patient account number (PAN), medical record number (MRN), and patient name:

```
PID|1|12345678^^^^PAN~987654^^^^MRN||Doe^Jane|||
|||||||||||
```

The patient visit segment will not be detailed here as it normally applies to patient admission, transfer, and discharge applications. Instead, we will focus on the details of the observation reporting segments.

The observation request segment, or OBR, identifies the observations to follow, detailed via the OBX segments. More than one OBR segment may appear in a typical R01 event. Multiple OBX segments can be associated with a single OBR segment, and there is no limitation or constraint on the number of OBX segments per OBR. The OBR summary in Table 3-8 represents only a subset of the total fields that can

Table 3-8 Abridged OBR segment

Field Number	Required/ Optional/ Not Used	Field Name	Notes
1	R	OBR Set ID	Increments the OBR number
2	O	Placer order number	
3	O	Filler order number	
4	R	Universal service identifier	Order identifier or order code
5	Not Used	Priority	Retained for backward compatibility
6	Not Used	Requested Date/Time	Retained for backward compatibility
7	O	Observation Start Date/Time	
8	O	Observation End Date/Time	
9	O	Collection Volume	
10	R	Collector Identifier	User identifier (identifier of individual making observation)

be used. A limited set of fields are presented as relate to order fulfill-ment and are not pertinent to communicating the result itself[76].

The following represents an example of an OBR segment that might be used within this ORU:

```
OBR|1|||abcdefg|||20071229071523|||Zaleski
```

The final component of the segment is the observation, OBX. The observation result segment communicates a single value and repre-sents the atomic or lowest level of granularity within the ORU. An example OBX segment follows in Table 3-9[77]. Note that this is not a complete segment but, rather, representative of a typical OBX associ-ated with the communication of vitals data.

The following OBX segments represent examples of pulse (symbol: HR) and temperature (symbol: T):

```
OBX|1|NM|8889-8&HR||77|/min|||||F|||2007122907
1523|||PULSE OXIMETRY|MED/SURG MONITOR||APICAL|||

OBX|2|NM|20091-5&T||100.2|C|||||F|||200712290715
23|||TEMP PROBE|MED/SURG MONITOR||ORAL|||
```

The findings are communicated as numeric values (NM). The symbols are HR and T, respectively. Preceding the symbols are coded values based on the Logical Observation Identifiers Names and Codes data-base[78]. The date and time stamps are precisely the same as those iden-tified in the OBR, PID, and MSH segments above. The source of the measurements are via pulse oximetry cuff and temperature probe, respectively. The equipment used to determine the findings was a Medical/Surgical Monitor—a portable vitals collection device nor-mally found in post-acute or medical/surgical units. The site for the HR and T measurements on the patient were the Apical and Oral, respectively.

As stated previously, many medical devices communicate serially (that is, they communicate through a serial port). Virtually all devices using serial port communication adhere to the EIA232 standards.

---

[76] HL7 SEDES Chapter 7.4, Section 7.4.1

[77] HL7 SEDES Chapter 7, Section 7.4.2

[78] Logical Observation Identifiers Names and Codes (LOINC) Users' Guide. Copyright 1995-2007, Regenstrief Institute, Inc.

Table 3-9 OBX component definitions

Field Number	Required/ Optional/ Not Used	Field Name	Notes
1	O	Set ID	Sequence number.
2	R	Value type	Finding type. Typical values in the context of device interfacing include numeric (NM), date (DT), string data (ST), structured numeric (SN)
3	R	Observation identifier	Unique finding identification label. Could be a coded value.
4	O	Observation sub-ID	
5	R	Observation value	
6	R	Units	
7	O	Reference range	
8	O	Abnormal flags	
9	O	Probability	
10	O	Nature of abnormal test	
11	O	Observation result status	C—correction; D—deletion; F—final; I—results pending, specimen in lab; N—nor asked; O—order detail description only, no result; P—preliminary results; R—results entered, not verified; S—partial results (only retained for backward compatibility); X—results cannot be obtained for this observation; U—results status change to final without retransmitting; W—post original as wrong or incorrect.
12	O	Effective date of reference range	
13	O	User-define access checks	
14	R	Date/time of observation	
15	O	Producer's ID	
16	O	Responsible observer	
17	O	Observation method	
18	O	Equipment instance identifier	
19	O	Date/time of the analysis	
20	O	Observation site	
21	O	Observation instance identifier	

Table 3-9 OBX component definitions *(continued)*

Field Number	Required/ Optional/ Not Used	Field Name	Notes
22	O	Segment instance identifier	
23	O	Mood code	INT—intent; APT—appointment, planned for specific date/time/location; ARQ—appointment request; PRMS—promise; PRP—proposal; RQO—request-order; EVN events, actually happening or happened or continuing; EVN.CRT—event criterion; EXP—expectation

Many devices publish existing serial communication interfaces so that healthcare enterprises may develop their own custom communication mechanisms for their internal, proprietary purposes[79]. However, those devices that support standardized communication via HL7 can be interfaced more easily to EMRs.

3.4 Other Medical Device Data

The market for medical device communication is expanding. To this point I've focused on the communication of discrete event data: findings or values that are transmitted to the EMR. Yet, in discussing data the story is incomplete without addressing those data that are available at the point of care and which are used for real-time clinical diagnosis and intervention. In the next chapter I discuss the use of real-time data and their communication.

---

[79] Examples include the GE Dinamap, LifeScan glucometers, Nellcor Puritan Bennett Ventilators, Siemens and Magnet Servo[i] ventilators, Welch Allyn Spot Vitals monitors, etc.

4 Real-Time and Non-Real-Time Data Management

4.1 Real-Time Vital Signs Monitoring & Telemetry

There are differences between real-time, high frequency, continuous data, such as that displayed on the critical care monitor of Figure 4-1, and findings data communicated at discrete intervals from a medical device or Medical Device Gateway with the EMR. In this chapter I will discuss approaches to "integrating" live, real-time vitals findings and waveform information into the clinical record. The term "integrating" is shown in quotes because this term is used loosely to define an approach for showing real-time data, whether it involves communicating raw telemetry data through the EMR for storage and subsequent display, or a more superficial approach such as an externally-accessed display tool that merely shows the data in context with a patient's EMR.

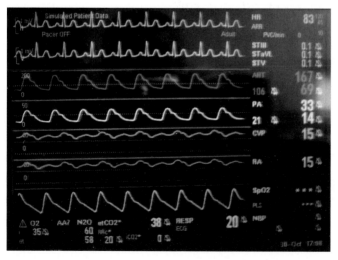

Figure 4-1 Example of a real-time waveform from a patient monitor
normally used in critical care (Photo by author)

In order to better understand the difference between data communicated at discrete intervals and real-time data, let's first understand what is meant by real-time data.

Real-time data collection translates into those data that are measured live (or near-live) and continuously as in the telemetry monitoring of patients. Such data typically comprise waveforms, video, and audio: data in which individual signal elements or data points are transmitted in intervals of milliseconds or tens of milliseconds. When we normally think of discrete data, such as findings communicated via a standard HL7 result transaction, it is normally implied that these data are communicated in intervals ranging from seconds to minutes to hours. Thus, these data can fall into the non-real-time or near-real time category. I offer the following definitions in the interest of promoting clarity:

Real-time data are those data that can be communicated unmolested from a source to destination without undo impedance. These data can include waveforms, video, and audio. Real-time data can also include discrete findings as opposed to waveform data. However, the same requirement on unimpeded delivery applies.

Non-real-time data are those data that may include waveforms but for which there is a measurable delay between the communication source and destination related to impeding factors (e.g.: network congestion) that impinge on the ability to accurately predict the delay. Non-real-time data can also include discrete findings.

Real-time data convey information for which each data element carries valuable content; for example, an electrocardiogram (ECG) waveform in which the structure (amplitude, timing) of individual segments of the signal (PQRST segment) provide information relative to patient health and survival. Discretely sampling such a waveform at intervals of seconds, minutes, or hours would convey no valuable information. This is illustrated in Figure 4-2 in which the time scale of an ECG signal P wave (approximately 100 milliseconds) is shown in comparison with a discrete sampling interval of 500 milliseconds (0.5 seconds). As can be seen, even with a discrete sampling interval of under 1 second, important information is lost, thus necessitating real-time data communication.

In order to ensure no loss of content it is necessary to provide for sampling down to the 10s of milliseconds or less. Thus, because of the need to communicate real-time data at high frequency (i.e., 10-200 data points per second), and because the timing of these data are key to intervention, it is important that the communication of such data

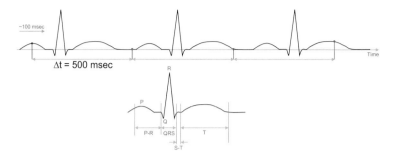

Figure 4-2 Notional ECG waveform showing time scale of signal in relation to discrete sampling during a typical time window

not be impeded unnecessarily. Access to real-time data, especially in high-acuity environments such as emergency departments and critical care, is essential for intervening in the life-and-death matters of patients:

"...for an ECG, the sampling rate should be at least 200 measurements per second...sudden heart stoppage or severe dysrhythmias are the most frequent causes of sudden death. Therefore, heart-rate and rhythm monitors must function continuously and should sound alarms within 15-20 seconds after detecting a problem.[80]"

Occurrences of catastrophic events, such as asystole (i.e., heart stoppage) requires communicating this event immediately to sustain life. While such monitoring can occur anywhere in the health enterprise and at any point in patient care depending on the ordering physician's prescriptive requirements, perhaps the most common locations in which live patient monitoring occurs are the operating room, the emergency department, and the intensive care unit.

One aspect of real-time data is that the time between actual measurement and display is minimal. What is meant by the qualifying adjective 'minimal? Essentially, it implies without undo delay. Such is the case in which the existing network over which the real-time data are communicated experiences no congestion so that the data are delivered unfettered from source to destination.

One way to visualize the concept of real-time versus non-real-time transmission and receipt of data is through the graphic illustrated in

---

[80] Edward H. Shortliffe, Ed. and James J. Cimino, Assoc. Ed. Biomedical Informatics Computer Applications in Health Care and Biomedicine, 3rd Ed. Springer Science & Business Media, LLC: 2006 Pages 616-17

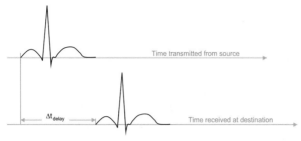

Figure 4-3 Illustration of delay between source and destination transmission of a real-time waveform

Figure 4-3. The delay between the time at which the signal (here, an ECG waveform) is transmitted and when it is received is represented as a delay,

$$\Delta t_{delay} = t_{received} - t_{transmitted} \tag{4.1}$$

Yet, the delay is not the only difference between real-time and non-real-time data. One obvious question that must be answered is what value of delay constitutes real-time versus non-real-time?

Figure 4-4 illustrates the time delay during an off-peak period (e.g.: 6 am on a Sunday morning) from a remote location outside of a controlled network (i.e., wide area network), through a wide area (WAN) network connection, in comparison to the delay between a monitor and a gateway server within a controlled local area network.

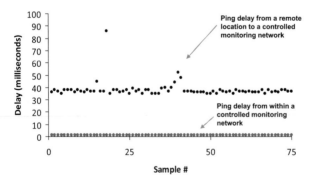

Figure 4-4 Comparison between ping delays within an isolated telemetry LAN and from outside the LAN, through a WAN operating over a virtual private network

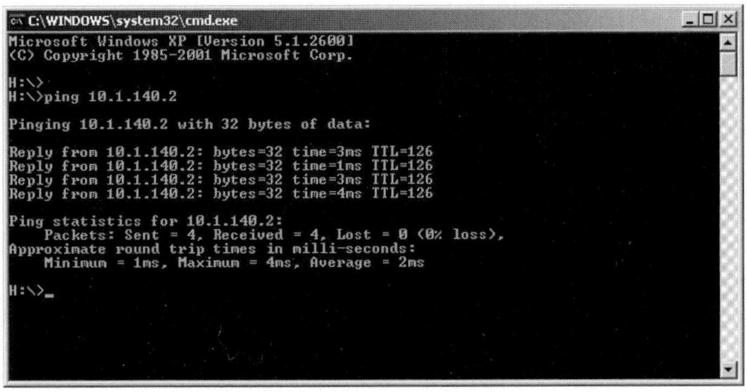

```
C:\WINDOWS\system32\cmd.exe                                        _ □ ×
Microsoft Windows XP [Version 5.1.2600]
(C) Copyright 1985-2001 Microsoft Corp.

H:\>
H:\>ping 10.1.140.2

Pinging 10.1.140.2 with 32 bytes of data:

Reply from 10.1.140.2: bytes=32 time=3ms ITL=126
Reply from 10.1.140.2: bytes=32 time=1ms ITL=126
Reply from 10.1.140.2: bytes=32 time=3ms ITL=126
Reply from 10.1.140.2: bytes=32 time=4ms ITL=126

Ping statistics for 10.1.140.2:
    Packets: Sent = 4, Received = 4, Lost = 0 (0% loss),
Approximate round trip times in milli-seconds:
    Minimum = 1ms, Maximum = 4ms, Average = 2ms

H:\>_
```

Figure 4-5 Use of ping command to verify network connectivity to a server, workstation, or network-enabled device

The delay reported is approximate and includes the processing time on both platforms as well as the network delay round-trip across the network. As such it is only an approximation. However, in comparing from within and outside a local area network, it is a telling measure of performance.

While it is obvious that the delays will vary between a WAN and an isolated LAN, noteworthy is the variability demonstrated between the two. If the only difference were a fixed delay (some value, t_{diff}), then it would be possible to approximate and compensate for this difference using this rather simple (and simplistic) model:

$$\Delta t_{WAN} = \Delta t_{LAN} + t_{diff} . \qquad (4.2)$$

Yet, the difference between the two delays is not predictable. The WAN delay can vary greatly depending on factors that cannot be controlled (or predicted with accuracy). Meanwhile, the LAN delay remains constant and predictable at any time of day and is independent of network traffic outside of the LAN because it is isolated. Indeed, the WAN delay can vary with time of day and day of week. This is quintessential. If the delay cannot be predicted with accuracy, how can we rely on the delivery of a telemetry signal for which a patient's life may be dependent? The answer is that we cannot comfortably do so. Furthermore, even though the signal can be transmitted using an assured delivery mechanism (i.e., TCP/IP) we have no control over whether the WAN will be operating. For instance, if we are relying on the distribution via a commercial Internet Service Provider (ISP) then it is unpredicatable as to whether some systemic delay or traffic pattern will interrupt the transmission of these data. Again, we cannot accurately predict the Quality of Service (QoS).

The delays shown in Figure 4-4 were measured using a simple ping command (i.e., involving transmission of a 32 byte message), in which the ping <IP address> command is executed on one machine within a network, to determine both connectivity to a given compute platform as verified by an acknowledgement received from the target compute platform at the transmitting compute platform. An example of the use of the ping command is illustrated in Figure 4-5.

Outside of these environments, ambulatory patient monitoring can occur in patient transit from one location to another within the hospital or outside, including emergency transport and home-health[81]. Many portable telemetry devices incorporate pulse oximetry, pulse, plus at least one-lead ECG monitoring[82].

These real-time monitoring functions sometimes employ embedded analytics, including rules-based processing algorithms that enable real-time assessments of values for the purpose of generating and transmitting alarms along with the raw measurement data from the monitors to a central point of connection, such as a monitoring station.

Perhaps the main yet obvious difference between real-time and non-real-time monitoring is captured within the scope of the name: real-time. The adjective associated with the name is also a good example of its definition. The term real-time implies that results and findings are available as soon as they are measured and are provided to a delivery point with a minimum of latency. The latency is typically determined by the limitations on the requisite communication and processing necessary to transmit and render the real-time data on the remote reporting device or devices.

4.2 Communication Protocols & Networking

Up to this point I have discussed communicating ad-hoc results asynchronously: pulse and blood pressure, for example. These were shown to be processed using a standards-based transaction such as HL7. These results were collected in 'bundles' called findings. In

---

[81] Dorothy W. Curtis et al., "SMART—An Integrated Wireless System for Monitoring Unattended Patients," JAMIA. 2008;15:44-53.

[82] Dorothy Curtis et al., "SMART: Scalable Medical Alert and Response Technologies." Computer Science and Artificial Intelligence Laboratory; Cambridge, MA. 2006.

many real-time monitoring environments the data communication mechanism is via a User Datagram Protocol (UDP), in which data are transmitted on a best-effort basis (no acknowledgement for assured delivery) from a specific client to a specific server, or multicast protocol, in which data are transmitted on a best-effort basis from a client to many clients and servers within a subnetwork on a best-effort basis. For those knowledgeable in communications protocols, this mechanism differs from the Real-Time Streaming Protocol (RTSP) standard[83] in several ways. The RTSP was recommended as an application protocol for the delivery of data to include video, audio, and other data. The key to RTSP is the synchronization of data. The client requests data from a media server and a virtual circuit is established between the client and the server.

In multicast transmissions, as is typical with many critical care monitors nowadays, the monitors communicate via a separate subnetwork to a MDG or standalone server, to nursing station monitors, or to each other. The transmissions are not acknowledged by the receiving system: the client merely transmits in the "hopes" that data will be received by the server or the listening clients. The transmissions using multicast operate within an IP range preceded by the 224 octet: 224.0.0.0. This range is reserved for all multicast transmissions. UDP transmission is similar to multicast from the perspective that the transmission from client to server is on a best-effort "fire-and-forget" basis, in which there is no acknowledgement or verification of receipt. These protocols both differ from the assured delivery mechanism under the Transmission Control Protocol / Internet Protocol (TCP/IP) in that this latter mechanism requires transmission acknowledgement and a re-transmission will occur if the acknowledgement is not received by the client within a specific period of time.

Multicast transmissions can be problematic because, in networks containing many monitors all communicating in this manner, quite a bit of traffic can result—another reason for maintaining these monitors on a separate subnetwork from any hospital or enterprise network. Transmitting such large quantities of data can quickly flood a network which can have a serious impact on network performance. Thus, in hospital health information and standard communication networks, it is undesirable to allow transmissions of this sort.

Another reason for maintaining separation between these and a hospital information network is these subnetworks are controlled from

---

[83] The Internet Society Network Working Group RFC 2326. Copyright 1998.

the perspective of the known traffic: only monitors are transmitting within these subnetworks and, therefore, the networking performance can be gauged accurately as well as the estimate of their impact on real-time transmission. In a standard enterprise health information network in which health information systems operate as well as standard Internet traffic, utilization and available bandwidth can vary depending on time-of-day. This type of network variability can impact the predictability of real-time transmissions and potentially result in delayed availability of data. In situations where real-time traffic (e.g.: waveform data) are necessary for the maintenance or monitoring of patient information directly related to sustaining human life, it is dangerous to operate in a networking environment in which performance variability can occur. This is especially true in intensive care, where monitoring traffic is communicated to central nursing stations whereby clinical staff can maintain constant watch over patient vital signs, and alarms associated with substantial deviations in vital signs can be transmitted for audible reporting to clinical staff. A simple rendering of this networking topology is shown in Figure 4-6.

Of course, deviations in network topology and design can and do exist. The actual design can vary by enterprise requirements and bandwidth availability. The ability to transmit the resulting real-time data to an EMR is limited for the aforementioned reasons. EMRs and their accompanying Health Information Systems which provide access to data typically will operate with discrete information that will

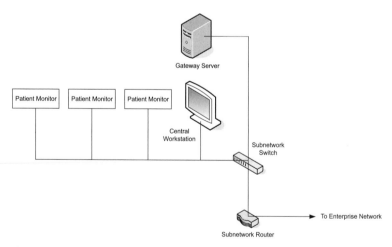

Figure 4-6 Simple two-tier network illustrating separation between monitoring and health information networks

be text-based. These data arrive at the EMR using a standard format such as an HL7 observation result (an R01 transaction). Real-time data in the form of waveforms will stress the EMR from the perspective of utilization, storage, display rendering speed, and retrieval in an enterprise network. That is, continuous feeds of information will cause excessive consumption of computing and database resources. Especially when combined with normal data retrieval requests and arriving discrete data, this can translate into systems with large latencies or may be unresponsive altogether. Clearly, if clinical users wish to record waveform data for display within the clinical record, an alternative to direct data feeds is needed.

4.3 End-User Display

Some manufacturers of monitoring equipment offer software components in the form of Web-enabled applications (e.g.: Java Applets or Windows ActiveX components) that can communicate with medical device MDGs within existing subnetworks in order to display a near-real-time feed of data that can be shown within a standard Web browser. However, the software components are proprietary to the specific manufacturer and therefore necessitates acquiring these software components for each system employed. These client-side components can communicate outside of the real-time subnetwork through the existing enterprise information network. As such, they will display waveforms in near real-time, or on a best-effort basis, because assured delivery outside of the controlled network cannot be guaranteed.

Another approach is to use video as a proxy or alternative for proprietary communication with an existing proprietary monitoring network. Video of patient monitors or other medical devices provides a medium for displaying images of waveforms remotely independent of the monitoring or device technology. What is being communicated, after all, is an image. A second benefit to using video is the ability to save off image segments (using the Moving Picture Experts Group, MPEG-4, compression methods, for example). These saved video images can then be linked to EMR Web pages for display and playback within the user interface.

Depending on the camera technology (that is, the digital resolution) and the distance between camera and the device, it is possible to pick up very accurate and clear images of waveforms and other live patient data for remote display within a Web browser. These images can be shown remotely (physician home, for example). While guaranteed service delivery cannot be claimed outside of an existing medical device monitoring subnetwork, the data and waveforms can be displayed on a best effort basis limited only by the latency in the existing public network infrastructure, the speed of connection to the remote location, and the processing speed of the computing device which renders the video. Alternatively, the video may be saved off into files which can be associated with the EMR on a particular patient for display after the fact. These video clips can be attached to the EMR as either hyperlinks to the EMR database or as a live link to a remote repository using patient-specific information as a linkage mechanism between the health information system and the current clinical record.

4.4 Real-Time Data and the EMR

Data display to the user is, perhaps, more important than storage because these data are used to intervene in patient care. Their storage, while interesting and of value, are of secondary importance from the perspective of the life-and-death scenario. Yet, that is not to say that real-time data cannot or should not be stored for later retrieval. It is unlikely that real-time data can be co-mingled with discrete findings, partly because of the demands on networking bandwidth, and partly because of the processing required to continually receive, store, and display the data in real-time. Thus, there are practical reasons why real-time and discrete, non-real-time data should not be stored in the same location or processed on the same computing platform. In the next chapter I will discuss the concept of the computer-based patient record and the mechanism for storing data for adequate retrieval by an end user. These data can include any type of information that convey findings and are not restricted to discrete data, whether real-time or non-real-time.

5 Computer-Based Patient Record

5.1 EMR: What's in a Name?

The acronym EMR is a legacy term: one that carries different distinctions (and names) depending on the focus and purposes for which the data are intended. I will use the term "Computer-based Patient Record" intentionally as a specialization of the concept EMR, primarily because it is more descriptive, if only superficially. This is the more common, modern terminology that has evolved over time[84]. My reason is that I wish to distinguish between the more generic term that befits the legacy repositories of medical information.

The American Health Information Management Association (AHIMA) published the results of an Internet search relating to patient health information management[85]. The rudimentary Internet search returned the following most frequently cited or addressed terms, including Electronic Health Record (EHR), Electronic Patient Record (EPR), Electronic Medical Record (EMR), Personal Health Record (PHR), Continuity of Care Record (CCR), Computer-based Patient Record (CPR), Computerized Medical Record (CMR), and others. Many of these are used interchangeably. Definitions of the CPR/EMR typically identify it as a repository for both episodic and longitudinal patient health information. The article suggested that

"Although there are differences between EHR, CPR, EMR, and EPR, all these terms describe systems that provide a 'structured, digitalized and fully accessible [patient] record.'"[86]

The Health Information Management Systems Society (HIMSS) offers the following definition for the Computer-based Patient Record (CPR),

---

[84] "Understanding Electronic Medical Record Systems," Future Healthcare (http://www.futurehealthcareus.com); 4Q2006.

[85] Kamila Smolij and Kim Dun, "Patient Health Information Management: Searching for the Right Model," Perspectives in Health Information Management 2006, 3L10 (December 12, 2006).

[86] Marietti, C. "Will the Real CPR/EMR/EHR Please Stand Up." Healthcare Informatics Online. May 1998; as quoted in Kamila Smolij, Jim Dub, "Patient Health Information Management: Searching for the Right Model." Perspectives in Health Information Management 2006, 3:10 (December 12, 2006).

Electronic Health Record (EHR), Electronic Medical Record (EMR), and Electronic Patient Record (EPR)[87]:

"The *Electronic Health Record (EHR)* is a secure, real-time, point-of-care, patient-centric information resource for clinicians. The EHR aids clinicians' decision-making by providing access to patient health record information where and when they need it and by incorporating evidence-based decision support. The EHR automates and streamlines the clinicians' workflow, closing loops in communication and response that result in delays or gaps in care. The EHR also supports the collection of data for uses other than direct clinical care, such as billing, quality management, outcomes reporting, resource planning, and public health disease surveillance and reporting."

Furthermore, the CPR provides access to tools (e.g.: clinical decision support) that can be used to develop a holistic view of the patient. This includes the capture, depiction, analysis and outcomes assessment associated with the information available from labs, radiology, bedside assessments, and medical devices. HIMSS' definition further defines that any system identifying itself as a CPR must meet specific requirements. I've summarized several key requirements related to data capture in Table 5-1[88].

Others[89] define the EMR/EHR/CPR simply as the all-encompassing records of patient information and treatment. EMRs are also referred to as CPRs in the literature[90]. Gartner[91] defines five generations or tiers of EMR technology. Of particular interest from the medical device data incorporation perspective are in the first through third generations. First generation health information technology systems provide for data capture and display. Second generation EMRs are those that provide for the inclusion of documents—both scanned and transcribed and limited collection of discrete data at the point of care.

---

[87] Prepared by HIMSS Electronic Health Record Committee. Thomas Handler, MD et al. "HIMSS Electronic Health Record Definitional Model, Version 1.1" September 24th, 2003. Available at http://www.himss.org/content/files/ehrattributes07073.pdf.

[88] Ibid.

[89] Diann Daniel, "Four Tall Hurdles to a Meaningful Electronic Medical Records (EMR) System," CIO Magazine, October 16th, 2007.

[90] David B. Meinert, "Resistance to Electronic Medical Records (EMRs): A Barrier to Improved Quality of Care." Informing Science and Information Technology education Joint Conference. Flagstaff, Arizona. June 16-19 2005; pages 493-504.

[91] Thomas J. Handler, "Only Two Vendors Reach Generation 3 in the Gartner 2007 North American Enterprise CPR Generation Evaluation." Gartner Industry Research ID Number G00151566, 9 October 2007.

Table 5-1 HIMSS's minimum requirements and evidence that a health information system rises to the definition of a CPR/EMR

Required Attribute	Measure of Effectiveness or Evidence that Requirement is Satisfied
"Provides secure, reliable, real-time access to patient CPR information at the time of need and at the point of care"	Provides access to data on an as-needed basis with an availability of 99.999%.
"Captures and manages episodic and longitudinal electronic health record information"	Conforms to clinical messaging standards on communication and coding (i.e., HL7, DICOM, LOINC, etc.) Accepts and integrates information from wide-ranging external systems.

Third generation EMRs are intended to represent clinical data more flexibly and to facilitate interaction with those data.

When I speak of the CPR in relationship to medical devices, I am referring to the communication of data from these devices to the medical record, and the typical input and output mechanisms. I am also referring to the assured or reliable transmission of these data via a reliable communication mechanism (TCP/IP, for instance). Mechanisms for communicating data to the electronic patient record have been discussed, both generally and in detail. However, in terms of the content of the EMR, I will limit my focus to the posting of findings, their access for clinical use, and dynamically changing data (such as monitored waveforms and electrocardiograph signals).

In standard practice, a flow sheet (or assessment sheet) is maintained in which a clinician (anesthesiologist, nurse, respiratory therapist, etc.) enters important patient state information, such as heart rate, respiratory rate, and many other key parameters. While I will discuss features and considerations associated with the design of these displays in a later chapter, it is worthwhile to consider the underlying framework for data storage, timeliness, and retrieval performance, and then the meaning of the data themselves.

5.2 EMR Data

Two specific classes of data related to medical device monitoring can be stored within the EMR. These fall into the category of either discretely monitored findings or continuously monitored waveforms. Discrete findings can either be recorded in an ad-hoc manner, asynchronously, on a given patient or they can be monitored continuously, synchronously. As information technology has been brought into the healthcare enterprise, much of the paper-based record is being supplanted by an electronic record, in which clinicians either record information manually or, in addition, automatically from clinical systems. The electronic medical record is maintained by the health care enterprise and follows the patient throughout all phases of diagnosis and treatment. Furthermore, this medical record is accessible to all authorized clinical personnel. An obvious benefit of this approach is that, unlike the paper record, the electronic medical record can be accessed from many different locations without physically retrieving the patient's hardcopy information from particular departments. The possibility of loss of information is minimized, and use of the electronic medical record establishes a uniform approach for recording of patient information, so that each department must conform to specific standards in terms of the types and quality of information recorded on each patient, thereby mitigating many errors in recording and transcription. Also, with Web-browser-based medical record access, convenience in terms of viewing, together with the reduced delays associated with retrieving the paper recording, ensure that clinicians can readily obtain patient information when required. In addition, two-way communication between the enterprise information system and clinical systems enable the error-free retrieval of patient demographic and administrative information (such as medical record number and insurance information) without adding further delay or introducing errors into the patient's record within the departmental system.

One key difference between the legacy paper record and the electronic medical record is that the paper record remained an intimate device by which the attending nurse monitored and recorded status on the patient: it stayed within close proximity to the patient and the nurse until the patient left the unit. With the introduction of the electronic medical record, data transmitted to that record and viewable by authorized individuals outside of the unit can lack the context of the actual situation in interpreting patient flow sheet findings. As society and healthcare move toward a completely automated and electronic medical record environment, it must be mindful of the fact that the introduction of new technologies must never impede quality healthcare[92]. In this context quality implies attentive and responsive care providers. The electronic medical record is but a tool to assist the care provider in their primary function: the care of the patient. Technolo-

---

[92] Patricia Benner, "Beware of Technological Imperatives and Commercial Interests That Prevent Best Practices," American Journal of Critical Care; 12(5): 469-471, 2003

gies facilitate and enable patient care. But, they cannot replace the human being who has a complete understanding of the patient that includes years of experience which no algorithm in this day and age can replace.

While legacy "systems" involving paper charting required the manual recording of these data by a nurse, respiratory therapist, or physician in discrete increments, the advent of medical device interfacing assists this process by enabling the intake of these data. In many if not most cases, the workflow involves receiving and displaying medical device data wherein a clinician is allowed (or required) to "validate" the findings. This validation process provides a mechanism—and checkpoint—whereby the clinical user can verify the efficacy of the data (i.e., that they are a true and valid record of the patient's telemetered state at the time of the measurement) and—as a requirement—must also provide the clinician with the capability to augment the findings with caveats (usually in the form of notes) that establish the conditions under which the findings were recorded.

For instance, if patient pulse and blood pressure are recorded and displayed continuously throughout the day then the user can validate that the findings at any particular time (say, during normal rounds) are valid during a typical interval of time, and to indicate that if an anomaly occurs an explanation is provided as to the cause or possible cause, thereby capturing the validity conditions of the measurements. Thus, the CPR must provide the clinical user with the capability to view monitored findings, to validate said findings, and to select which findings should be entered as formal documentation within the patient record.

I emphasize the importance of the validation step since every piece of information captured for the patient record has the potential to influence treatment and the concomitant writing of physician orders, to include (perhaps most obviously) the administration of drugs. Any system which permits the recording of telemetered values on patients must provide the capability to verify that said findings are valid as they can have a direct impact on patient treatment. The only "entity" at the point of care that has the complete system view of the patient (i.e., visual, audio, history, and state) is the live clinician—not the technology at the bedside. Hence, it is the clinician who must make the final call as to which findings are valid or not. Too often a patient may be adjusted within the bed or changes in medication administration may be made which could immediately affect the patient's state. Without the understanding of cause and effect these simple findings collected from medical devices could be misinterpreted and misapplied in treatment.

We can view the findings as a representation of the state of the patient at a particular time. Each finding has associated with it a time stamp that establishes the point at which the measurements were valid. In automated (or synchronous) monitoring, the medical devices typically "push" findings to the CPR where they can be displayed and maintained in a temporary buffer until validated by the clinician. These "pushed" findings are transmitted at the time of measurement (or in close proximity thereto), thus the time stamp associated with them cannot be misinterpreted nor will there be a concern over the "staleness" of the findings with respect to the time of collection. Situations in which this is normally the case are postoperative or intraoperative settings. Emergency department monitoring also falls into this category. However, in more "relaxed" settings, such as recovery wards, monitoring can be rather asynchronous—nursing or nursing technologists will visit patients on rounds throughout their shifts (perhaps three times per shift) in order to collect findings such as respiratory rate, blood pressure, pulse, and temperature. In these situations it is possible that findings will not match with the actual time of collection. One reason for this depends on whether the findings are collected automatically or interpreted and entered manually.

Consider the scenario in which a nurse enters a patient room with an ad-hoc portable vitals monitor (critical care monitors are usually tethered or associated with the room in which they are initially located). The nurse may measure several parameters as part of the overall finding using the device. The nurse may then become distracted or may need to assist the patient in some way. Once the distraction has been dealt with the nurse will write the finding on a paper flow sheet in order to capture the specific finding within the clinical record. Depending on whether the nurse made a note as to when the original findings were made, it might be possible the he or she will write the values at the current time rather than the time of actual collection. In this particular case the findings do not match strictly with the time stamp recorded in the clinical record. While in some cases this is of minor concern (perhaps the patient's respiratory rate is not a key finding at the moment), in other cases the acuity of the finding (blood pressure, pulse) may dictate intervention which is linked to the administration of a particular drug, and the administration time is important for care. While time stamp differentials of a few seconds or even a few minutes may be inconsequential, situations in which nursing must collect all findings within a ward before returning to a nursing station, whereby a physician can review the chart and write an order, or a laboratory finding can be consulted prior to administration of a drug, may impact patient care. A ward with 20 beds might require thirty minutes to one hour in order to complete a round. Thus, findings determined to be "stale" by this amount of time may actually be rather meaningless once they are recorded within the CPR.

5.3 EMR Architecture

For a simplified rendering of the CPR physical and logical architectures, we turn to Figure 5-1, Figure 5-2 and Figure 5-3, respectively.

The simple network topology of Figure 5-1 is intended to illustrate the relative location of computing hardware within an enterprise containing a CPR. The CPR is embodied in Web, Application, and Database servers. Here, the Web and Application servers are shown combined into one—not a bad assumption in a relatively small enterprise (perhaps no more than several dozen simultaneous users). The Database server provides access to requests from the Application server based upon user queries initiated through a Web-based instance of the CPR application. The client-components are illustrated by the existence of

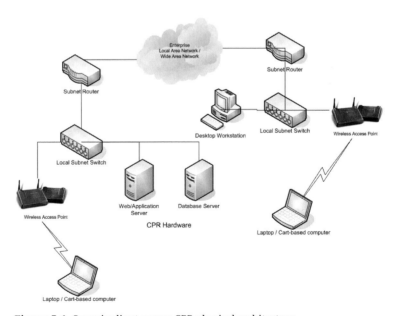

Figure 5-1 Generic client-server CPR physical architecture

wireless laptop computers—either roaming throughout the enterprise or, perhaps, on a mobile cart used by clinicians at the point of care. One Desktop Workstation client is shown to communicate the possible use by individuals in offices (physicians, for instance), at nursing workstations, or individual departments. The tacit assumption is made that the CPR application is indeed Web-enabled so that a clinical client can access via a simple Internet page. In such instances pages can be served to users as static Web pages or can employ some dynamic components such as those that can provide for plotting of data or other client-side processing.

Start with a simple query. In Figure 5-2 we have a Web-client which requests some content from the CPR system. The request is received by the Web/Application server via a simple post or "get" as in standard form processing. The request is serviced by the application server which, through its processing, determined the specific data item to be retrieved per the user request and then transmits it to the Database server, which manages the physical data repository and communicates with the database software via Structured Query Language (SQL). Ultimately, data are retrieved, returned to the Application server for appropriate processing and formatting and a Web page is then displayed to the client. Now, we can extend this diagram to include the inbound data which is stored within the CPR.

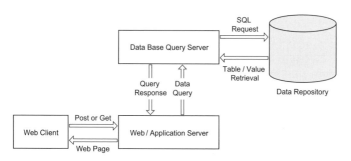

Figure 5-2 Web-enabled client data request from CPR

Medical devices can interface with the CPR via a standards-based format, such as HL7, or may communicate in a proprietary format using some type of intermediary processor to translate the data into an appropriate and universal interface. The dashed outline between the Medical Devices block and the Medical Device Interface Server in Figure 5-3 is shown to underscore the point that both may be part of the same subsystem (for example, a Medical Device Gateway, as was

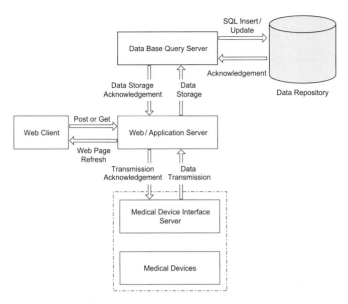

Figure 5-3 Medical device data transmission to CPR logical view

described in preceding chapters). Alternatively, the medical devices might communicate with an interface server that translates the proprietary data between the medical device and the device server into a more standardized format and transmits it to the CPR Application Server. Upon transmission to the Application Server they can, for instance, be presented to the user via a synchronously updated user interface. This provides the user with a mechanism for reviewing them prior to validation. The user can then indicate which data values are to be transmitted into the CPR for permanent storage by submitting a post or "get request" which then triggers specific findings to be transmitted to the Database Server in preparation for inserting or updating the data in the data repository. In this model the Application Server must maintain a buffer or a temporary storage location so that all results arriving from the Medical Device Interface Server can be buffered from which the user can select prior to validation and storage.

Data findings stored within the CPR will be available for query on an as-needed basis. In a critical care flowsheet, updates can occur once every 15 minutes, in which nursing would review results and validate for permanent storage. However, data can arrive from monitors more than once a minute. Hence, the user has the opportunity to view many data values prior to validating and can select those to validate based upon interventions or events. Each finding has a time stamp associated with it, thereby unambiguously associating findings when they were measured.

Database updates resulting from arriving medical device data are therefore blended with query traffic. The CPR physical and logical architectures must, therefore, be sufficiently robust to provide the capability to receive and serve data simultaneously while meeting data retrieval and processing latency requirements. In general, the CPR must be designed such that

1) data are not lost as they arrive from the medical device to the Application and Database Servers;

2) the server utilizations are sufficiently small so that data retrieval latencies are manageable and acceptable (typically on the order of no more than 2-3 seconds);

3) the compute hardware and network are sized appropriately to accommodate enterprise-wide traffic from many simultaneous sources; and,

4) ample storage is available to retain the data anticipated based on the arrival rate and the number of patients in all affected units within the healthcare enterprise.

For instance, assuming data arrive through the Medical Device Interface Server in the form of an HL7 transaction, the average size of these transactions will vary according to the type and quantity of data being transmitted. Consider Table 5-2 which shows an HL7 transaction containing four observation, or OBX, segments.

Storage within the CPR typically involves parsing the individual transaction for specific findings (in this case, oxygen source, minute venti-

Table 5-2 An example of an HL7 vitals transaction (unsolicited observation result) containing 420 bytes of data

```
MSH|^~\&|Source_Device||Destination_CPR|Test|2008021313073
5||ORU^R01|20080213130735|P|2.3
PID|1||61000396^^^^PN-400609^^^^MR||Surname^Fore-
name||||||||||||61000396
OBR|1||||||20080213130735|||Clinical_User_Identifier||||||
|||||||||||
OBX|1|TX|O2 SOURCE||OXYGEN|||||F|||20080213130735
OBX|2|TX|LPM||3|||||F|||20080213130735
OBX|3|TX|FIO2||24|%||||F|||20080213130735
OBX|4|TX|DEVICE||TRACH|||||F|||20080213130735
```

lation, inspired oxygen fraction, and gas delivery device). The arrival of findings at the interface to the CPR Application Server may be rather frequent. Therefore, the ability to receive, process, and display them must be supported and care must be taken to ensure that the client can see these findings refreshed regularly (that is, synchronized with the actual time of arrival of the finding). As described earlier, the user will validate a portion or all of the findings so that they may be stored in the permanent record. The Application Server in this example instance must provide the capability to process and retain all of the arriving data until the clinician has had the opportunity to select and validate them for permanent storage. In practice this can become quite complex in terms of the feature, function, and support requirements associated with a fairly simple CPR:

1) the CPR must provide the capability to accept inbound transactions from a medical device or its requisite interface information system;

2) the CPR must provide the capability for users to retrieve and view findings on an as-needed basis;

3) the CPR must accept inbound findings and provide the user with the capability to validate these as required;

4) the CPR must provide the capability to retrieve stored findings and render them in a display to the user;

5) the latency associated with the acceptance, processing, and retrieval of findings by a clinical user must not exceed 3 seconds as measured from the time the request is made by the user (via mouse click within a form, for example) to the time the data are rendered or painted on the screen;

6) the CPR must allow for the validation of results displayed within the user interface screen so that only those findings determined to be clinically relevant, true, and pertinent to patient care may be incorporated into the permanent record;

7) time and date stamps associated with each measurement must be displayed prominently with the findings;

8) the ability to enter text-based clinical notes must be provided so that the clinical user may record information and explanations that will have relevance to the veracity of a particular measurement, or to identify anomalistic or deviant behavior; and

9) the ability to mark a previously entered result as invalid in the instance of a user error must be provided, together with the ability to enter an update to a corrected finding for a given date and time stamp.

The last of these points is quite important! The CPR user interface and logic **must** provide for corrective action in such a case so that a finding, if validated in error (for instance, the patient was moved during a blood pressure measurement thereby rendering a particular value invalid), is understood to be anomalous and should not be used for clinical assessment. Other situations apply that underscore this need. One such case is the instance in which a clinical user inadvertently selects the record on the wrong patient, and retrieves or otherwise associates a finding with that patient. This type of error can be mitigated to a degree with technology. In the chapter on associating medical device data with patients I will discuss some mechanisms for doing so. Nonetheless, no process is foolproof. Hence, an approach must be taken to allow for the marking of the erroneous result at a minimum, together with the capability to enter a corrected value.

5.4 Make-versus-Buy Decisions

Today there are many EMR vendors offering health information technology. The decision to buy an EMR system versus developing one's own within a healthcare enterprise hinges on a number of things: cost, return on investment, ability to achieve desired functionality within the timeframe of the enterprise versus that of the vendor from whom an existing system is to be purchased, etc. Most, if not all, of the major health information system developers provide mechanisms for receiving external data, whether from devices, lab, radiological, or other ancillary systems. A benefit to purchasing such systems is evident in the fact that the developers of these must ensure that they can interact with a wide array of communication and device architectures so as to be able to support many customer environments. Developing a custom EMR and communication system is not subject to the requirement that it be able to be tailored to any customer environment, but it does mean that the enterprise is responsible for maintenance, future development, testing, and support.

It is frequently more cost-effective to have commercial vendors and manufacturers support these aspects of the EMR since they can be done more cheaply, do not require the enterprise to maintain a dedicated development staff, and can ensure that quality be designed into the process, particularly in regard to regulatory requirements. I have worked with enterprises which have developed their own enterprise health records. In such instances it is often possible to tailor these to support clinical research interests of the enterprise, including clinical trials. To me, the primary benefit of custom development is being able to design the user interfaces in a manner that best suits the enterprise clinical user environment. In either case (make versus buy), a balance must be struck among the variables of cost, maintenance, usability, custom feature/function, supportability, availability, and other factors.

For smaller healthcare enterprises which do not have or cannot afford to maintain robust clinical engineering and information technology development staffs to meet the aforementioned needs, the make versus buy decision is simple as the resources do not exist to pursue the former option. However, in large-scale healthcare enterprises—university-based medical centers, for instance—the custom development of an electronic health record system may be desirable to the clinical staff, especially if engaged in sophisticated clinical research whereby the interaction between the operational clinical environment and research teams mandates developing unique applications that are not used anywhere else in the commercial world.

6 Correctly Associating Device Data With Patients

6.1 Identifying the Patient

Data association and positive patient identification techniques have, as their objective, assigning the right data to the right patient. Retrieving raw data from medical devices is insufficient: it is necessary to tag it with information that positively identifies the patient, and how to use that information to ensure patient safety, privacy, and assured delivery to the computerized patient record is the goal. The Joint Commission on Patient Safety reported that incorrect patient identification was involved in 13% of surgical errors and 67% of transfusion errors[93]. As part of this report, the Commission identified Patient Safety Goal 1A for 2005, with two identifiers required when

1) administering medication or blood products;

2) collecting blood or specimen samples; or,

3) providing of treatments or procedures.

Various techniques can be used to identify patients. Inpatients fitted with wrist bracelets containing Universal Product Code (UPC) symbols can be identified using a barcode scanner. Similar bands containing Radio Frequency Identification (RFID) chips can use scanners that are quite similar to the traditional barcode units. Technologies such as barcodes and RFID and fingerprinting (e.g.: biometrics) can be procured which do not require specialized interfaces to EMR systems, thereby saving development effort, time, and cost. While most applications of positive patient identification techniques typically apply to functions such as medication administration checking (e.g.: for infusion therapy), the use of barcoding and RFID for patient identification have been shown to have a real impact on patient safety. The Food and Drug Administration (FDA) estimated that 25,000 medical errors amounting to $4.5 billion could be prevented each year using an ID

---

[93] "Technology in Patient Safety: Using Identification Bands to Reduce Patient Identification Errors." Joint Commission Perspectives on Patient Safety, April 2005, Volume 5, Issue 4. Copyright 2005 Joint Commission on Accreditation of Healthcare Organizations. Page 1.

band.[94] This is significant: in one study of the Pennsylvania Safety Reporting System (PSRS) over a 1 year period from November 2003 to April 2004, approximately 2% of incidents involving significant or temporary harm to patients were attributed to patient identification problems.[95]

Examples of RFID and barcode readers are shown below in Figure 6-1.

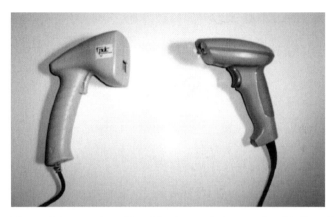

Figure 6-1 Examples of Precision Dynamic Corporation (PDC) Radio frequency Identification and IT 3800 barcode reader (right) (Photo by author)

Using these technologies mitigates the likelihood of making an error in identifying or selecting a patient from within an EMR. Despite this, it is somewhat puzzling that these technologies are not uniformly required across all healthcare enterprises, save for those that do not employ EMRs at all.

Whatever method is used, it is first necessary to record the patient's unique identifying information within the EMR registration system in order to positively associate medical device data with specific patients. Consider this process with the aid of Figure 6-2.

A patient arriving within the hospital will begin by visiting the registration desk. Regardless of whether this is an initial or repeat visit, the

---

[94] "Technology in Patient Safety: Using Identification Bands to Reduce Patient Identification Errors." Joint Commission Perspectives on Patient Safety, April 2005, Volume 5, Issue 4. Copyright 2005 Joint Commission on Accreditation of Healthcare Organizations. Page 2.

[95] "Patient Identification," Pennsylvania Patient Safety Authority. Copyright 2004.

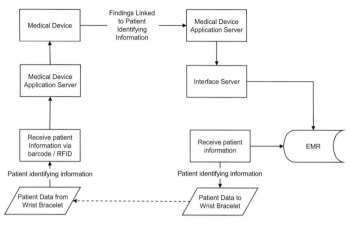

Figure 6-2 Patient identifying information flow to medical device and results flow to EMR

patient will receive a new visit identifier and possibly a medical record number assignment. The workflow in Figure 6-2 assumes that a patient will be admitted and will receive an identifying wrist bracelet. The patient identifying information is simultaneously written to the EMR and to a wrist bracelet in the form of a barcode, text, and/or an RFID chip.

6.2 A Patient Data Association Scenario

During normal rounds through a medical/surgical unit or elsewhere within the healthcare enterprise, patient information read from wrist-bracelets is verified using a barcode or RFID reader and may then be applied toward laboratory, pharmacy, and medication administration.

In the scenario depicted by Figure 6-2, the patient identifying information is used to associate a patient with a medical device. An instance of this could be the passing of patient information to a telemetry monitor. The telemetry monitor would then produce outbound results (both waveforms and findings) that fuse the patient identifying information with these findings for transmission back to the EMR.

An example of specific patient-identifying information (PII) is shown in Table 6-1.

While these data are not completely representative of all patient identifying information, they do form a good basis of estimate from which

Table 6-1 Example of data used to uniquely identify patients

Identifier	Definition
Name	Patient last, first, middle initial
MRN	Medical record number
PTN/ACN	Patient number / Account number
DOB	Date of birth
Gender	M/F/variant
Blood Type	Self-explanatory
Height	Measured in cm
Weight	Measured in kg
Location	Patient room and bed information

to establish a unique association of a medical device with a patient. Once provided, these data can be used within or by a medical device to associate subsequent results with that patient.

Table 6-2 shows a sample HL7 results record produced by medical device interface software—either a telemetry gateway (MDG) or a dedicated application that communicates directly with a vitals collection

Table 6-2 Example HL7 results transaction

```
MSH|^~\&|Source_System||Destination_EMR||YYYYMMDDhhmm||ORU^R01|
YYYYMMDDhhmmss|P|2.3|||||||||

PID|1||123456^^^^MRN~123456789^^^^ACN||Last_Name^First_Name||||||||
|||||ACN

OBR|1||||^Vitals|||200403130304|||||||||||||||||||||||||||||||||||||||||

OBX|1|ST|^Resp||20|/min|||||R||||||||

OBX|3|ST|^Pulse||65|/min|||||R|||||||

OBX|4|ST|^Pulse Location||Monitor||||||R|||||||

OBX|5|ST|^Temp||29.3|ºC||||R|||||||

OBX|6|ST|^Temp Site||Oral||||||R|||||||

OBX|7|ST|^NIBP Systolic||122|mmHg|||||R|||||||

OBX|8|ST|^NIBP Diastolic||80|mmHg|||||R|||||||

OBX|9|ST|^NIBP Location||Left Arm||||||R|||||||   OBX|10|ST|^NIBP

OBX|10|ST|^NIBP Source||Monitor||||||R|||||||   OBX|11|ST|^NIBP

OBX|11|ST|^NIBP Position||Sitting||||||R|||||||
```

Table 6-2 Example HL7 results transaction (cont.)

```
OBX|12|ST|^Weight||52|kg|||||R|||||||

OBX|13|ST|^Scale Type||Bed||||||R|||||||

OBX|14|ST|^Height||120|cm|||||R|||||||

OBX|15|ST|^O2 device||Mask||||||R|||||||

OBX|16|ST|^lpm||5|L/M||||R|||||||

OBX|17|ST|^O2Sat||98|%|||||R|||||||

OBX|18|ST|^Pain Scale||2||||||R|||||||
```

device such as an ad-hoc vitals monitor. In Figure 6-2 the outbound results are shown flowing to an interface server—a software component that resides functionally between the medical device and the EMR—and then onward to the EMR. The data in Table 6-2 are tied explicitly to the patient whose identity is established via identifiers in the PID segment. This is possible because the identifying data were sent earlier to the medical devices (telemetry monitors in this case) which then communicated this information together with the patient findings outbound to the EMR.

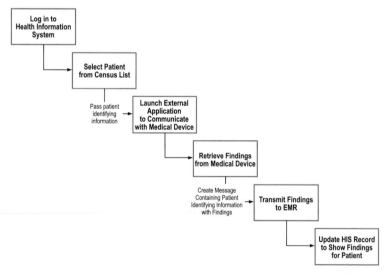

Figure 6-3 Suggested process for associating patient findings with patient identifying information: case in which medical device cannot receive identifying information directly

But, what happens when a medical device has no means of receiving unique patient identifying information? In this case a scenario must be created (and an application) that allows patient identifying information to be positively associated with the findings from the medical device. I'll describe one approach, which is illustrated in Figure 6-3. The assumption here is that the user can access a health information system (HIS) and select a patient from a census list of all patients for a given ward. Selecting a specific patient causes that patient's health information from the health record to be displayed within a user interface. An assumption is made that an external application link is provided that enables the user to execute a method that communicates directly with the medical device retrieving data directly from the patient.

When this application is executed, patient identifying information is passed from the patient record to the external application that communicates with the medical device. The clinical user retrieves the data (findings) from the medical device and then transmits them upon visual inspection to the EMR, where they can be retrieved for viewing.

6.3 Associating Data with Patients During Normal Rounds

Several variants on this approach can further reduce the possibility of incorrectly associating patient findings with the wrong patient. While the personally identifying information (PII) can be readily associated with the findings using this approach, the possibility still exists for the clinician to select the wrong patient from the census because of the manual selection process. This workflow would be applicable to the situation in which a clinician is collecting findings in an ad hoc manner from patients within a ward.

One task for nursing or allied health professionals within the health care enterprise is measuring patient findings (specifically, pulse, blood pressure, temperature, oxygen saturation, respiratory rate, etc.) several times per day (most often at clinical shift changes). These "collections" occur using mobile vitals monitors, some of which provide no means for providing direct association between the monitor and the patient (i.e., they do not provide a mechanism for retrieving or retaining such information). The nurse moves from room to room, bed to bed taking these vitals measurements. The nurse then records this information within the clinical record. The record can be completed electronically given the nurse collects information automati-

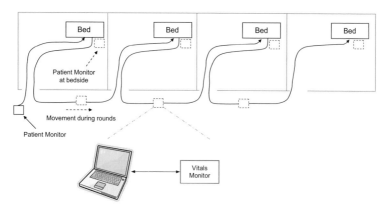

Figure 6-4 Patient vitals collection workflow for nursing staff during normal rounds

cally at the bedside using a laptop computer or similar device. This workflow is illustrated in Figure 6-4.

The movement from room to room can involve the manual selection of each patient from the census list within the HIS. The possibility exists for the nurse to simply select the wrong patient. The subsequent launching of the application that communicates with the medical device will then perform correctly—that is, it will retrieve medical data and transmit these findings together with whichever patient is selected, albeit the wrong one.

Using a barcode or RFID tag system to launch the medical device communication application directly would help mitigate this kind of error. The application would remain restricted unless and until patient identifying information is retrieved. In the process of collecting vitals data the nurse must also validate information measured at the bedside to ensure that it is a true and accurate representation of those vitals attributed to that patient at this specific time. In an ideal scenario, the nurse would transmit these vitals as a finding into the EMR using an automated mechanism accessed through a user interface such as a Web portal or client application on a laptop or other computing hardware that accompanies the nurse.

In the situation depicted in Figure 6-4, the local computing platform with which the nurse launches or otherwise accesses the method for vitals collection would be attached directly or through some mechanism to a medical device. Such a mechanism could be via a fixed and hard-wired cable connection (RS232 serial, for example). This establishes a one-to-one association between the local computing platform and the device used to measure the patient vitals. However, other connectivity options exist. Several of these include wireless access via 802.11 networking ("Wi-Fi"), direct connection via infrared ("IrDA"), or wireless connectivity via 802.15 connectivity ("Bluetooth"). In all cases care must be taken to associate the device with the local compute platform with which the nurse is collecting the vitals on a given patient. Wi-Fi networks are becoming more commonplace within the hospital enterprise (more so in newer hospitals). These networks provide access to the local area network, wide area networks, and telemetry networks within the hospital. This makes the use of Wi-Fi an enticing and potentially inexpensive option because the connection to the vitals monitor can be "piggy-backed" off of the existing wireless infrastructure.

One drawback to this approach is that in the event the vitals monitor contains no wireless networking capability on its own (i.e., a built-in network card), then the device must be augmented with a standalone bridge—a device that converts a serial interface into a connection that can be networked over a LAN—that converts the serial connectivity to a standard Ethernet-based connection (wireless LAN, WLAN). While devices of this type are relatively inexpensive (several hundred dollars), the software used to communicate between the local computing device and the vitals monitors must contain logic that establishes positively which device should be associated with the current patient. While this connection may be static, it is still necessary to assure that positive identification of the device to the patient medical record is achieved. Furthermore, it is necessary to configure the wireless bridge on the medical device to conform to existing hospital or enterprise requirements on wireless security within the environment. This latter requirement is not so difficult, as most of the modern devices manufactured comply with 802.1x Extensible Application Protocol (EAP), Wi-Fi-Protected Access (WPA) and WPA2 (which implements the full 802.11i standard) certification programs.

Another drawback to this approach is that the connectivity between the local computing platform and the medical device through its wireless networking bridge is susceptible to network dropouts, latency, and availability issues. For this reason an 802.15 networking approach might be considered because the network can indeed be local and will not be dependent on the existing 802.11 networks. In this approach a pairing must be done between the local medical device and an associated Bluetooth adapter that converts a serial to a Bluetooth-capable client computing device (examples include tablet PCs and laptops that contain Bluetooth adapters).

In the case of Bluetooth connectivity, the typical approach requires pairing the compute platform (i.e., the laptop) with the Bluetooth-serial adapter. This is manual and is outside the normal workflow of nursing: clinicians should not be required to configure technology—they are focused on patient care management. Therefore, a mechanism for performing an automatic association between a Bluetooth-to-Serial port adapter on a medical device is needed. This enables associating the compute platform with the device automatically. One of the challenges of performing this association in general is that Bluetooth is a local, short range network (typically under 30 meters in effective range). A scenario that presents a concern and a risk for accurately recording vitals data from a monitor is the situation where medical devices are affixed at the bedside of the patient, and the computing platform is moved from room to room via a mobile cart by the nurse. Here it is necessary to re-associate the Bluetooth adapter on the mobile computing platform with the Bluetooth-to-Serial port adapter. In a medical/surgical ward, many such medical devices can exist and their proximity to one another will be rather close. Due to the range of Bluetooth, this means that the Bluetooth adapter on the local compute platform may "see" multiple adapters which can be associated. This poses a potential hazard from the perspective that the wrong monitor may be associated with the local patient in proximity to the nurse.

This point is illustrated in Figure 6-5 in which overlapping circles indicate the communication range of the two Bluetooth adapters. This figure shows a typical ICU (approximately 10 rooms) of modest size

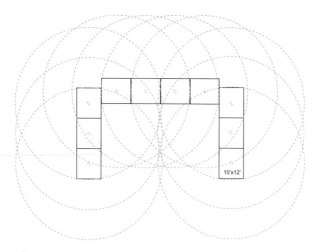

Figure 6-5 Example of overlap between two transmitting Bluetooth adapters

(10 feet by 12 feet). The circles represent Bluetooth transmitter ranges of radius 30 ft. Shown here, the amount of overlap is significant. Therefore, other mechanisms must be used to correctly associate the local vitals monitor (a.k.a. "Medical Device") with the medical record of the local patient. Fortunately, as with standard Ethernet Network Interface Cards (NICs), Bluetooth adapters possess unique Media Access Control (MAC) identifiers or addresses. This provides a handle with which to associate a Bluetooth adapter with a medical device. The exact mechanism for selecting and using the MAC address of the specific Bluetooth adapter can be accomplished using a supplementary technology, such as barcoding or RFID. The mechanism would involve the nurse arriving at the bedside of the patient and using a barcode scanner to scan an inventory or serial number barcode on the medical device itself. The barcode scan provides a unique device identifier which is then mapped to a table of MAC addresses. A list of MAC addresses is compared with the MAC addresses available for pairing as determined by the Bluetooth adapter on the local compute platform. The barcode data are then used to select the appropriate MAC address which is compared with the list of MAC addresses available for pairing. A match between the available list of MAC addresses and the MAC address associated with the barcode identifier results in an automatic pairing of the two, thus enabling communication between the medical device and the application on the local compute platform.

To illustrate this implementation, refer to Figure 6-6.

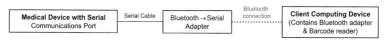

Figure 6-6 Bluetooth connectivity between computing platform and medical device

Commercially available Bluetooth-serial adapters contain a serial port profile (SPP). This means that, when paired with a client Bluetooth device, the client Bluetooth device (Laptop computer, tablet, PDA) will recognize the adapter as a virtual Serial port connection. The virtual Serial port will be assigned a Serial COM port identifier (e.g.: COM 40). The client device will then be able to communicate with the Serial port on the medical device. The Bluetooth transmission will then simply be interpreted as a serial connection. By combining with barcode it is possible to identify the medical device using some unique identifier (e.g.: a barcode UPC symbol attached to the medical device itself).

The communication mechanism can be written in a number of languages. However, regardless of the programming language, the program must interface with the local device using a Bluetooth stack. Common stacks are Winsock, WIDCOMM, and Bluesoleil. The Broadcom software development kit enables developers to write Bluetooth enabled applications for personal computing platforms and personal digital assistants (PDAs)[96]. BlueCove, the Java library for Bluetooth, currently interfaces with WIDCOMM, BlueSoleil and Microsoft Bluetooth stacks on Microsoft Windows mobile platforms[97].

In this implementation the barcode reads the unique UPC symbol on the device which is then matched with a table of previously populated media access control (MAC) addresses. The MAC address is then used by the program to identify the desired Bluetooth adapter pairing.

6.4 Summary

Patient identification methods such as wrist bracelets containing a barcode UPC symbol or embedded radio frequency identification chips are keys to positively associating medical device data with a patient. Once we have positively identified the patient and provided the capability to associate medical device data, we can then focus on how to use the data to the benefit of the patient.

---

[96] http://www.broadcom.com/products/bluetooth_sdk.php

[97] http://www.bluecove.org

7 Balancing Data Quantity with Quality: Techniques for Data Analysis and Reduction

7.1 Analyzing Medical Data

Perhaps a natural consequence of automating the data acquisition process is the quantity of data that can be downloaded from the medical devices. When data are entered manually into electronic records or even on paper it becomes more difficult to perform long-term trending and analysis because of the inability to apply techniques rapidly to the information at hand and because a natural consequence associated with the relative tedium of manual data collection is the variability with which it is collected. With automated measurement it is much easier to collect medical device data over long periods of time in regular intervals. But, the ability to automate also means that information lacking valuable clinical content may be downloaded. For example, clinically significant events may not occur very often and the data collected between the occurrences of events may be uneventful and contain minimal content. Yet, in order to capture those events it is necessary to sift through large quantities of information, should it all be stored for real-time or posteriori analysis. So, a balance must be struck: what are the right data and what types of tools, functions, and methods can aid the user—both clinical and otherwise—in culling these to arrive at only essential information? Otherwise, analysis paralysis can result. The old adage that work expands to fill the time allotted has an analog here: the data expand to fill the hard drive space allotted.

The cheap cost of storage enables capturing and archiving enormous quantities of information that are difficult to sift or mine through in a timely manner. While the ability to measure, collect, and store data can be made simple, once this is accomplished the question becomes, "now what?" Part of what I will focus on here is to offer a sampling of techniques on how to reduce and analyze medical device data for the purpose of providing clinical value to the end user.

There are a number of techniques I have used over the years for data reduction and analysis. By no means do they represent the totality of techniques that can be applied to reducing and evaluating patient-specific medical device data. However, they are a good start; I've used these approaches and they define what I term a starter set for temporal data reduction from which the reader may jump to alternative or expanded approaches and techniques. They are offered as a means of sparking creativity in the analyst to answer the "what if" questions that arise. Aside from the "usual" computation of expected values and sample variances, parametric tests of significance are very useful in analyzing, comparing, and determining the significance of data in comparison with known distributions or other samples. These are briefly described. Yet, a most widely used non-parametric test is the chi-square (also written χ-square). I delve into this test and its application in some detail as it is most aptly applied to goodness-of-fit testing, tests of contingency (i.e., testing the statistical independence of two separate populations), tests of homogeneity (i.e., testing of two samples to determine whether they arose from like or the same distributions), and tests to determine whether a sampling of data is random.

7.2 ICU Patient Data

I have already talked about the process of validating results entering the EMR, in which a clinician determines what and whether certain data should be stored for long-term archival and assessment. This process works well in cases in which data are collected relatively infrequently and are based on asynchronous events; that is, when findings are measured and collected as the result of an order like a ventilator setting change or the measurement of vitals at a shift change within a ward. However, there are other data which do not fit this model as they are synchronous; they are not solicited, but rather are measured continuously, oftentimes over long periods of time. Examples of this type of information include telemetry obtained from patient monitors both within the operating room and the critical care unit. Telemetry data, including ECG waveforms, respiratory data, etc. are necessary for patient assessment, diagnosis, and treatment, especially in high-acuity wards like critical care where patients are technologically dependent over extended periods. Partially due to the nature of these data (that is, changes tend to occur more gradually) and due to the fact that collected manually, the clinician would have to be present as a sentinel to ensure that no event is missed, most information such as pulse, cardiac data, mechanical ventilation settings, infusion pump rate, and volume delivered would have to be collected over relatively extended periods in order to find a meaningful trend.

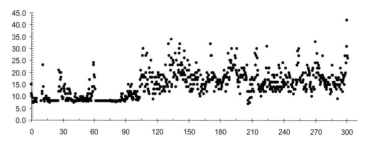

Figure 7-1 Spontaneous respiratory rate (breaths per minute) versus time (minutes)

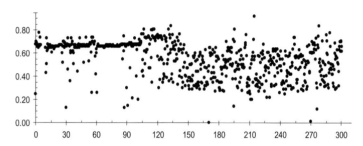

Figure 7-2 Spontaneous tidal volume (liters) versus time (minutes)

Let's begin by considering the following example[98]. Figure 7-1 and Figure 7-2 are plots of respiratory rate and tidal volume of a single patient. These data were collected from a mechanical ventilator via serial interface over the course of 5-6 hours. Having been collected automatically, these data reflect discrete values measured from the mechanical ventilator and amount to just over 750 data points per plot. That computes to 125 data points collected per hour—far more than a nurse or respiratory therapist could reasonably collect and record within any given hour owing to the vast amount of energy and time this would require. It can be seen that between 90 and 105 minutes the data appear to become more scattered. This is due to the fact that the ventilation mode was switched from intermittent mandatory ventilation (IMV) to continuous positive airway pressure (CPAP) so the patient could begin breathing spontaneously in anticipation of

---

[98] All sample data representative of actual patient findings were collected under protocol #570-0 approved by the Committee on Studies Involving Human Subjects. Measurements conducted during graduate work at the Hospital of the University of Pennsylvania. Letter dated February 23rd, 1996.

weaning trials. The patient's breathing indicates both variability in tidal volume (breath volume) and respiratory rate. During weaning trials, a measure often used to determine the viability for successful weaning (that is, extubation) is the rapid-shallow breathing index, or RSBI. This is the ratio of the respiratory rate to the tidal volume. As a rule of thumb, a value of RSBI > 105 indicates potential problems in weaning. As a clinical measure, the RSBI is but one indicator of the efficacy of weaning mechanically ventilated patients[99,100,101,102].

Should a value of tidal volume or respiratory rate continuously move in a direction detrimental to the patient, then the temporal trending of the information presented in these two figures would provide the clinician with the evidence to assist in making important decisions as to appropriate interventions. The density of the information taken together with their suggested evolution over time (that is, trending) shows both the values and their rate of change. This information can be associated with other data (e.g.: medication infusions) to help establish causal relationships between events occurring in the patient's condition. Furthermore, the density of the data provides important details that may be missed by a sparsely populated data set.

7.3 Simple Statistics Modeling

The RSBI—also referred to as the Tobin Ratio after Martin J. Tobin—is computed as the ratio of the respiratory rate to the tidal volume. Tobin has put forward that a simple measure of weaning efficacy is determined via the RSBI threshold value of 105 breaths/minute/liter: values in excess of 105 are indicative of possible failed weaning attempts, while values less than 105 are indicative of successful weaning.

From the data above, the RSBI can be computed point-by-point for the period of time in which the patient is breathing spontaneously—essentially, from about 120 minutes on. This is shown in Figure 7-3.

---

[99] K.L. Yang, M.J. Tobin, "A prospective study of indexes predicting the outcome of trials of weaning from mechanical ventilation," NEJM, Volume 324:1445-1450; May 23, 1991; Number 21.

[100] Maureen Meade et al., "Predicting Success in Weaning From Mechanical Ventilation," Chest 2001; 120; 400-424

[101] Paul L. Marino, The ICU Book, 2nd Edition, Williams & Wilkins, Baltimore, MD. 1998. Page 470.

[102] Robert M. Bojar, Manual of Perioperative Care in Cardiac Surgery, 3rd Edition, Blackwell Science, Inc., 1999, Page 192.

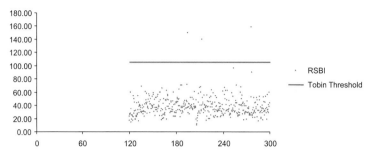

Figure 7-3 RSBI (breaths/minute/liter) versus time (minutes)

In the plot I show the Tobin Threshold (bold line). As can be seen, most of the individual data points are well below the threshold, 105/min/liter—an encouraging finding. The data above provide a measure of patient readiness to wean. Interspersed within the ensemble of patient data are what appear to be outliers that are either close to or are located outside of the Tobin Threshold. Let's summarily analyze these data to establish a measure of statistics in regard to these outliers.

We can begin our analysis by looking at the expected value of RSBI values—the mean of all of the data points. The expected value of the sample of data is given by (7.1):

$$E[X] = \hat{X} = \frac{1}{n}\sum_{i=1}^{n} X_i \qquad (7.1)$$

The X_i are the individual data points within the sample set—in this case, each of the n RSBI measurements. Next, the variance describes the mean of the variability of the individual measurements with respect to the mean. The sample variance of each measurement with respect to the mean is given by (7.2):

$$S^2 = \frac{1}{n-1}\sum_{i=1}^{n}(X_i - \hat{X})^2 \qquad (7.2)$$

Computationally, the sample variance can be represented in the following way:

$$S^2 = \frac{n}{n-1}\left(E[X^2] - E[X]E[X]\right) \qquad (7.3)$$

135

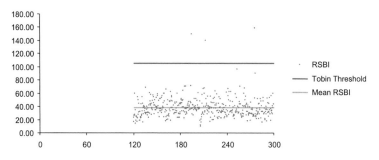

Figure 7-4 RSBI showing mean value

The expected value of the sample data is shown in Figure 7-4. The calculation indicates that the mean RSBI value is approximately 40/min/liter.

The sample standard deviation can be overlaid with respect to the data points and the mean value.

To assist us in understanding the standard deviation let's consider the Gaussian, or Normal probability density function of Figure 7-5. Under the assumption of a normally-distributed sample set, the standard deviation (±) defines the range in which approximately 68.3% of values reside within ±1 standard deviation of the mean. Approximately 95.4% of all values reside within ±2 standard deviations of the mean. Approximately 99.7% of all values reside within ±3 standard deviations of the mean.

The Normal distribution is a reasonable approximation for estimating distributions of variations in many natural phenomena and processes found in everyday life (e.g., distribution of height of children; variability of the size of bolts in manufacturing processes, etc.) and is governed by the following density function:

$$f(x) = \frac{1}{\sigma\sqrt{2\pi}} e^{-(x-\mu)^2 / 2\sigma^2} \tag{7.4}$$

where μ is the mean value of the distribution and σ is the standard deviation.

Random values drawn from a normally-distributed random number generator can approximate large quantities of sample measurements, given the measurements come from an unbiased distribution and the sample size is large. The behavior of the sample set as it relates to or approximates a normally distributed random variable must be deter-

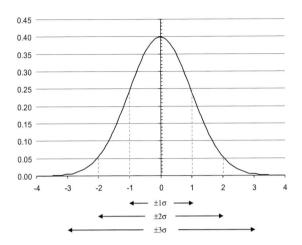

Figure 7-5 Normal probability density function

mined before making the assumption as to the likelihood that data within a single sample standard deviation of the mean are likely to be found with a probability of 68.3%. I will discuss momentarily this process as it relates to comparing two distributions. Before addressing this, we overlay the sample standard deviation to show the variability of the raw measurements with respect to the mean. Upon overlaying the standard deviation (±S), Figure 7-6 results.

Note that several values exceed the RSBI threshold value, and a larger quantity of data points reside beyond ±1 sample standard deviation. So, one question is to what degree are these "outliers" significant with respect to the mean and ±1 standard deviation?

Returning to the question of whether two distributions are alike, this is often raised in statistics as a quantitative assessment of whether or

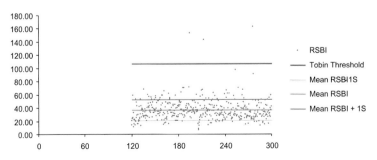

Figure 7-6 RSBI with mean and sample standard deviation overlaid

not any two variables within a sample or distribution have a tightly or loosely coupled relationship with one another. In statistics, the hypothesis as to whether two samples are drawn from the same distribution is typically estimated using the *chi-square test* for significance.

To begin, let's visualize the RSBI data in a manner similar to the normally-distributed density function curve. We can see from Figure 7-7 and Figure 7-8 the distribution of data points from the sample above. The highest RSBI value occurrence within this sample set of over 760 data points is in the range of values between 20 and 40. This is supported by the cumulative distribution curve which shows that more than 90% of values are less than approximately 50.

We can see from this latter figure that the two distributions have a similar shape but there are significant differences in terms of amplitude and width of the distribution. The normal distribution has the same mean and variance as the measured data. Later on in this chap-

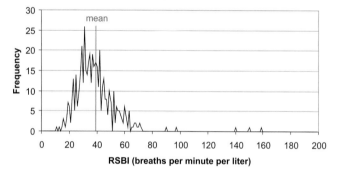

Figure 7-7 RSBI Frequency distribution

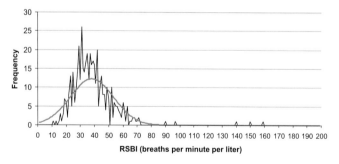

Figure 7-8 Overlay of RSBI measurements and normal distribution of same mean and variance

ter I will discuss calculating the significance of the differences between these two distributions to establish a quantitative measure as to similarity.

From these data we can demonstrate the use of simple statistics to analyze relationships among data. But why do we care whether two distributions are similar to one another? Because if we can demonstrate similarity then we can extend the validity of assumptions relative to modeling of those measurements based on the assumption that a known model (e.g., normal distribution) correctly represents the original data.

In the preceding analysis I show sample calculations of the mean, standard deviation, and frequency distributions of sampled data. The benefit of collecting these data automatically is quite clear when considering the large quantities that make up the types of sample sets described here. Simple statistics can be used to estimate variability of these measurements, thereby providing a basis for determining the significance of outliers with respect to the mean value.

7.4 Nonparametric Tests for Significance

We can hypothesize whether the plot of the raw RSBI data shown in Figure 7-8 is represented accurately by a normal distribution of equal mean and variance. To do this we call upon a test of statistical significance. One such method for comparing measurements of one distribution with those of another (or a model) to determine "appropriateness" or sameness is the chi-square test. Other nonparametric tests for significance, such as Student's t, which is typically used for testing differences between and among pairs of mean values, can be employed to similar effect. Another test is the F-test, which tests the hypothesis that two samples have different variances by evaluating whether the null hypothesis can be rejected (i.e., their variances are consistent). Other statistical tests can be applied which are outside the scope of this text. However, chi-square (or χ-square) is most appropriate when comparing two different distributions to establish likelihood that they are drawn, or represented by, the same statistical model.

We will use χ-square to test the hypothesis that two samples of data are from the same distribution. The null hypothesis, H0, is accepted for two samples of data if the χ-square statistic is small. That is, for a given level of significance, if the value of the χ-square statistic compared with the critical value associated with the level of significance exceeds this value, then the null hypothesis is rejected.

χ-square for two discrete data samples may be computed most simply with the aid of (7.5):

$$\chi^2 = \sum_{i=1}^{N} \left(\frac{ObservedFrequency_i - ExpectedFrequency_i}{ExpectedFrequency_i} \right)^2 \tag{7.5}$$

When comparing measured data with a model of measured data, this can be expressed as:

$$\chi^2 = \sum_{i=1}^{N} \left(\frac{y_i - y(x; \beta_1 ... \beta_M)}{\sigma_i} \right)^2 \tag{7.6}$$

in which N is the number of data points and M is the total number of coefficients. We can compute a probability distribution for values of χ^2 given $v = M - N$ degrees of freedom. The probability of "goodness-of-fit" (i.e., that the two samples are taken from the same distribution) can then be approximated. This is based on the assumption that all measurements have the same standard deviation:[103]

$$\sigma^2 = \sum_{i=1}^{N} \frac{\left(\tilde{y}_i - y_i(x_i) \right)^2}{v} \tag{7.7}$$

As an example, consider the following hypothesis: given the RSBI distribution of Figure 7-9, in which a Gaussian distribution sample frequency (being proffered as a model) is shown in comparison with the actual measurements, what is the likelihood that this distribution can be represented by a normally-distributed (i.e., Gaussian) random variable with mean centered at the sample mean and having some variance? To the eye, the two frequency distributions look similar. However, can we quantitatively determine using a robust method whether both distributions are alike? One benefit would be if we can show that the measurements adhere to a known distribution within

---

[103] William H. Press, Saul A. Teukolsky, William T. Vetterling, Brian P. Flannery, Numerical Recipes in C: The Art of Scientific Computing, 2nd Ed. Cambridge University Press: 1992. Page 661.

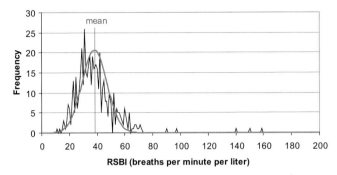

Figure 7-9 Overlay of RSBI data on Gaussian density function.
Gaussian mean and variance: $\mu = 38.19$; $\sigma^2 = 81$

an acceptable confidence level, then we can take advantage of the mathematical benefits associated with that distribution and extrapolate.

If N_i represent the number of observed events in bin i, and n_i is the number of expected events in bin i, then the χ-square statistic is:[104]

$$\chi^2 = \sum_i (N_i - n_i)^2 / n_i \tag{7.8}$$

The χ-square probability function, $Q(\chi^2, v)$, evaluates the null hypothesis (i.e., that two distributions are alike) and quantifies statistically the degree of difference between two or more sets of data. The variable v is the number of degrees of freedom (i.e., data bins). Thus, the χ-square probability function tests whether the observed χ-square statistic for a correct model should be less than the computed value of χ^2. The complement to this function, $P(\chi^2, v)$, tests whether the observed χ-square for a correct model should be less than the computed value of χ^2. The functions are related rather trivially by:

$$P(n, x) = 1 - Q(n, x) \tag{7.9}$$

P and Q are computed via the incomplete Gamma function. One computational method is described in the text *Numerical Recipes*[105]:

---

[104] William H. Press, Saul A. Teukolsky, William T. Vetterling, Brian P. Flannery, Numerical Recipes in C: The Art of Scientific Computing, 2nd Ed. Cambridge University Press: 1992. Page 621.

[105] Ibid. Pages 216-222.

$$P(a,x) \equiv \frac{\gamma(a,x)}{\Gamma(a,x)} \equiv \frac{1}{\Gamma(a)} \int_0^x e^{-t} t^{a-1} dt \qquad (7.10)$$

The χ-square probability is computed computationally by substituting the values:

$$a = \frac{v}{2} \text{ and } x = \frac{\chi^2}{2}$$

In the example above, the following values were computed using an Excel spreadsheet calculator based on an approximate method described independently by Pezzullo[106] and Yahya *et al*[107].

$v = 199$

$\chi^2 = 5.5134$

$Q = .999 +$

It is interesting to note that the characteristics of the Gaussian chosen for this test have the characteristics

Gaussian:

$\mu = 38.19$

$\sigma^2 = 81$

While the mean is the same as that of the sample distribution, the variance differs:

Sample:

$\mu = 38.19$

$\sigma^2 = 227.88$

The principle reason for this is because of the relatively wide distribution of samples, as is illustrated in the plot of Figure 7-9.

I have "forced" the two samples to appear similar to one another by giving the Gaussian density function a higher peak and narrower width. However, statistically, the Gaussian is not the same as the sample density function.

---

[106] John Pezzullo, http://statpages.org/JCPhome.html & http://statpages.org/pdfs.html

[107] Waheed Babatunde Yahya, Philip Iyiola Farayola, Daniel Eni, "A Numerical Procedure for Computing Chi-Square Percentage Points." InterStat Journal: April 2007 (http://interstat.statjournals.net/)

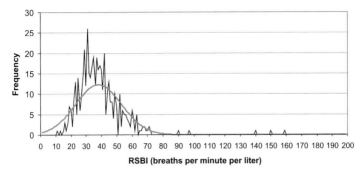

Figure 7-10 Overlay of RSBI data on Gaussian density function. Gaussian
mean and variance: $\mu = 38.19$ and $\sigma^2 = 227.88$

If we were to reconstruct the normal distribution curve using the
same variance as that of the sample set, then the plot of Figure 7-10 is
created. Note that the height of the distribution is much smaller now.

In terms of visual appeal, the distribution "seems" to misrepresent
the data, although, based on the computed mean and variance, the
two distributions are the same. In all cases, care must be taken to
avoid errors in applying statistics incorrectly to sample sets.

One characteristic of the χ-square distribution is that as the number
of data points (bins) increases, the density function approaches that
of a normal distribution. Hence, the interpretation that the sample
can be represented using the Normal distribution curve can be misleading from the perspective that the sample size is large and tends to
offset the significance of the variability in the measurements. Let's
look at our example again with fewer data points, as in the plot of Figure 7-11.

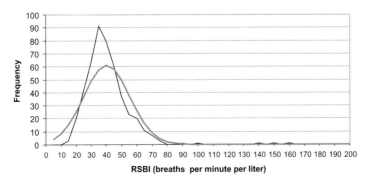

Figure 7-11 Frequency versus RSBI with $v = 40$

143

Fewer bins (degrees of freedom) make for a coarser representation of the data frequency. It is more obvious in this plot that the two distributions (sample versus Normal) are indeed different. I include a Visual Basic macro in Chapter 11 that can be used inside of an Excel spreadsheet to compute the $P(\chi^2, v)$ and $Q(\chi^2, v)$.

We can also apply this technique to the study and comparison of data within the same sample sets.

Consider the plot of Figure 7-12, respiratory rate versus time.

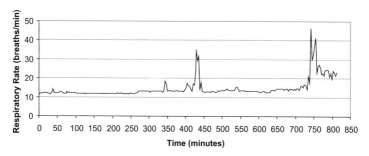

Figure 7-12 Spontaneous patient respiratory rate versus time

This figure illustrates the spontaneous breathing profile of a mechanically ventilated patient through the time of extubation. One can see respiratory rate spikes of 25 and 35 breaths per minute occur at approximately 430 and 750 minutes, respectively. These data identify what appear to be deviations from the baseline values (approximately 12 breaths per minute) throughout the duration of the time on mechanical ventilation. These data were measured in discrete intervals approximately once every 3 minutes throughout the period indicated in the plot, or just shy of 260 individual data points. A key task in critical care nursing workflow involves recording patient findings at regular intervals. Depending on the interval, values of interest may be overlooked or not recorded simply because they have not been captured within the EMR. Alternatively, recording all information retrieved from medical devices can be a tedious task of limited value except for those situations in which events occur. As illustrated, two such events occur within the span of more than 12 hours. One question that arises is: when representing large quantities of data containing only several key events, is it possible to identify only those events of interest to the clinician? The obvious answer is yes. However, there are many techniques for doing so. One mechanism which is widely used in clinical decision support (CDS) is to raise a flag or notification when an event—measured by exceeding some threshold or meeting some specific condition—arises. Such techniques involve comparing measured quantities with thresholds, such that when some threshold on a specific value, x_{thresh}, is exceeded a notification is triggered.

A number of techniques exist to accomplish this. I will show several that I have employed to good result. To begin, let's return to the plot of Figure 7-1. In reviewing this plot it seems intuitive that there are at least two different behaviors occurring in terms of the locus of data points. By inspection, it appears that two different data distributions are evident occurring in the approximate ranges of 0-100 minutes and 101-300 minutes, respectively. The statistics and shape of these two distributions are shown in Figure 7-13.

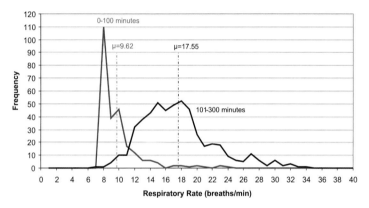

Figure 7-13 Frequency functions for respiratory rate data for two different time spans

Quantitatively, the means of the two segments of the distribution are quite different. This supports the hypothesis that the characteristics of the samples change or evolve over time. In actuality, the physiological reason the data are different is because at the time interval between the two segments, the respiratory settings on the ventilator were changed from intermittent mandatory ventilation (IMV) at a support level of approximately 8 breaths per minute to spontaneous breathing. Hence, the lack of variability of the distribution below 100 minutes is due in large part to the fact that ventilatory support was being supplied to the patient that mandated a minimum breathing rate and the patient's spontaneous breathing was also somewhat inhibited by the use of sedatives. Beyond 100 minutes, this patient

145

was breathing more spontaneously over time, resulting in the possibility of wider variability in breathing rate (evidenced by the broadness of the frequency distribution). The χ-square statistic to test the hypothesis of whether these two sets of samples are drawn from the same distribution is determined to be $\chi^2 = 375$ with $v = 40$. The probability of the null hypothesis, P, is approximately 0, indicating that it is highly unlikely that the two sets of measurements were drawn from the same distribution. This supports the earlier suspicion that the data were indeed different. It is noted that when comparing two different samples of data, as is the case here, the χ-square statistic used is slightly different from that of equation (7.5):

$$\chi^2 = \sum_i \frac{(R_i - S_i)^2}{R_i + S_i} \tag{7.11}$$

where R_i and S_i are the number of samples contained within the ith bin of each sample set, respectively.

While the respiratory rate sample data in the plot of Figure 7-1 were broken into only two subsets in this example, the method can be extended by segmenting the original sample into further subsets. This is illustrated in Figure 7-14. The frequency distributions are normalized to facilitate comparison along the y axis as the total number of samples differs within each subset.

As we see with this further decomposition of the data set into parts, the selection of the time point 100 minutes appears to be a logical breakpoint for an "event"—the change in a basic characteristic of the distribution of samples. The data from 101-300 minutes, even when

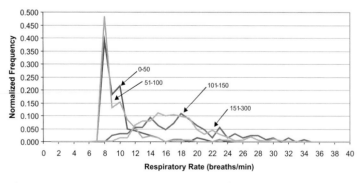

Figure 7-14 Normalized frequency densities for samples from respiratory rate distribution

separated into two additional subsets, support the hypothesis that they are indeed similar in behavior.

The method outlined above can be used to detect statistically significant changes or patterns in data. The χ-square statistic is very useful, and can serve as a method for determining whether such changes are likely to be representative of normal behavior, artifact, or are genuine changes or variations in patient findings.

7.5 Least Squares Regression

Least squares regression is most often used for fitting polynomials, or models, of known functions to sampled measurements, and in the context here, for modeling data with respect to time as the independent variable. This allows for temporally trending medical device data.

The objective of trend analysis is to determine the trajectory of a dependent variable with respect to an independent variable for the purpose of identifying a possible relationship (either causal or associative) using the "simplest function that would describe the data adequately[108]." As such, the mathematical modeling of data involves representing the behavior of the dependent variables in terms of independent variables and establishing a functional form that adequately describes the nature of this relationship. Stated in another way, this means that the model that is developed to represent the behavior of the measured data with respect to the independent variable must be determined in accord with some measure that defines quantitatively (if not rigorously) the "goodness" of fit between the model and the measured data. Functionally, the model is usually represented in the following way.

$$y_{\mathrm{model}} = g(x; \beta_1 ... \beta_K) \tag{7.12}$$

One model that is frequently used is that of a power series, in which:

$$y_{\mathrm{model}} = \sum_{k=1}^{K} \beta_k x_k \tag{7.13}$$

---

[108] James F. Zolman, Biostatistics: Experimental Design and Statistical Inference, Oxford University Press, 1993, Page 122.

Expanding, this can be written more explicitly as[109]:

$$y_{model} = \beta_0 + \beta_1 x + \beta_2 x^2 + \beta_3 x^3 + ... + \beta_k x^n + \varepsilon \qquad (7.14)$$

where

$$g(x, \beta_k) = \beta_0 + \beta_1 x + \beta_2 x^2 + \beta_3 x^3 + ... + \beta_k x^n \qquad (7.15)$$

The coefficients, β, are computed in a manner that determines their value such that the sum of least squares is minimized. This method is based at its core upon maximum likelihood estimation.[110] The coefficients are determined such that the sum-of-squares error (SSE) differences between measured and fit values of the independent variable, y, are minimized. The resulting model will then be optimal. Mathematically, we can express this statement by:

$$SSE = \sum_{i=1}^{n} \{\tilde{y}_i - g(x_{ik}, \beta_k)\}^2 \qquad (7.16)$$

where $\tilde{y}_i$ represents the individual measurements and k represents the coefficient number preceding the order of the dependent variables, x. The choice is made as to the model desired (e.g., constant, linear, quadratic, cubic, etc.). This process of selecting the best model can also be optimized based upon the best correlation coefficient of the resulting model or other criteria, such as χ-square. However, given a specific model form, the multiplications are carried out as suggested above. Following this, the derivative of the SSE is computed with respect to each of the coefficients β_k. This results in the constraint equations that are set equal to zero to satisfy optimality conditions:

$$\frac{\partial g(x_{ik}, \beta_k)}{\beta_k} = 0 : \qquad (7.17)$$

$$\frac{\partial g(x_{ik}, \beta_k)}{\beta_k} = 2 \sum_{i=1}^{n} - x_{ik}(y_i - g(\tilde{x}_{ik}, \beta_k)) = 0 \qquad (7.18)$$

---

[109] Ibid., Page 124.

[110] William H. Press, Saul A. Teukolsky, William T. Vetterling, Brian P. Flannery, Numerical Recipes in C: The Art of Scientific Computing, 2nd Ed. Cambridge University Press: 1992; Page 657.

In vector-matrix form, the model can be expressed as follows:

$$Y = X\beta + \varepsilon \tag{7.19}$$

where the column vector, β, holds the k coefficients associated with the order of the model and ε is the column vector of residuals, or differences (errors) between the model and the individual measurements. A unique solution to the column vector is determined by isolating these in the above expression. This process begins by normalizing both left and right sides of the general model equation by multiplying by the transpose of the independent variable equation:

$$X^T Y = X^T X \beta \tag{7.20}$$

Multiplying both sides by the inverse of $X^T X$ matrix yields:

$$\left\{ X^T X \right\}^{-1} X^T Y = \left\{ X^T X \right\}^{-1} \left\{ X^T X \right\} \beta \tag{7.21}$$

This, in turn, yields:

$$\left\{ X^T X \right\}^{-1} X^T Y = I \beta \tag{7.22}$$

Or, simply:

$$\left\{ X^T X \right\}^{-1} X^T Y = \beta , \tag{7.23}$$

where I is the identity matrix.

Consider a simple linear model of the form:

$$y_{model} = \beta_0 + \beta_1 x. \tag{7.24}$$

The SSE can be expressed as:

$$SSE = \sum_{i=1}^{n} \{\tilde{y}_{ij} - \beta_0 - \beta_1 x_i\}^2 \tag{7.25}$$

Consider each element, i:

$$\varepsilon_i^2 = \{\tilde{y}_i - \beta_0 - \beta_1 x_i\}^2 = \{\tilde{y}_i - \beta_0 - \beta_1 x_i\} \times \{\tilde{y}_i - \beta_0 - \beta_1 x_i\} \qquad (7.26)$$

Expanding:

$$\varepsilon_i^2 = \tilde{y}_i^2 - 2\beta_0 y_i - 2\beta_1 x_i y_i + 2\beta_0\beta_1 x_1 + \beta_0^2 + \beta_1^2 x_1^2 \qquad (7.27)$$

Take the derivative with respect to each coefficient:

$$\frac{\partial \varepsilon_i^2}{\beta_0} = 2y_i + 2\beta_1 x_1 + 2\beta_0^2 = 0 \qquad (7.28)$$

$$\frac{\partial \varepsilon_i^2}{\beta_1} = 2x_i y_i + 2\beta_0 x_1 + 2\beta_1 x_1^2 = 0 \qquad (7.29)$$

Collecting terms:

$$\beta_0 + \beta_1 x_i = y_i \qquad (7.30a)$$

$$\frac{\partial \varepsilon_i^2}{\beta_1} = 2x_i y_i + 2\beta_0 x_1 + 2\beta_1 x_1^2 = 0 \qquad (7.30b)$$

In matrix form:

$$\begin{bmatrix} 1 & x_i \\ x_i & x_i^2 \end{bmatrix} \begin{bmatrix} \beta_0 \\ \beta_1 \end{bmatrix} = \begin{bmatrix} y_i \\ x_i y_i \end{bmatrix} \qquad (7.31)$$

In the general case, we sum over all measurements, or:

$$\begin{bmatrix} 1 & \sum_{i=1}^{N} x_i \\ \sum_{i=1}^{N} x_i & \sum_{i=1}^{N} x_i^2 \end{bmatrix} \begin{bmatrix} \beta_0 \\ \beta_1 \end{bmatrix} = \begin{bmatrix} \sum_{i=1}^{N} y_i \\ \sum_{i=1}^{N} x_i y_i \end{bmatrix} \qquad (7.32)$$

This model is easily extended. We show without proof the case of a quadratic model. However, this can be derived using the same technique as outlined above:

$$\begin{bmatrix} 1 & \sum_{i=1}^{N} x_i & \sum_{i=1}^{N} x_i^2 \\ \sum_{i=1}^{N} x_i & \sum_{i=1}^{N} x_i^2 & \sum_{i=1}^{N} x_i^3 \\ \sum_{i=1}^{N} x_i^2 & \sum_{i=1}^{N} x_i^3 & \sum_{i=1}^{N} x_i^4 \end{bmatrix} \begin{bmatrix} \beta_0 \\ \beta_1 \\ \beta_2 \end{bmatrix} = \begin{bmatrix} \sum_{i=1}^{N} y_i \\ \sum_{i=1}^{N} x_i y_i \\ \sum_{i=1}^{N} x_i^2 y_i \end{bmatrix} \qquad (7.33)$$

Returning to the plot of Figure 7-1, we seek to find a model that represents these data. One approach is to assume a model of some form (e.g., quadratic) and proceed by solving for the coefficients of (7.33). For the data comprising this figure, we determine the coefficients as follows:

$$\begin{bmatrix} 767 & 116919.25 & 23470468 \\ 116919.25 & 23470467.92 & 5296953813 \\ 23470467.92 & 5296953813 & 1.27512E+12 \end{bmatrix} \begin{bmatrix} \beta_0 \\ \beta_1 \\ \beta_2 \end{bmatrix} = \begin{bmatrix} 11452.4 \\ 1941434.86 \\ 403329732 \end{bmatrix}$$

Solving for the coefficients, we have:

$$\begin{bmatrix} \beta_0 \\ \beta_1 \\ \beta_2 \end{bmatrix} = \begin{bmatrix} 0.01285519 & -0.00017 & 4.7061E-07 \\ -0.0001702 & 2.94E-06 & -9.065E-09 \\ 4.7061E-07 & -9.07E-09 & 2.9781E-11 \end{bmatrix} \begin{bmatrix} 11452.4 \\ 1941434.86 \\ 403329732 \end{bmatrix} = \begin{bmatrix} 6.506771779 \\ 0.095197117 \\ -0.000198917 \end{bmatrix}$$

The resulting model becomes:

$$y_{\text{model}} = 6.506 + 0.0952x - 0.00019892x^2 \qquad (7.34)$$

Plotting, Figure 7-15 results:

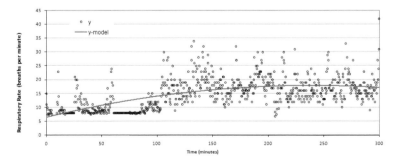

Figure 7-15 Quadratic model fit to raw respiratory data

151

However, the use of linear regression for general curve fitting can be misapplied. The plot illustrates the fact that while a quadratic model can be used to represent the data, the "goodness" with which the model and the data are associated is less than adequate. Mathematically, we can represent this curve using any number of variables we wish (up to the total data points minus 1). We have chosen to use a quadratic model and, therefore, are using three coefficients. But, from the quality of the suggested model in comparison with the original measurements, to claim that this model represents the data well would be misleading. One method of illustrating this is by computing the linear correlation coefficient between the fit model and the raw data. The linear correlation coefficient is given by:

$$r = \frac{\sum_i \left(x_i - \hat{x}\right)\left(y_i - \hat{y}\right)}{\sqrt{\sum_i \left(x_i - \hat{x}\right)^2}\sqrt{\sum_i \left(y_i - \hat{y}\right)^2}} \qquad (7.35)$$

The value of r varies between -1 and 1 (inclusive). The implication of this value: when $r = 1$, or complete positive correlation, all measured data points lie directly along a line given by the model in which increasing x implies increasing y. When $r = -1$, or complete negative correlation, all measured data points lie directly along a line given by the model in which increasing x implies decreasing y. When $r = 0$ or is close to zero, this implies no correlation between the x and y values[111]. Values of r between 0 and 1 or 0 and -1, respectively, imply varying degrees of strength associated with the correlation between the x and y values.

In the case of Figure 7-15, the correlation coefficient was determined to be 0.518. This indicates a relatively weak correlation between respiratory rate and time. In situations where weak correlations exist, using linear regression to predict or propagate future trends can be rather misleading: the implication that y varies with x may certainly be the case and demonstrated by the data. However, whether y behaves in a manner given by a well-defined relationship is another matter. It is somewhat obvious from Figure 7-15 that the respiratory rate values (y) are indeed changing and even increasing over time.

---

[111] William H. Press, Saul A. Teukolsky, William T. Vetterling, Brian P. Flannery, Numerical Recipes in C: The Art of Scientific Computing, 2nd Ed. Cambridge University Press: 1992. Page 636.

However, in the range of values selected (that is, the ensemble), suggesting a quadratic model for the overall set is seemingly inappropriate.

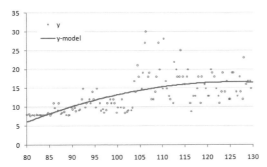

Figure 7-16 Spontaneous Respiratory Rate (breaths/minute) versus time: 90-120 minute segment

Consider Figure 7-16, which plots a subset of the original data. Here, the subset of data from 90-120 minutes is shown. The quadratic equation representing these data becomes:

$$y_{model} = -63.337 + 1.27236x - 0.005059x^2 \qquad (7.36)$$

The correlation coefficient associated with these data is recomputed to be 0.598. This clearly shows that in this region a higher positive correlation exists between respiratory rate and time.

7.6 Spatial-Temporal Methods for Data Filtering

One approach to representing aperiodic data that preserves both temporal and spatial characteristics of these data is the wavelet transform. This differs from traditional periodic signal representation, so aptly represented by the Fourier series, as explained below[112].

While many measurements from medical devices vary temporally (i.e., vary with time), not all behave periodically or pseudo-periodi-

---

[112] C. Sidney Burrus, Ramesh A. Gopinath, Haitao Guo, Introduction to Wavelets and Wavelet Transforms: A Primer, Prentice Hall: 1998. Page 3.

cally (e.g., sudden changes in RSBI or respiratory rate, pulse, stroke volume, etc.) As a result, the use of signal processing techniques such as Fourier transforms to detect signal frequency variation will have limited utility. An alternative tool that can aid in detecting, quantifying, and filtering measurements from medical devices is the wavelet transform. The wavelet transform method enables representing a signal both temporally and spatially. A wavelet is a functional representation of a continuous-time signal that can be used to determine spatial and temporal characteristics of that signal. This is beneficial in the field of medicine because it is frequently of interest to understand how a signal changes temporally, where the change occurs in time, and what the change looks like (amplitude, location within the temporal field, as well as the frequency characteristics of the changed signal). In so rendering, the wavelet transform provides the analyst with a capability to analyze segregate artifact from actual events.

Returning to the plot of Figure 7-12, we see two occurrences of spikes—behavior that deviates from the normal or standard behavior of the overall "signal." All of these data are recorded automatically from a medical device (mechanical ventilator). While the plot of the actual data comprises nearly 130 data points, the events associated with the two respiratory rate changes can be detected using a Haar wavelet reconstruction comprising only 6 data points. This is illustrated in Figure 7-17.

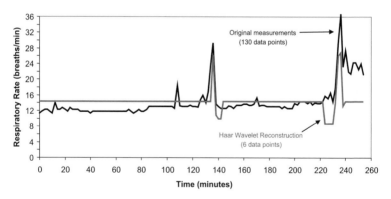

Figure 7-17 Haar wavelet reconstruction of original respiratory rate

Although many types and applications of wavelet transforms exist, particularly in the fields of image analysis, compression, and reconstruction, I will focus on the use of the wavelet transform for data compression, change detection, and reconstruction. The Haar representation, developed by Alfred Haar, is recognized as the first wavelet and is unique in that it comprises a series of step functions and lends itself to rapid computation. These step functions are used to "build up" the original data in the form of coefficients having the same order as those data but which lend themselves to straightforward analysis—such as evaluation of significance of the contributions of each coefficient to the makeup of the original data.

The Haar wavelet is based on a scaling function, $\psi(t)$, which is described by this step function over the range of $0 \le t \le 1$ such that

$$\varphi(t) = 1 \text{ when } 0 \le t \le 1, \tag{7.37a}$$

$$\varphi(t) = 0 \text{ otherwise.} \tag{7.37b}$$

The original data, represented by the function $f(t)$, which, we hypothesize, can be recreated via a series comprising a known set of coefficients multiplying a scaling, or basis, function that spans the space of the original data series.

Therefore,

$$f(t) = \sum_j a_j \varphi_j(t). \tag{7.38}$$

Derivation of the scaling and wavelet functions is beyond the scope of this book. However, it can be shown that the scaling function, $\varphi(t)$, equates to:[113]

$$\varphi(t) = \sum_j h(j)\sqrt{2}\varphi(2t - j). \tag{7.39}$$

The scaling function, (7.39), is satisfied when the coefficients, $h(j)$ are:

$$h(0) = 1/\sqrt{2}, \text{ and} \tag{7.40a}$$

$$h(1) = 1/\sqrt{2} \tag{7.40b}$$

---

[113] C. Sidney Burrus, Ramesh A. Gopinath, Haitao Guo, Introduction to Wavelets and Wavelet Transforms: A Primer, Prentice Hall: 1998. Pages 11-12.

The wavelet coefficients themselves, perhaps more subtly, describe the differences in the space spanned by the scaling function. The continuous form of the wavelet coefficient is described by:

$$\psi(t) = \sum_j (-1)^j h(J-1-j)\sqrt{2}\varphi(2t-j)$$

(7.41)

Expanding for $j = 0, 1$:

$$\psi(t) = (-1)^0 \left(\frac{1}{\sqrt{2}}\right)\sqrt{2}\varphi(2t-0) + (-1)^1 \left(\frac{1}{\sqrt{2}}\right)\sqrt{2}\varphi(2t-1)$$

(7.42)

$$\psi(t) = \varphi(2t) - \varphi(2t-1)$$

(7.43)

Equation (7.43) spans $j = 2$. The larger the space (i.e., as j increases), the more coefficients are required to represent the original function from the wavelet decomposition.

The Haar wavelet lends itself to rather simple computation and involves decomposing signals into a series of high- and low-pass filters. This decomposition serves to "root out" the averages and the differences that together describe the details of the signal being decomposed. The average is calculated according to the standard convention. Difference calculations are one-half the difference between any two consecutive values.

Thus,

$$s_i = \frac{f_i + f_{i+1}}{2}$$

(7.44a)

$$d_i = \frac{f_i - f_{i+1}}{2}$$

(7.44b)

For example, consider the following "signal," represented by the vector $\underline{f} = \langle 5,-2,3,1,7,9,-3,5\rangle$. The calculation of the sums and differences proceeds as shown in Figure 7-18 below, using the expressions of (7.44a) and (7.44b) successively, taking sums and differences to arrive at the set of discrete wavelet transform (DWT) coefficients.

The averages of all of the values within the vector represent the first value in the DWT. Successive differences of these values result in the vector of filter elements which remain, as illustrated above. This method of computation is well described in the literature[114, 115].

Computations proceed accordingly: the average of each raw sample is computed with respect to its immediate neighbor, together with the difference (divided by 2). Once these are computed, the average and difference of these results are then computed. This process is continued until the complete ensemble (that is, the single value and difference) corresponding to the entire signal is determined. The first wavelet coefficient is given by the ensemble average corresponding to the longest scale value over the entire interval. The next wavelet coef-

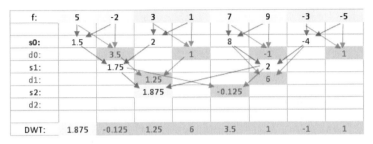

Figure 7-18 Example of a DWT calculation

ficient corresponds to the size of the difference of averages at the next scale up. The remaining coefficients follow the pattern of the differences between the averages at finer and finer scale (in general). Thus, the vector of wavelet coefficients given the data sample above appears as follows:

$$b^T = \begin{bmatrix} 1.875 & -0.125 & -0.25 & 6 & 3.5 & 1 & -1 & 1 \end{bmatrix} \qquad (7.45)$$

The creation of the Haar matrix follows a predictable pattern as the number of rows and columns increases. However, by applying the Haar wavelet transform, the size of the matrix increases according to 2^n scale, where n is a positive integer. In the Haar basis, the quantity of data must conform to this scale as well. We can expand this Haar basis to an H_8 basis, illustrated here:

---

[114] C. Sidney Burrus, Ramesh A. Gopinath, Haitao Guo, Introduction to Wavelets and Wavelet Transforms: A Primer, Prentice Hall: 1998. Page 3.

[115] Tommi Vuorenmaa, "The Discrete Wavelet Transform with Financial Time Series Applications". Seminar on Learning Systems at the Rolf Nevanlinna Institute, University of Helsinki, April 9th 2003.

$$f = H_8 b, \tag{7.46}$$

where H_8 is described by:

$$H_8 = \begin{bmatrix} 1 & 1 & 1 & 0 & 1 & 0 & 0 & 0 \\ 1 & 1 & 1 & 0 & -1 & 0 & 0 & 0 \\ 1 & 1 & -1 & 0 & 0 & 1 & 0 & 0 \\ 1 & 1 & -1 & 0 & 0 & -1 & 0 & 0 \\ 1 & -1 & 0 & 1 & 0 & 0 & 1 & 0 \\ 1 & -1 & 0 & 1 & 0 & 0 & -1 & 0 \\ 1 & -1 & 0 & -1 & 0 & 0 & 0 & 1 \\ 1 & -1 & 0 & -1 & 0 & 0 & 0 & -1 \end{bmatrix} \tag{7.47}$$

The Haar matrix may be inverted using standard methods. Then, the wavelet coefficient which may be determined directly from the raw data vector follows directly:

$$b = H_8^{-1} f \tag{7.48}$$

A method was developed to accomplish this automatically, and is included in Chapter 11. The inverse of H_8 can be accomplished using linear decomposition. I have found and used a number of different methods for this. Yet I am sensitive to the user's dilemma from the perspective that authors sometimes simply state that this must be calculated but then defer to other sources for the actual method. I provide a matrix inverse method written in Java in Chapter 11. The original method was written by Pang in C[116].

Another benefit of using the wavelet transform method is that it establishes the relative scale of the signal differences with respect to the raw data. This is important and a key condition because the signal may be reconstructed at varying levels of granularity based on the number of wavelet coefficients employed. The implication here is at least twofold: (1) data may be represented in a compressed manner by using only a subset of wavelet coefficients to represent any given set of raw input data, and (2) data may be filtered by omitting components of the wavelet coefficients that correspond to small changes—potentially representative of artifact or noise. While the discarding or

---

[116] Tao Pang, An Introduction to Computational Physics. Cambridge University Press: 1997. Version written in C date 10/24/2001.

exclusion of wavelet coefficients does indeed translate into a lossy form of data compression, in certain situations this may be acceptable. From the perspective of omitting coefficients from the data reconstruction process, we can also evaluate whether changes in the data are substantive or representative of noise. Thus, as in the previous examples wherein we evaluated the significance of changes in data characteristics to determine significance of these changes with respect to other data within the same sample set, we can do the same by comparing wavelet coefficients from (at least) two different segments of data within the same sample (or even different samples) to determine significance.

The threshold level that defines the inclusion of wavelet coefficients for raw data reconstruction may be based on statistical significance levels (defined previously) or via arbitrary thresholds on the amplitude of wavelet coefficients. Defining the statistical significance level of this threshold can be done in accord with well-documented practices, especially relative to setting confidence intervals with respect to a known distribution[117,118,119]. Wavelets are a tool to filter data so that (1) communication of all data elements between medical devices and the EMR will not become overwhelming in terms of quantity and (2) data can be reconstructed from a subset of the wavelet coefficients and to provide a lower resolution, initial representation of those data, which are useful for display on lower bandwidth devices (e.g., PDAs), and finer detail can be added should the user (clinician) require higher resolution.

One way to illustrate these concepts is by applying an exclusion threshold on the smallest values of coefficients: the magnitude of the wavelet coefficients provides insight into the level of contribution they make to the character of the overall raw signal. By omitting certain coefficients it becomes possible to exclude noise, artifact, or other components that are judged to have minor influence on the overall raw data sample. For instance, the plot of Figure 7-19 shows the raw signal data with two overlays: one with a 10% and another with a 30% exclusion threshold. This means that wavelet coefficients with values less than either 10% or 30%, respectively, of the maxi-

[117] James F. Zolman, Biostatistics: Experimental Design and Statistical Inference; Oxford University Press, 1993; pp 77-99.

[118] Christopher Torrence, Gilbert P. Compo, "A Practical Guide to Wavelet Analysis," Bulletin of the American Meteorological Society; Vol. 79, No. 1: 69-71, January 1998.

[119] Sheldon Ross, A First Course in Probability, 3rd Ed.; Macmillan Publishing Company, 1988; pp 336-357.

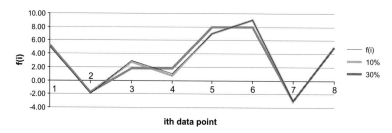

Figure 7-19 Raw data reconstruction with 10% and 30% wavelet exclusion thresholds

mum wavelet coefficient value are set to zero, indicating that their contribution in raw data reconstruction is removed.

While a statistical determination as to the significance of the differences between the reconstructed signal and the original can certainly (and must be) employed to establish accuracy of the reconstruction, casual inspection of reconstruction even with a 30% exclusion threshold indicates a reasonable correlation between the original data and that based on the 30% wavelet exclusion.

Depending on the characteristic shape, periodicity, and complexity of the original data, the degree of loss vis-à-vis discarding wavelet coefficients may or may not be acceptable to the end-user. In the case of a predictable or repetitive signal, the discarding of wavelet coefficients can have a trivial effect on the reconstruction of the original signal.

In a clinical departmental environment, such as an intensive care unit or operating room, vast quantities of patient data are normally collected. Most of this raw information is not retained for use by clinicians or for post-operative analysis. The bulk of the data are discarded. The clinical assessment sheet (or flow sheet) provides the primary means for collecting and retaining information within the long-term clinical record. These data are normally updated at discrete intervals, and the recording of these data are normally not associated with significant clinical events, but are rather based on a temporal update (every 15 minutes, for instance). In a telemetry environment, though, data and events recorded within these data can occur at any instant. An analogy would be "drinking from a fire hose" in terms of the quantities and frequencies of data arrival. Data can arrive from bedside monitors at relatively high frequencies with respect to the clinical assessment sheet update interval. Furthermore, the quantity of patient results available can measure into several hundred unique findings. Sending data at high rates from many monitors into the

EMR can be prohibitively expensive from the storage, networking, and compute processing perspectives.

Consider a hypothetical situation illustrated by Table 7-1, in which findings arrive continuously from a patient bedside monitor at the rate of one set every 15 seconds. In the span of one hour, 240 individual findings are recorded. For patients who are monitored over many hours, where many parameters are normally collected (typically several dozen), this translates into tens of thousands of findings arriving at the EMR over the course of an 8 hour shift. Multiply this by the number of patients and it becomes clear that data management is challenging!

Table 7-1 Typical data quantities for vitals findings, assuming an update rate of 4 transactions per minute

Monitor duration (hours)	Total quantity of data points measured per result	10 Results	20 Results
1	240	2,400	4,800
2	480	4,800	9,600
4	960	9,600	19,200
8	1920	19,200	38,400

An argument can be made that the intention is never to store all of the patient telemetry: that one of the clinician's roles is to weed out unimportant information and only record that which is necessary for proper care of that patient. However, it can be difficult to draw the line as to what information is necessary and that which is spurious: clinicians are frequently moving from patient to patient and their primary focus is on patient care, not on dedicating their time and energies to full-time data collection. Clinical decision support tools and rules methodologies based on such standard approaches as the Arden Syntax do provide some mechanisms for the filtering of repeated information. On the other hand, data that are not periodic or contain artifact are not always accommodated by filtering approaches. In these cases there is no substitute for the trained eye and situational context.

Results stored in an assessment or flow sheet for the purpose of clinical reporting can be inadequate as well. To illustrate this point, consider the pulse data recorded from a bedside monitor as illustrated in Figure 7-20. Results recorded continuously from a critical care monitor are displayed and overlaid with discrete sampling points over a

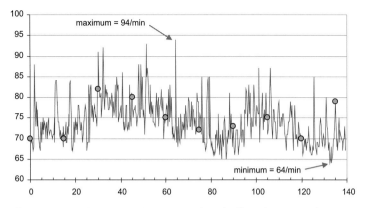

Figure 7-20 Pulse versus time. An overlay of a flow sheet recording
at 15 minute intervals is shown

140-minute period. Overlaid on this plot are the associated record-ings that would typically be taken during normal assessment sheet updates of a telemetry patient. These data points reflect those value recordings that normally are taken given a 15-minute update of the clinical assessment sheet. To the casual observer, it is quite evident that the assessment sheet recordings omit a large amount of patient telemetry. Furthermore, these recordings provide very little true indication as to the typical value of heart rate, its maximum and min-imum during the course of this entire recording interval, or episodes indicative of range of expected values. For instance: the raw data col-lected at 15 second intervals show that a minimum pulse rate record-ing of 64 beats per minute was measured at approximately 132 min-utes, 30 seconds. The maximum pulse of 94 beats per minute was measured at approximately 64 minutes, 30 seconds. It is entirely pos-sible, even likely, that important events may be missed in the process of recording discrete observations at such wide intervals.

One response to this observation might be that by maintaining a run-ning record of the minimum, maximum, and the mean signal value, the issue just identified can be resolved. This additional information, while providing more insight into the range of the values over the course of the measurement interval, does not provide insight into the character (that is, behavior and trend) of the measurements over time. The ensemble average value, together with signal minimum and maximum, add three additional data points at each of the assess-ment sheet recording times. If the time of minimum and maximum measurements are added then an additional two data points become part of the record for this patient. However, variation in signal behavior, and short-term response to stimuli (such as drug interactions) are still missing from the assessment sheet, even with this additional information.

Pose a hypothetical question: is it possible to represent these same results, possibly with some loss of specificity, but with fewer data points than the full set, while still providing insight into the character and trend of the original signal data? The answer is yes. Let's define the degree of acceptability of the compressed representation of the original measurements as to how accurately they capture the major trends in the data, including maximum and minimum values. Therefore, if we can at least represent these values, then we are not providing any less information to the long-term record than we already had. However, any more information can be treated as beneficial for describing the overall characteristics of the data. From the mathematical discussion in the previous section, the wavelet coefficients provide a characterization of the signal in space and time. The total number of wavelet coefficients is equal to the total number of data points contained within the original signal. The benefit afforded us by the use of wavelet coefficients is that they provide a means of determining the relative contribution of each measurement. We can observe that by excluding certain of these coefficients we can approximate the original signal. The wavelet coefficients for the measurements are shown in the plot of Figure 7-21.

These coefficients can take on both positive and negative values. Let us begin our analysis by specifying a threshold, below which wavelet coefficients will be omitted from signal reconstruction. The wavelet

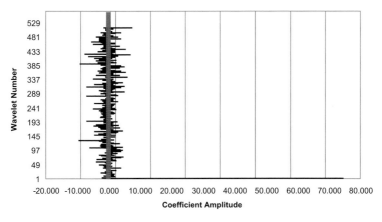

Figure 7-21 Magnitude of wavelet coefficients

coefficient exclusion threshold is defined exactly as described in the previous section. Mathematically, we can state this threshold as:

$$b_{thresh} = \alpha \times b_{max} \tag{7.49}$$

where α is a constant wavelet exclusion threshold (fraction, < or = to 1) and b_{max} is the largest wavelet coefficient within the total range of coefficients under consideration. A wavelet exclusion threshold of 4% implies that any coefficient with an amplitude less than 0.04 x b_{max} will be excluded from consideration when reconstructing the original measurements from the wavelet coefficients.

Use a relatively small wavelet exclusion threshold: 1%. Figure 7-22 shows the reconstructed signal associated with this case. Note that by setting this threshold level, 164 coefficients are excluded from the wavelet basis. Thus, the original signal is reconstructed using 348 wavelet coefficients. Therefore, we are representing the original 512 data point signal using approximately 68% of the total data points we started with. Contrasting these values with the original signal we can see that, to the casual observer, the two are quite close.

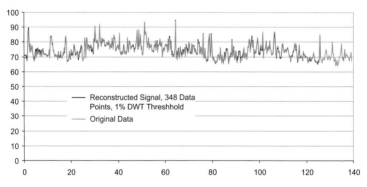

Figure 7-22 Reconstructed signal with $\alpha = 1\%$; 348 data points used for signal reconstruction

I developed a wavelet compression tool that computes and compares the raw data with the wavelet-reconstructed measurements. The source code is provided in Chapter 11. The user interface showing the reconstructed and original measurements is illustrated in Figure 7-23.

Figure 7-24 illustrates the reconstructed signal when the wavelet exclusion threshold is doubled: that is, set to 2%.

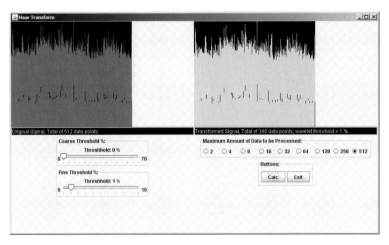

Figure 7-23 HaarXform.java user interface window $\alpha = 1\%$

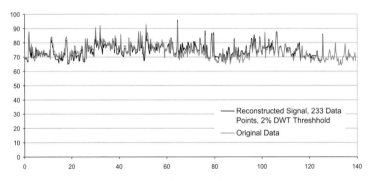

Figure 7-24 Reconstructed signal with $\alpha = 2\%$; 233 data points used for signal reconstruction

Now 279 wavelet coefficients are discarded from the signal reconstruction. We are approximating the original 512 data point signal using 233 wavelet coefficients, or 46% of the original data points. Again, the casual observer can see that the original assessment sheet data are contained within the span of the reconstructed signal. Furthermore, measurement reconstruction still captures the maximums and minimums associated with the variability of the original data. From the program, *HaarXform.java*, we can view the resulting interface for this case in Figure 7-25.

Continue this process with different levels of exclusion threshold to evaluate the impact on the overall data reconstruction process. At

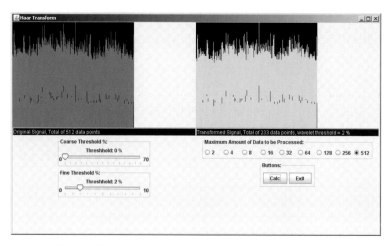

Figure 7-25 HaarXform.java user interface window $\alpha = 2\%$

some point enough coefficients will be excluded that the original data reconstruction will become meaningless. However, this serves to illustrate that it is possible to consider a substantially reduced subset of the data in order to evaluate behavior of the original data points. Potential benefits of this approach include rendering data on a device that does not have a robust processing capability or lacks sufficient memory for display and visualization of information, or lacks sufficient bandwidth to retrieve large quantities of data across a wireless network. A trade-off exists (naturally) between what level of data are necessary clinically to properly and adequately visualize in a way that enables accurate clinical decision making. Discussion of this topic in more detail is covered in Chapter 8.

The mean variability between the original measurements and the reconstruction with a 2% exclusion threshold is 4.36 beats per minute with a sample standard deviation of 5.5 beats per minute. This is computed by determining the mean root-sum-square (RSS) error between the original measurements and the reconstructed measurements at that threshold. Intuitively, as the discard threshold increases, the error increases (that is, the ability to reconstruct a true representation of the original signal degrades). Compare this result with the mean RSS error and for the 1% exclusion threshold, which calculates to 0.54 beats per minute with a sample standard deviation 0.85 beats per minute. A plot of the variation between RSS error and number of wavelet coefficients used in reconstructing the original data set is shown in Figure 7-26. The value of RSS error could provide a quantitative measure of reconstruction accuracy and the level of error that could be tolerated in terms of clinical use. Clearly, the balance in this case exists between what is acceptable for clinical decision making versus the cost of storage, retrieval, and processing of the information at hand. While the clinical answer to this might be always to err on the side of providing the most information possible, the question as to whether any data are spurious or lack key information for decision making must be posed, since today the EMR only contains a subset of data from the complete sample. Even at the reduced level of data afforded via this compression technique, this still translates into much more information being provided than is available via discrete collection every 15 minutes over the same duration.

Thus, by compressing the data using a lossy method such as a wavelet transform, potentially relevant patient information may be excluded from the reconstructed raw signal data. This is a valid argument. The purpose of the method proposed here is not to present the clinician with an alternate means of storing the data, but rather to present the clinician (and researchers) with a tool to analyze the data for comparison with other patients. By reducing the overall quantity of information that is retrieved across a hospital network and stored within an EMR, we provide the capability to reduce the storage requirements and speed the local processing. We can archive the data in one location, and retrieve only that much necessary for adequate analysis of the patient, as opposed to retrieving all data. Furthermore, a clinician may wish to have some notification of changes in behavior in a particular finding during the course of patient monitoring. Applying a threshold to the wavelet coefficients, and excluding those coefficients that are relatively small (i.e., basically, removing artifact from the signal), we are left with only those peaks that are significant. The implication for clinical decision making is significant: we have effectively defined a method for performing change detection on the original

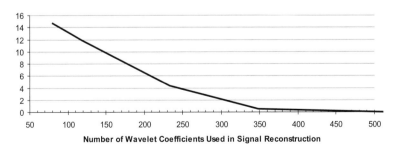

Figure 7-26 Variation in RSS error between original and reconstructed data set versus number of wavelet coefficients used in reconstruction (vertical axis units in beats per minute)

data, using a significantly reduced quantity of information with respect to the original data sample, while preserving the key features of the original data set.

We could foresee, for example, recording the wavelet coefficients in the EMR and allowing the user to identify a threshold to remove artifact or otherwise analyze the data. The reconstruction of the data could occur on a server platform that is remotely located with respect to the user, and the rendering could occur on a local device (tablet PC or PDA). The data processing required to display the signal would be less due to the reduced quantity of data. Thus a user could query the flow sheet to retrieve specific data on a patient, and these data could be returned in whatever level of resolution desired simply by selecting the threshold imposed on the wavelet coefficient reconstruction process. The reconstructed data would then be returned. Maintaining the Haar basis matrix locally would be unnecessary since it is computed independently of the actual data set.

The discrete wavelet transform (DWT) was selected as a possible filtering mechanism because the DWT preserves both spatial and temporal behavior of a raw data signal. This is a very important feature in the study of medical telemetry, because many processes are not stationary, making the application of traditional signal processing methods (such as Fourier Series) inappropriate. The creation of a DWT processing method that exists as an adjunct to the existing departmental information system imposes no additional software requirements on the existing telemetry system, and operates off of the existing clinical network. Furthermore, the benefits of using the DWT processor as both a noise filter and as an automatic data filter are affirmed inasmuch as both stationary and non-stationary signals are processed appropriately using the DWT method: stationary signals can be represented by relatively few overall data points in the form of wavelet coefficients, whereas threshold filtering of non-stationary signals can provide accurate reconstruction of raw signals with even a factor of two fewer data points than the original signal. This benefits a potentially congested network and speeds recreation of the original signal by requiring fewer overall calculations to be performed by that enterprise information system.

This approach lends itself quite readily to automation. The process described above was developed into a method written in the Java programming language called *HaarDB.java*. This method also operates with an MS Access database so that raw data obtained from the bedside monitors are transmitted via the network through a Java listening utility into the database. The database is therefore updated continuously with patient data. The *HaarDB* utility can be run at any point in time during this process and will automatically select the available data from the database, and sequence it using the patient medical record number. Presently, the method is limited to 512 discrete data points. Assuming a 15 second update interval per data point, this translates into slightly more than two hours worth of raw data. The method can be easily expanded to support much more. The source code is supplied in Chapter 11.

7.7 Kalman Filtering

Kalman filtering can be employed for both smoothing and estimating the future trajectory of data versus time. It has been applied in fields ranging from signal processing to the military, especially in the tracking of moving objects such as missiles, aircraft, and spacecraft. The basis for, benefits of, and implementation of it is very well defined in the literature. I will discuss its application to telemetry data because it is often collected in both the operating room and critical care units and is quite important in establishing and monitoring patient vital signs.

Figure 7-27 shows a plot of a sampling of arterial blood pressure (systolic component) in a patient undergoing coronary artery bypass grafting (CABG) surgery.

The plot shows discrete measurement points collected throughout a portion of CABG surgery around the cross-clamp phase (in which the heart is stopped and the patient is on the bypass machine). What is shown is the systolic blood pressure at the point at which the heart is

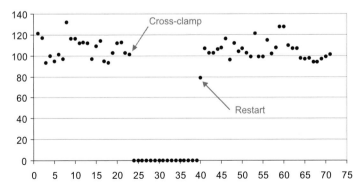

Figure 7-27 Systolic blood pressure in a patient undergoing CABG surgery

stopped and where it is restarted. The horizontal axis represents the measurement number, used in order to remove the temporal component. The time component is not important in terms of the application of the mathematical development.

Devised by Rudolph E. Kalman circa 1960, Kalman filters are termed linear estimators of process state. Their purpose is to estimate the current state of a measurement based upon the previous estimate and the current measurement. As stated above, they have been typically applied in the aerospace field for such applications as missile, aircraft, or even spacecraft tracking. The Kalman filter is unique and unlike typical state estimation (akin to least squares estimation) in that the estimate of the current state (and the propagation to a future state estimate) does not require knowledge of all prior estimates—only that of the previous time step.

The time-dependent model of state is well-described in the literature. I list these equations here to provide an easily-accessible reference point for them. I have used a number of texts on the subject in the past, and books such as those by Bar-Shalom and Gelb provide a solid theoretical background as well as practical implementation examples[120]. One purpose for using the Kalman filter is to model the state of a particular physiological variable (or the collective state of such variables) over time. I'll demonstrate this by example. Consider the discrete measurements of Figure 7-27. The Kalman filter defines a discrete-time model in the form of a difference equation:

$$x_k = Ax_{k-1} + Bu_{k-1} + w_{k-1} \qquad (7.50)$$

in which the estimated state, x_k, is defined in terms of the previous state and a transition function (or matrix) A, subject to a control input, u, with its accompanying transform function B and a process noise term, w_{k-1}. Future measurements or observations are represented by the measurement equation,

$$z_k = Hx_k + v_k \qquad (7.51)$$

---

[120] Examples: (1) Yaakov Bar-Shalom & X. Rong Li, Estimation and Tracking: Principles, Techniques and Software. Artech House: 1993. (2) Yaakov Bar-Shalom (Editor), Multi-target-Multisensor Tracking: Applications and Advances, vol. I. Artech House: 1990. (3) Yaakov Bar-Shalom (Editor), Multitarget-Multisensor Tracking: Applications and Advances, vol. II. Artech House: 1992. (4) Arthur Gelb (Editor), Applied Optimal Estimation. The MIT Press: 1974

where z_k are measurements of the parameter, x, at discrete time step k. The measurements are represented as a transformation from the parameter space represented as x to the observer's frame of reference via a transformation matrix H. The possibility that the measurements of the actual state will only be approximate is represented in the form of the random variable, v_k, which is an estimate of measurement noise. Both process and measurement noise are typically modeled as either white, zero-mean, or uncorrelated white noise and have covariance represented by Q and R, respectively[121, 122]. However, the probability distributions for process and measurement noise are typically represented as covariance matrices, Q and R, respectively.

Process noise is typically added to make up for inaccuracies or inadequacies in the state model. Measurement noise reflects the inaccuracy in the observer measuring the actual state or value of the parameter being observed. Various methods for enumerating the state estimate are available. I will discuss a simplified model for a single parameter (that of the plot above)[123]. In practice, the filter comprises a set of temporal transition equations and measurement update equations. The process involves estimating the future state, k, of a parameter, obtaining a measurement at a new time, refining the estimate based on the measurement, and then using the new state estimate to project the next estimate. The process is then repeated for each measurement. A subtlety must be understood as it is essential to the discrete computational process. These are *a priori* and *a posteriori* state estimates. The *a priori* estimate (subscript j–1) represents the estimate of parameter state based on the knowledge of the state at a time prior to time t_k. The *a posteriori* estimate (subscript j) represents the estimate of the state given the measurement at time t_k. The *a posteriori* state estimate, $\hat{x}_{k,j}$, is related to the *a priori* state estimate, $\hat{x}_{k,j-1}$, as follows:

---

[121] Treating noise terms as uncorrelated white noise is, actually, naïve. Most processes in nature do not actually conform to this assumption. A better approximation would be a Gauss-Markov process in which the noise term is represented as a white noise component in which each random draw is also dependent on the previous value based on a time 'period' by which the previous noise term can exert its influence on the current value of the noise. So, for example, one such model is $v_k = v_{k-1}e^{-t_c} + w_{k-1}$, where the random number, w_k, is drawn from a normally-distributed random number generator and added to the previous noise level which is multiplied through an exponential term attenuated by a time period, t_c, typically referred to as the *correlation time*, which is equal to $t_k - t_{k-1}$. The correlation time defines the influence of the previous random number on the current one.

[122] Arthur Gelb et al., Applied Optimal Estimation. The MIT Press: 1974. Pages 81-82.

[123] Computational method based in part on a method originally developed by Greg Welch and Gary Bishop, "An Introduction to the Kalman Filter," UNC-Chapel Hill, TR 95-041. July 24th, 2006.

$$\hat{x}_{k,j} = \hat{x}_{k,j-1} + K_k(z_k - H\hat{x}_{k,j-1}) \qquad (7.52)$$

The concept of *a priori* and *a posteriori* state estimates and their relationship to one another is adapted from an illustration by Simon[124] and is illustrated in Figure 7-28.

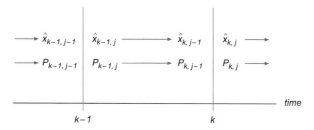

Figure 7-28 Illustration showing *a priori* and *a posteriori* state estimates and covariance

In summary, the *a posteriori* estimate of the state, subscript j−1, represents the expected value of all measurements up to and including the current estimate, whereas the *a priori* estimate represents the estimate of the state up to but excluding the current state, subscript j[125].

The term K_k is the gain that multiplies the innovation (i.e., the residual between measurements and *a priori* estimate of the state). As stated earlier, the details of the underlying mathematical theory is beyond the scope here. However, the computational method will be presented so that the user may reproduce the calculations as desired. The Kalman gain is computed as follows:

$$K_{k,j} = P_{k,j-1}H^T(HP_{k,j-1}H^T + R)^{-1} \qquad (7.53)$$

where *P* is the state covariance estimate, with *a priori* and *a posteriori* components computed as follows:

---

[124] Dan Simon, Optimal State Estimation: Kalman, H∙ and Nonlinear Approaches. John Wiley & Sons: 2006. Page 126.

[125] Dan Simon, Optimal State Estimation: Kalman, H∙ and Nonlinear Approaches. John Wiley & Sons, Inc.: 2006. Pages 124,125.

$$P_{k,j-1} = E\left[(x_{k,j-1} - \hat{x}_{k,j})(x_{k,j-1} - \hat{x}_{k,j-1})^T\right] \tag{7.54}$$

$$P_{k,j} = E\left[(x_{k,j} - \hat{x}_{k,j})(x_{k,j} - \hat{x}_{k,j})^T\right] \tag{7.55}$$

We are now prepared to begin the calculation process for our sample systolic blood pressure measurement set. It is possible to address some limiting cases and to simplify based on our knowledge of the problem. First, the generalized Kalman filter equations are written in matrix-vector form. In our case we are measuring a single scalar value. Hence, we can simplify (7.53) as follows:

$$K_{k,j} = \frac{P_{k,j-1}H}{HP_{k,j-1}H + R} \tag{7.56}$$

When measurement error is small (i.e., $R \to 0$),

$$K_{k,j} = \frac{1}{H} \tag{7.57}$$

When the observations (or measurements) are made in the same frame of reference as the state, then $K_{k,j} = 1$. However, when the covariance approaches zero, then $K_{k,j} = 0$. The significance of these statements is that in the former case higher confidence is placed in the measurements, whereas in the latter case higher confidence is placed in the state estimate. We will see the significance of this in a moment.

The algorithm proceeds typically as follows. We first look at general discrete time Kalman filter.

The Kalman filter is initialized by establishing an initial estimate of the *a posteriori* state and covariance:

$$\hat{x}_0 = x[0] \tag{7.58}$$

$$P_0 = P[0] \tag{7.59}$$

Then, the filter proceeds as follows:

$$P_{k,j-1} = AP_{k-1,j}A^T + Q_k \tag{7.60}$$

$$K_{k,j} = P_{k,j} H^T (R_k)^{-1} \tag{7.61}$$

The *a priori* state estimate is given by:

$$\hat{x}_{k,j-1} = A \hat{x}_{k-1,j} + B u_{k-1} \tag{7.62}$$

The *a posteriori* state estimate is given by:

$$\hat{x}_{k,j} = \hat{x}_{k,j-1} + K_{k,j} \left(z_k - H \hat{x}_{k,j-1} \right) \tag{7.63}$$

The *a posteriori* estimate of the covariance is given by:

$$P_{k,j} = (I - K_{k,j} H) P_{k,j-1} \tag{7.64}$$

For our sample problem we can begin by first applying our assumptions:

- we are working with scalar variables only;
- there are no outside control or forcing functions (i.e., $B = 0$);
- the state transition matrix is unity; that is, there is no specific computational model for projecting ahead ($A = 1$); and,
- the observations are performed in the same space as the measurements themselves (i.e., $H = 1$).

Applying these assumptions to equations (7.60)-(7.64) reduces these to:

$$P_{k,j-1} = P_{k-1,j} + Q_k \tag{7.65}$$

$$K_{k,j} = \frac{P_{k,j}}{R_k} \tag{7.66}$$

$$\hat{x}_{k,j-1} = \hat{x}_{k-1,j} \tag{7.67}$$

$$\hat{x}_{k,j} = \hat{x}_{k,j-1} + K_{k,j} \left(z_k - \hat{x}_{k,j-1} \right) \tag{7.68}$$

$$P_{k,j} = (I - K_{k,j}) P_{k,j-1} \tag{7.69}$$

We define the process noise and measurement noise as the expected variance in these sources:

$$Q = \sigma_Q^2 \tag{7.70}$$

$$R = \sigma_R^2 \tag{7.71}$$

We begin the iteration with the initial state $\hat{x}_{k-1,j} = 120$. The value selected here is not critical within a reasonable range of initial values (e.g., an initial systolic blood pressure = 1,000 is not reasonable). The initial state covariance estimate, P_0, is not critical, either. I have opted to set this to 1. So, for instance, we can study the case in which the measurement noise, σ_R^2, is very small ($= 0.0001$) and the process noise, σ_Q^2, is large ($= 100$). Figure 7-29 shows the Kalman filter track of the systolic blood pressure measurements. In the case of Figure 7-30 the values are reversed (i.e., $R = 100$, $Q = 0.0001$, respectively). There is a startling difference in the filter performance between these two cases.

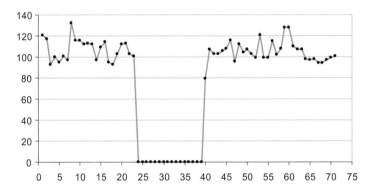

Figure 7-29 Systolic blood pressure Kalman filter model, $R = 0.0001$, $Q = 100$

In the first plot, the measurement noise is very small and the process noise is very large, thereby causing the filter to follow the measurements very closely. In the latter case, the measurement noise is very large and the process (or state) noise is very small, thereby reducing the importance of the measurements on the state estimate.

As the measurement noise is increased, the filter follows the measurements more sluggishly, resulting in a smoother response curve.

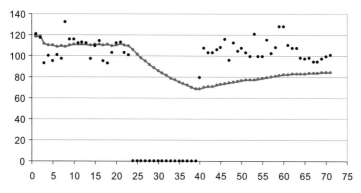

Figure 7-30 Systolic blood pressure Kalman filter model, $R = 100$, $Q = 0.0001$

This Kalman filter model was instantiated in a Microsoft Excel spreadsheet. Several of the calculations are shown in Table 7-2, should the reader wish to recreate.

Table 7-2 Kalman filtering calculation table

	time update		measurement update			Truth state		= x[k] + measurement noise		
measurement, k	xhat[k][j-1]	P[k][j-1]	K[k]	xhat[k][j]	P[k]	x[k]	Measurement Noise	z[k]	xhat[k][j] + sqrt(P[k])	xhat[k][j] - sqrt(P[k])
1	120.00	10.10	0.76	123.42	2.41	121.00	3.4885	124.4885	124.97	121.87
2	123.42	2.51	0.44	120.33	1.40	117.00	-0.5662	116.4338	121.51	119.15
3	120.33	1.50	0.32	112.44	1.02	93.00	2.7806	95.7806	113.44	111.43
4	112.44	1.12	0.26	108.28	0.83	100.00	-3.4792	96.5208	109.19	107.37
5	108.28	0.93	0.23	103.12	0.72	95.00	-9.5246	85.4754	103.96	102.27
6	103.12	0.82	0.21	103.26	0.65	101.00	2.8171	103.8171	104.07	102.46
7	103.26	0.75	0.19	102.30	0.61	97.00	1.2577	98.2577	103.08	101.53
8	102.30	0.71	0.18	108.23	0.58	132.00	2.8056	134.8056	108.99	107.47
9	108.23	0.68	0.18	110.17	0.56	116.00	3.2304	119.2304	110.92	109.42
10	110.17	0.66	0.17	111.01	0.54	116.00	-0.9433	115.0567	111.75	110.27

The 'truth state' represents the actual values of the measurements. These are the values of the parameters "unknown but to God," as any measurement contains some "noise" based on the process of measurement. In order to create the measurements, $z[k]$, the truth values are "dirtied" by adding Gaussian noise. The Gaussian noise is represented as a random number drawn from a normal distribution having standard deviation equal to the square root of R and zero mean. The measurement noise is added to the truth state resulting in the measurement at each time step, k.

7.8 Summary

In this chapter I have presented a selection of analytical techniques for processing and reducing medical device data. My objective here has been to promote creative thinking in this area as opposed to an exhaustive mathematical treatment of data reduction techniques. Most of the techniques that I've discussed relate to analysis of temporal data—that is, data that are time-varying, or time-dependent. Time-dependent data are apt for analytical consideration as they relate to data that are collected from devices and displayed in the flowsheet of a patient during treatment. Of course various relationships exist that are not temporal in nature. However, the temporal evaluation of data are often used in assessing and predicting (or trending) the state of a patient's health over time. This is especially true of patients in technologically-dependent states, such as surgical intensive care. In cases such as these the patient is monitored closely and continuously. In such environments, changes in physiological, respiratory, and cardiovascular state over time are indicative of whether the patient is "evolving" normally or is experiencing an adverse event. The measurement and actions taken as a result of the accompanying assessment of patient state is important knowledge when considering intervention. This is especially important for implementing methods for automatically controlling medical devices in response to patient state. Here, changes in data over time define the concomitant responses from medical devices and equipment. Thus, analytical techniques for reducing, processing, and managing medical device data are essential for patient care. This topic of automatic control will be addressed in more detail in Chapter 10.

8 How to Display Data in a Flowsheet

8.1 Guidelines for Effective Displays of Data

"Graphical excellence is the well-designed presentation of interesting data—a matter of substance, of statistics, and of design.
Graphical excellence consists of complex ideas communicated
with clarity, precision, and efficiency. Graphical excellence is
that which gives to the viewer the greatest number of ideas in
the shortest time with the least ink in the smallest space. Graphical excellence is nearly always multivariate. And graphical
excellence requires telling the truth about the data."

—Edward Tufte [126]

Throughout this chapter I will focus on the effective display of data.
Perhaps an obvious statement is that effective displays of data must
communicate information content in a way that provides the most
information within the eyespan of the viewer. Edward Tufte, of whom
I consider myself a student, makes this a basic tenet of data display
and information communication [127]. Medicine is among those fields
in which effective displays of data (information) are paramount and
critical, because they influence and even define clinical decision making. [128]

It is necessary to look at the display of data not as an afterthought or
treated as secondary but rather as second only to the data itself in
importance. Why? Because the display of data through the user interface (UI) is the mechanism by which the clinician makes key decisions
on patients. So, what must be displayed? Per Shortliffe & Cimino, we
can suggest foundational data upon which to build [129]. For each observation displayed to the user:

---

[126] Edward Tufte, The Visual Display of Quantitative Information, 2nd Ed., Graphics Press;
Cheshire, CT, 2001; page 51.

[127] Edward Tufte, Beautiful Evidence, Graphics Press, LLC: 2006. Page 159

[128] Edward H. Shortliffe, Ed. and James J. Cimino, Assoc. Ed. Biomedical Informatics Computer
Applications in Health Care and Biomedicine, 3rd Ed. Springer Science & Business Media,
LLC: 2006. Page 46.

[129] Edward H. Shortliffe, Ed. and James J. Cimino, Assoc. Ed. Biomedical Informatics Computer
Applications in Health Care and Biomedicine, 3rd Ed. Springer Science & Business Media,
LLC: 2006 Page 47

1) the patient identity, including name, date of birth, medical and visit information (e.g., medical record number, visit identifiers), gender, height, weight, family histories, ailments, etc. to which the parameter is associated must be established without a doubt and in a way that the user cannot (except through wanton neglect) falsely-identify said patient;

2) the parameter being observed must be defined clearly and must be readily visible to the user:

   • the observation value and its units;

   • the date and time of the observation; and

   • any qualifying notations that describe the conditions under which the observation is valid.

Those displays of statistical data which enable and encourage the viewer to compare different observations, avoid distortions, and reveal both their fine and broad structure are also tenets of good graphical design[130]. Comparisons between different observations also assist in the process of making clinical decisions (vis-à-vis, clinical decision support, CDS)[131]. Displays of comparative data enable the clinical user to evaluate the importance of deviations from expected trends.

In summary, show comparisons, contrasts, and differences[132]:

1) show causality—the mechanism, structure, and explanation

2) show multivariate data containing more than 2 variables where possible; and

3) completely integrate words, numbers, images, and diagrams.

8.2 The Data Story

What types of data need to be displayed to the clinical user, and how? Table 8-1 summarizes the types of data typically employed by physicians when making clinical decisions during treatment in a trauma-focused intensive care unit[133].

---

[130] Edward R. Tufte, The Visual Display of Quantitative Information, 2nd Ed. Graphics Press, Cheshire, CT. 2001. Page 13.

[131] Edward H. Shortliffe, Ed. and James J. Cimino, Assoc. Ed. Biomedical Informatics Computer Applications in Health Care and Biomedicine, 3rd Ed. Springer Science & Business Media, LLC: 2006 Pages 54-58.

[132] Edward Tufte, Beautiful Evidence, Graphics Press, LLC: 2006. Pages 126-130.

Table 8-1 Data use distribution within a shock-trauma ICU

Component	Value
monitor	13%
observation	21%
laboratory	33%
drugs I/O IV	22%
blood gas	9%
other	2%

At least 98% of data refer to measurable quantities upon which a clinician bases key decisions. Upwards of 77% of all data are associated with the areas of monitoring, laboratory, intake & output (I/O) and blood gases alone—vital measures key to ensuring patient survival. Clearly, their display influences use as their value is incalculable:

"Making Decisions based on evidence requires the appropriate display of that evidence. Good displays of data help to reveal knowledge relevant to understanding mechanism, process and dynamics, cause and effect. That is, displays of statistical data should directly serve the analytic task at hand."

—Edward Tufte[134]

Let's begin designing our candidate display of information taking into account the aforementioned guidelines. Furthermore, let's consider building this display relative to an actual case. For this example I'm going to refer to data I collected on one of my coronary artery bypass grafting patients (CABG)[135]. This individual was a male older than 60 years of age. This patient's height and weight were approximately 160 cm and 70 kg, respectively. Patient body surface area (frequently used in the titration of intravenous solutions) was computed to be approximately 1.7 m^2.

During the surgical procedure for a patient undergoing coronary bypass the patient is sedated by an anesthesiologist through the

---

[133] Edward H. Shortliffe, Ed. and James J. Cimino, Assoc. Ed. Biomedical Informatics Computer Applications in Health Care and Biomedicine, 3rd Ed. Springer Science & Business Media, LLC: 2006 Page 605

[134] Edward R. Tufte, Visual and Statistical Thinking: Displays of Evidence for Making Decisions. Graphics Press, LLC: 1997. Cheshire, Connecticut. Third Printing: 2005.

[135] Clinical trials conducted under Institutional Review Board approval at the Hospital of the University of Pennsylvania via study #570-0; 1996.

administration of drugs such as fentanyl. In traditional open-heart surgeries the heart is stopped to facilitate the grafting of a venous segment typically harvested from another location in the body (for instance, legs). The patient is administered paralyzing drugs to negate motion during the surgery. One of these drugs is pancuronium bromide. This drug acts as a muscle relaxant that facilitates intubation and mechanical ventilation. Breathing cessation occurs during CABG surgery, and this is accomplished through the administration of this drug. The effects can be reversed after surgery by administering drugs such as neostigmine.

The heart is then stopped. During this process, the heart is 'bypassed' literally by using cannulae to redirect the flow of blood from the vena cava to the aorta through a bypass machine that oxygenates the blood and returns it to the body. The harvested vein is sewed both to the aorta and to the coronary artery below the blocked region. The actual surgery from induction of anesthesia to movement of the patient from the operating room to the ICU can consume as much as 6 hours or longer depending on the complexity of the surgery (i.e., number of grafts and other complications).

The anesthesiologist makes a complete record of the surgery, identifying all drug administrations and vitals observations within a flow sheet. These flow sheets may be paper or electronic. Some of these parameters are shown and discussed below. We can experiment with ways to display these data most effectively to a user.

Figure 8-1 shows patient pulse over time. The reader will see several annotations on this plot; specifically, when drug administrations occurred, when cross-clamp occurred, and then when the patient's surgery was completed. Also shown is the post-operative pulse history in the surgical intensive care unit (SICU) from arrival through extubation, when the endotracheal tube (ETT) through which the

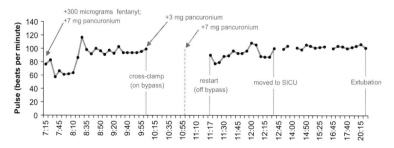

Figure 8-1 CABG patient intraoperative pulse

181

patient receives respiratory support via mechanical ventilation, is removed.

These data provide a complete record of pulse profile within the eye-span of the clinician. The obvious discontinuity—cross-clamp—is clearly identified. The viewer can visually distill the average pulse over time preoperatively. The data in this plot, together with other information that should be displayed concomitantly, will provide a clear picture of the goings-on around this patient from the telemetry and management perspective.

Complementary data include patient arterial blood pressure (ABP), Figure 8-2; oxygen saturation, Figure 8-3; core temperature, Figure 8-4; and cardiac output measured post-operatively, Figure 8-5.

Aside from the story these data tell, there are some basic formatting and display attributes that bear mentioning. First, all of these plots are displayed on the same abscissa: all are displayed with respect to a time axis having the same start and end points and increments. This enables for both easy comparison along the same axis in addition to removing the possibility of confusion.

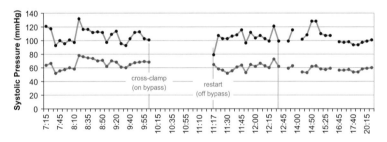

Figure 8-2 CABG patient intraoperative arterial blood pressure

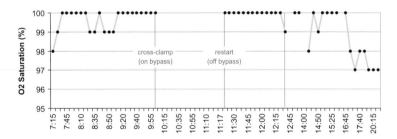

Figure 8-3 CABG patient intraoperative O$_2$ saturation

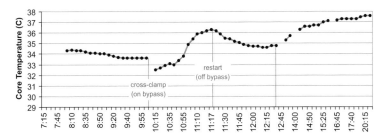

Figure 8-4 CABG patient intraoperative core temperature

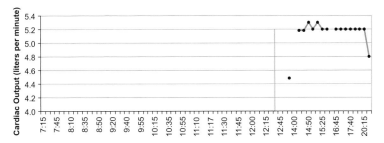

Figure 8-5 CABG patient postoperative cardiac output

This temporal and (seemingly) continuous information must be augmented with notes, orders, laboratory information, etc. to complete the picture of the 'state' of the patient at any point in time. This is important because each set of observations over time (e.g., pulse, or blood pressure, or temperature, etc.) describes only one scalar component. Separately they have little meaning. It is only together, in that context, in which they provide a full and meaningful representation of patient condition.

Consider the patient pH and partial pressure of carbon dioxide. These are illustrated in Figure 8-6 and Figure 8-7, respectively. Note the normal ranges are shown in these plots (the lower-bound normal range for pH is the axis itself: 7.35). These latter values are not collected automatically but are obtained through blood-gas laboratory analysis based on blood draws. The frequency of these laboratory reports are driven by clinical assessments and are performed on the order of the attending physician. Typically a blood gas assessment is made upon arrival in the ICU and then several times thereafter, including prior to extubation and, on occasion, when a decision to wean a patient from post-operative mechanical ventilation is made.

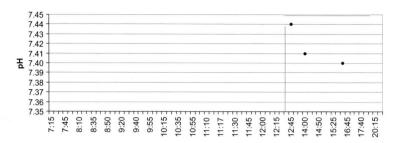

Figure 8-6 CABG patient postoperative pH

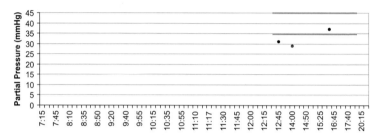

Figure 8-7 CABG patient postoperative partial pressure of carbon dioxide showing normal ranges

Patients are gradually weaned from post-operative mechanical ventilation. Two of the key parameters that are reduced as patients regain spontaneous respiratory function are the inspired oxygen fraction (F_iO2) and the respiratory rate, specified in terms of the number of mandatory breaths per minute with which the mechanical ventilator offers the patient during the period of time in which the patient is unable to breathe on his or her own.

The timing and amount of support reduction must be determined on a patient-by-patient basis. Figure 8-8 and Figure 8-9 illustrate the FiO2 and IMV support level reductions over time. These data can be

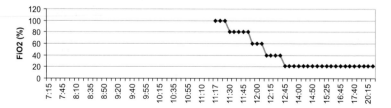

Figure 8-8 CABG patient inspired oxygen fraction

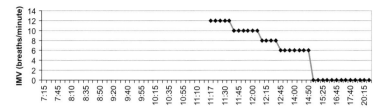

Figure 8-9 CABG patient intermittent mandatory ventilation

collected automatically from mechanical ventilators and displayed within the user interface so as to compare the mandatory level against the spontaneous.

The data presented in the several plots above include those observations that are manually obtained and those that can be automatically measured from medical devices. I will focus on the display of the medical data alone.

8.3 Displaying Medical Device Data

"...there are right ways and wrong ways to show data; there are displays that reveal the truth and displays that do not."

—Edward Tufte[136]

Anyone who uses a computer is a consumer of user interfaces. Every screen viewed through an Internet Web browser has experienced the display of information as created by a computer program which translates data or raw information into an aesthetically pleasing view that facilitates the human-computer interaction. Thus, as the visual mechanism for communicating information from the processor to the user, the user interface is critical: it operates as the information liaison between the world of the binary and the world of the visual. Yet, the architecture of that user interface is dependent on the specific needs of the user. For instance, the interface presented by computer programs such as Microsoft Excel spreadsheets may be appropriate for use by individuals performing mathematical or data analysis, but such an interface may not be appropriate for individuals using the interface to assess information on patients in an operational high acuity environment such as critical care or an emergency department.

---

[136] Edward R. Tufte, "Visual and Statistical Thinking: Displays of Evidence for Making Decisions." Graphics Press, LLC: 1997. Third Printing: 2005. Page 23.

185

Consider the plot of Figure 8-10. Here we have a comparison between the mandatory respiratory support level (IMV) and spontaneous (patient) values over time for a CABG patient. This plot satisfies several tenets identified earlier: show comparisons and causality. The spontaneous respiratory rate is an indicator of the patient's ability to assume increasing and independent support over the ventilator. This is supported by the clinical assessment that the patient can, indeed, sustain this support as evidenced by the reduction in mandatory support over time.

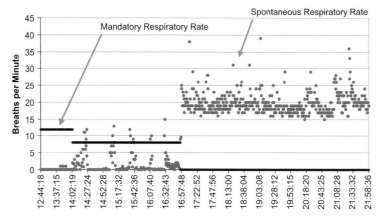

Figure 8-10 Mandatory and spontaneous respiratory rates

These data tell a story. It is important to show a comparative data story because it provides the user with a rapid and informative view of key observations all within the eyespan. The clinician can see what was ordered (vis-à-vis the reduction in IMV support) and the patient's response over time. The clinician can see just how the patient responded and the variability associated with the patient values. The clinician also can see the patient's spontaneous values near to the time of extubation, at which the patient is fully conscious and breathing on his or her own prior to extubation. Another important point: all of the data shown in Figure 8-10 were collected automatically from a mechanical ventilator via a serial connection.

So, how might data be presented to the clinician in an effective and helpful way? There is certainly more than one answer to this question. However, we can show several approaches that adhere to the tenets described earlier for good user interface design.

Figure 8-11 is a composite drawing showing multiple findings displayed over time. Several items of note:

1) All data are displayed along the same time axis. This enables consistent comparison of the findings and their changes to analyze and hypothesize on causal relationships among them;

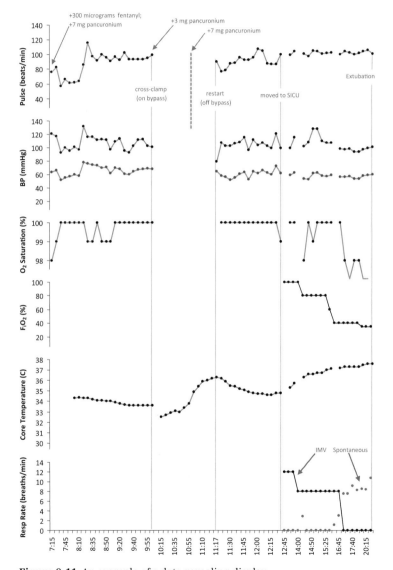

Figure 8-11 An example of a data-revealing display

2) All data are displayed within the eyespan of the viewing clinician. This enables the clinician to make the aforementioned comparisons without having to flip pages or commit data to memory prior to viewing other findings. In short, this facilitates rapid analysis;

3) The data provide a complete record from the beginning of surgery—the event at which data collection begins—through extubation from mechanical ventilation. This provides the clinician with the entire 'story' on the patient. Notes are added as overlays to provide context relative to events during surgery such as anesthetic administration and surgical events ("cross-clamp"). Postoperatively, we can look at the mandatory respiratory rate (i.e., mechanical ventilation) in comparison with the spontaneous values. The respiratory rate and inspired oxygen fraction are both adjusted during the postoperative weaning process and this is readily visible from the data.

This representation is not complete as is. Still missing from this user interface view is patient-identifying information. Look again at Figure 1-9 from Chapter 1, but with a redesign to display the findings within a single screen. The blood pressure, pulse, and temperature findings may be displayed using the data above. Figure 8-12 is a suggested interface for vitals observations. Note several items:

1) The patient identifying information is shown at top and is available for the clinician to see within the eyespan. This is important because it ensures that the clinician always knows who is viewed at all times. This mitigates risks (or hazards) associated with linking these data to the wrong patient;

2) The attending physician is identified so that any questions regarding the patient condition can be directed to that clinician;

3) The findings show a time frame that can be associated with a specific episode of care for a defined time window. The time window can be adjusted using arrows or a slider whose width is proportional to the amount of prior data outside of the given window; and

4) The values of the findings are displayed on the right side of the individual plots so that the clinician can see at a glance what those values are and then can see the trends peripherally to the left of those to gain a complete view of them.

Perhaps less optimal are other associated data which are shown to be accessible via tabs on the right side of this findings page. I am show-

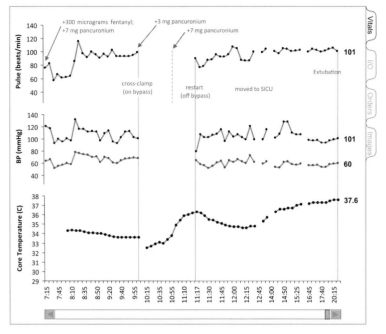

Figure 8-12 Sample user interface showing findings related to automatically collected findings

ing tabs for information such as intake and output (I & O) relating to infusion and excretion, images related to radiological information (X-Ray, MRI, CT, Ultrasound, etc.), and existing physician orders. Nursing and physician notes would also be included. However, my objective is not to define the perfect all-encompassing user interface but rather, to focus on the automatically collected findings on the patient. Therefore, I will accept that those items not directly related to automated data collection are excluded from the view—a failing. One exception to this statement is the intake and output information: some infusion data certainly can be measured and collected automatically. These data can be included in the plots shown in Figure 8-12.

While the view in Figure 8-12 is a start, it is incomplete both for the aforementioned reasons and because it is only displaying a limited set of data. There are those who might suggest that the user interface will become cramped and unreadable given too much information is displayed. My response to that is "only if we do not display the data correctly"—that is, in a manner that is unreadable to the clinical user. *If the data are required by the user to make assessments on the patient, then a claim that more data cannot be shown should be questioned as a failing of the design and architecture of the user interface.* The available tools for displaying data should not prohibit or deny the user from seeing all of the necessary information. We merely need to use the correct tools to do so.

Included in Figure 8-13 are 7 plots relating to patient state. The findings within this view are consistent with the previous figure in that they provide the values at the current time on the right side of each plot together with the scroll bar that lets the user adjust the time and date axis. The point to be made here is that the user interface must display the data as efficiently as possible in the smallest amount of user interface real estate. This implies, too, that other information (patient identifying information, for instance) must be shown in an efficient yet clear and unambiguous manner.

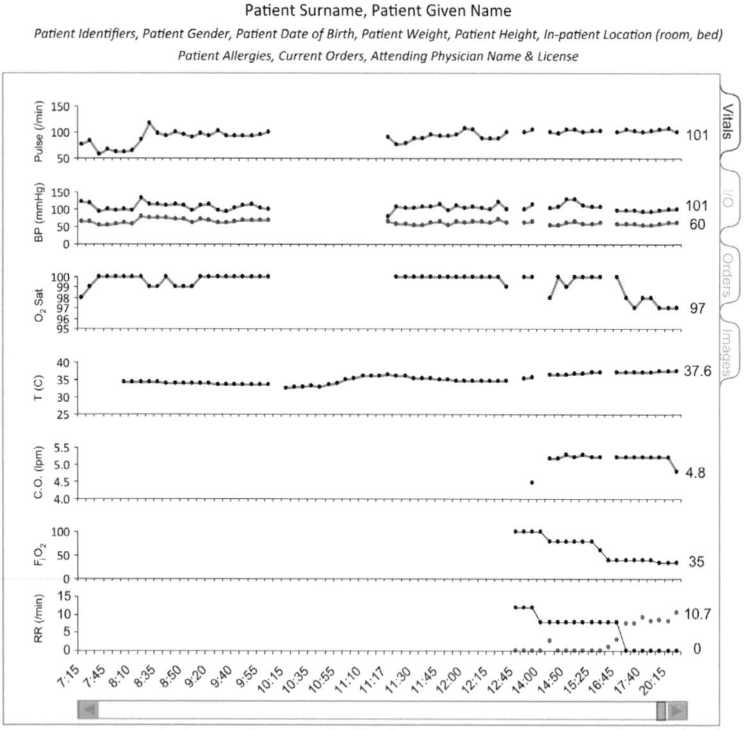

Figure 8-13 User interface showing additional observations within the findings user interface tab

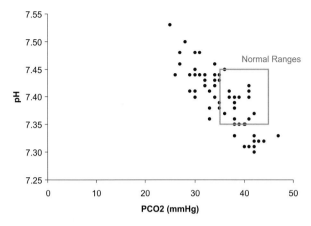

Figure 8-14 Comparison of the relationship between pH and PCO2
with normal ranges (67 data points; Source: Author)

Another important point is to provide the capability to show comparisons of measured data with normal ranges. One example of this is provided in Figure 8-14.

Several pieces of information are available from this graphical view. The relationship between pH and the partial pressure of carbon dioxide suggests causality. While pH is a measure of acidosis and alkalosis, defined by PCO2, the specific numerical relationship is shown in this plot. Furthermore, a comparison between the acceptable ranges for both pH and PCO2 reveal those values that are not normal. It is important to show and exploit comparisons between like data sets and within data sets so that relationships are revealed without requiring separate or offline analysis. This is key to the effective display of information.

8.4 A User Interface that Stresses Data Comparisons

A different type of user interface is shown in Figure 8-15.

This interface is not quite as informative as that in Figure 8-13. However, it provides for rapid viewing of multiple parameters. Shown are the current value, previous, and the time interval between prior and last values. The black, white and gray crosshairs describe thresholds beyond which current values of shown parameters will be flagged. The setting of these threshold values is established with the aid of the

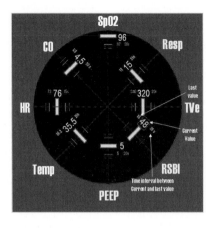

Figure 8-15
User interface "dashboard" design for multiple parameter viewing (US Patent 6,956,572)

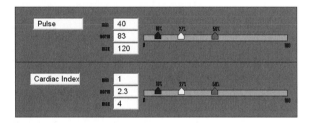

Figure 8-16 User interface threshold definition and selection

tool in Figure 8-16 which illustrates only two specific parameter values as examples.

The black slider indicates that if the current value of the parameter exceeds 10% of the mean value, a first notification will be identified. Similarly, the white slider identifies a normative value, 27% in this case, which establishes a second threshold. A third threshold, controlled by the gray slider, here set to 50%, establishes an outside value for threshold notification. Examples illustrating the cases in which the gray and white thresholds are exceeded are shown in Figure 8-17 and Figure 8-18, respectively.

In both cases the change in coloration of the current value bar establishes the notification to the user of a significant change in parameter value.

A collection of Java programs has been developed that approximates the function of this user interface. These are provided in Chapter 11.

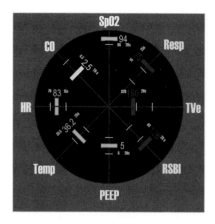

Figure 8-17
User interface example illustrating the gray threshold setting (Resp,Tve, RSBI)

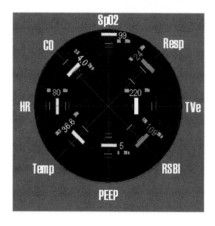

Figure 8-18
User interface example illustrating the white and gray threshold setting (Tve, Resp, RSBI)

8.5 Data Validation Mechanisms

We are still not complete in our data view representation of Figure 8-13. We can add the capability to edit the field values so that the user may validate or change values when necessary and then can select values to be transmitted to the EMR using a SEND button, as illustrated in Figure 8-19. This provides the clinician with control over what is transmitted into the EMR and how frequently.

The ability to add and remove values from the user interface is an additional feature that will allow clinicians to tailor their interfaces to them. Then, the user interface can be recalled each time the user accesses the system.

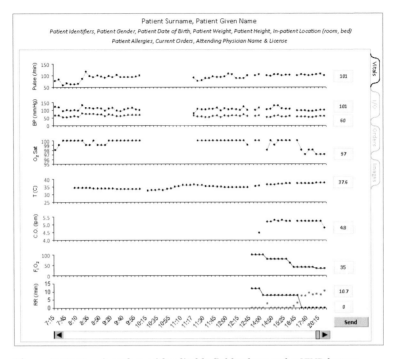

Figure 8-19 User interface with editable field values and a SEND button
to transmit results to the EMR

8.6 Key Points in User Interface Design

User interfaces must communicate data accurately and clearly. The preceding examples serve to illustrate this point from the perspective of providing the most complete view of the data. The key point is that the user should be presented with what is required to make clinical decisions. Artifacts of design and user interface architecture should always focus on this. Making the most of the given real estate before the clinician's eyes involves showing more, not less, data.

Frequently, opponents to this idea cite studies proffering the empirical idea that human beings can only remember a handful of items[137]. It seems that this rule-of-thumb has been applied (incorrectly, in my opinion) to everything from data to the number of bullet points within Microsoft PowerPoint slides. The importance of the user inter-

---

[137] George A. Miller, "The Magical Number Seven, Plus or Minus Two: Some Limits on Our Capacity for Processing Information." The Psychological Review, 1956, vol. 63, pp.81-97.

face is to display complete and accurate information regarding the state of the patient, not for the clinician to walk away remembering only a handful of incomplete data. To suggest that only seven parameters can or should be shown without comparison with other key information is presumptive arrogance on the part of the designer of the user interface.

Perhaps another aspect of the user interface that is very important to clinical users is that of non-productive interaction; for example, mouse clicks that do not result in immediate access to data or which require users to access other screens in order to obtain more information. Maximizing the amount of data within the eyespan of the user translates into the need for fewer mouse clicks and movement away from that screen, as well as data comparisons that require a clinician to memorize or commit certain data items to memory in order to make mental (versus visual) comparisons among findings.

9 Interface Software as a Medical Device

9.1 The Need for Quality and Regulatory Management

"As to diseases, make a habit of two things—to health, or at least to do no harm."

Hippocrates in *Epidemics*, Bk I, Sect. XI[138]

Ethical and legal issues abound in the areas of medical device and EMR regulations[139]. Medical devices that produce information or data vital to patient survival fall into the class of federally regulated monitoring hardware and software categories requiring pre-market notification[140]. These include commercially-developed, clinical information systems that represent medium risk in terms of the implications on patient safety or life.

The U.S. Food and Drug Administration (FDA) of the Department of Health and Human Services (HHS) establishes three device classes normally used to guide the development, management, and monitoring of medical device hardware and software. These include:

Class I, involving General Controls;

Class II, involving Special Controls; and,

Class III, involving Pre-market Approval.

All three classes conform and are subject to regulations listed under Title 21 of the Code of Federal Regulations (CFR) Part 807. General controls involve adhering to standards and manufacturing processes in accordance with 21 CFR Part 820. Device labeling is also required in

---

[138] Quoted in: Cedric M. Smith, "Origin and Uses of Primum Non Nocere—Above All, Do No Harm!" The Journal of Clinical Pharmacology, 2005; 45:371-377.
Hippocratic oath discussed in: Stephen Perles, "It's All Greek to Me," Dynamic Chiropractic, January 15, 2006, Volume 24, Issue 02.

[139] Edward H. Shortliffe, James J. Cimino, Eds. Biomedical Informatics: Computer Applications in Health Care and Biomedicine. Springer Science and Business Media: 2006. Page 395

[140] Ibid., Page 400

accordance with 21 CFR Part 801 or 809[141]. The FDA reports that most Class I medical devices are exempt from pre-market notification. Devices in this category typically include scalpels, sharps (a.k.a. needles for syringes), and surgical gloves. Pre-market notification follows the 510(k) process[142].

The 510(k) filing process requires the manufacturer to make the case for substantial equivalence. This point is of key importance. If the manufacturer proposes a device that involves some risk to the patient and has a clinical use that involves monitoring, affecting, or controlling functions imperative to the life of the patient, but for which no substantial equivalent can be determined, then it is likely that the proposed device involves pre-market approval (PMA).

Devices requiring pre-market notification are typically those of low or medium risk and require FDA approval and oversight prior to being marketed. Such devices typically fall into the Class II category. As part of the 510(k) pre-market filing and approval process, manufacturers compare their proposed devices and/or solutions (both hardware and software) with those existing in the market. If substantial equivalence to those devices currently within the market space can be established, then the case for classification of the new device within that category as a low- to medium-risk system can be affirmed. Devices in this category include non-invasive monitoring equipment and software used to communicate or process patient vitals data for use in clinical assessment and decision making.

Pre-market notification is differentiated from devices requiring pre-market approval as those falling in this latter category are typically Class III devices. Such devices normally require clinical trials prior to introduction to the marketplace. Devices in this category include invasive instruments such as pacemakers, defibrillators, or controllers. Automatically-controlled mechanical ventilation hardware and controlling software would reside in this category. Additionally, devices for which no predicates exist are typically in the Class III category. Clinical trials may be necessary to establish device efficacy and safety prior to pre-market notification approval.

Applying for pre-market notification via a 510(k) filing process can take months. In my experience, the process has taken approximately 6 months, depending on the maturity and complexity of the device, its documentation supporting substantial equivalence, the complete-

---

[141] http://www.fda.gov/cdrh/devadvice/3132.html#class_2

[142] Robert A. Greenes, Clinical Decision Support: The Road Ahead. Elsevier: 2007. Page 438.

ness and rigor of the manufacturing process, and the thoroughness with which the design has been validated, tested, and documented demonstrating the safety and operation of the device.

For me, creating and fielding medical devices in clinical environments is to assume a great and sacred responsibility. The question I ask myself in such situations is whether I have expended the effort and have, to the best of my ability, ensured that any device that comes into contact with patients—software or hardware—is indeed safe and will cause no harm. In such cases I ask myself whether I would trust such a device to be used in the service of care for a member of my family: my children, my wife.

9.2 Regulatory Requirements and Process

Organizations involved with developing hardware or software (or both) for use in patient care follow "best practices" if they assess the potential need for regulatory filing. Let me be clear: not every device requires classification, but an evaluation of any device for potential risk must be undertaken to aid the developer in determining whether any potential adverse effects can result from its usage. The Centers for Devices and Radiological Health (CDRH) of the U.S. Food and Drug Administration is a focal point for medical device pre-market notification (PMN) and approval (PMA) and oversees the process by which medical devices are evaluated for general market use. Several years ago the Director of the CDRH gave a presentation on the organizational structure and purpose of the CDRH[143].

The CDRH manages many offices and among these is the Office of Device Evaluation. Within this office are several divisions which focus on medical device evaluation and approval for general market use. These include the division of Cardiovascular Devices; Division of General, Restorative and Neurological Devices; Division of Anesthesiology, General Hospital, Infection Control, and Dental Devices; and Division of Ophthalmic and Ear, Nose and Throat Devices.

Most of the medical devices related to cardiovascular data collection detailed in this book would be associated with and evaluated by one or more of these divisions. In the process of seeking market notification clearance for sale, a pre-market notification must be sought. This

---

[143] Heather S. Rosecrans, "Medical Device Regulatory Update," The North Carolina Medical Device Organization Medical Device Forum. Monday, May 16, 2005.

involves filing what is known as a 510(k) application with the FDA. This enables the FDA to determine whether substantial equivalence exists in the current marketplace between the candidate and the existing field of devices available for general sale. The substantial equivalence process seeks to determine whether the device being considered for general sale has the same intended use and technological characteristics of existing, legally marketed devices or, given the same intended use, does not raise questions of safety and effectiveness relative to marketed predicate devices.

In order to make a decision in this matter a thorough and detailed understanding of the proposed device must be submitted to the FDA. Manufacturers, device specification developers who intend to have a device manufactured by a third party, repackagers or relabelers who make labeling changes to medical devices that significantly alter their usage, and foreign manufacturers introducing devices to the U.S. market are all required to submit 510(k) applications. The CDRH provides a link to a decision tree on its Web site[144] that codifies the process of ascertaining substantial equivalence in order to approve a device for market (PMN) or to determine whether PMA is required. The FDA publishes a guidance document as an offered standard in determining substantial equivalence[145]. A flow diagram is provided in Figure 9-1 which is based on the original published by the FDA. I have altered the diagram to make it more succinct.

As part of this guidance document the CDRH identifies some specific standards relative to classes of medical devices. For instance, 510(k) applications for infusion pumps should contain information on chemical formulation and biocompatibility of materials that contact the fluid path, and metal components must use ASTM material specification standards, whereas 510(k) applications for noninvasive blood pressure measurement systems should include performance testing data and should demonstrate conformity with the ANSI/AAMI SP10 standard. Furthermore, the 510(k) must be submitted at least 90 days prior to device introduction and is therefore typically submitted prior to final acceptance testing by the manufacturer.[146]

---

[144] http://www.fda.gov/cdrh/ode/dd510kse.pdf

[145] "Use of Standard in Substantial Equivalence Determinations." U.S. Department of Health and Human Services Food and Drug Administration; Center for Devices and Radiological Health—Office of Device Evaluation. Document issued on March 12th, 2000.

[146] "Use of Standard in Substantial Equivalence Determinations." U.S. Department of Health and Human Services Food and Drug Administration; Center for Devices and Radiological Health—Office of Device Evaluation. Document issued on March 12th, 2000. Page 4.

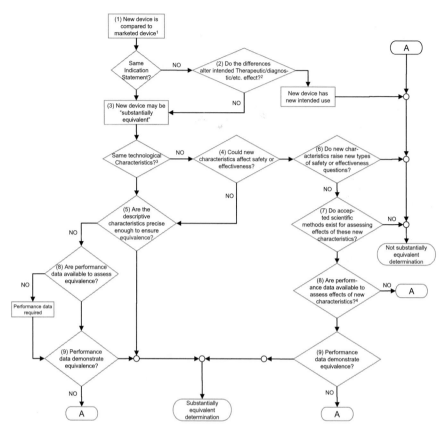

Figure 9-1 510(k) substantial equivalence decision-making process. Decision-making flow diagram is based on the original publication
(Used with permission of the Food and Drug Administration)

A 510(k) application is required when a device is being introduced to
the market for the first time or changes its intended use or significant
changes to existing devices with PMN are being considered. Medical
devices are subject to the FDA's authority under the Code of Federal
Regulations (CFR). Under the CFR, medical devices typically fall
within Title 21 under parts 800-1299[147]. The Quality System Regula-

---

[147] http://www.fda.gov/cdrh/devadvice/365.html

tions (QSR) mandate that all Class II and III medical devices be prepared in accordance with 21 CFR 820.30 design controls.

Average 510(k) review times have historically been about 75 days. This does not include the time required for the manufacturer to respond to questions from the FDA. Total days from first application to receiving PMN have been reported in the range of 100 days[148]. Title 21 CFR subchapter H provides the overall guidance for registering and listing medical devices for PMN. Specifically, under 21 CFR 807—Pre-market notification procedures—a summary of the information required for a PMN submission includes:

(a) device name, including trade and proprietary;
(b) registration number of the owner submitting the pre-market notification;
(c) proposed classification of the product being submitted;
(d) proposed labeling;
(e) a demonstration of substantial equivalence to predicate devices;
(f) indications for use and supporting data to demonstrate adherence to safety standards; and,
(g) supporting technical data to include design specifications, architecture, and verification & validation procedures and demonstrated adherence to same.

9.3 FDA Guidance on Software

The CDRH also publishes guidelines on principles of software validation[149]. Software is different from hardware in some obvious and not-so-obvious ways. Hardware is tactile: you can touch it. It has distinct and clear boundaries. Software can be analogous but also can have less well-defined boundaries. Software can contain unforeseen problems (such as branching, or other logical issues) that may not be anticipated during design. Methodologies for software standardization exist, but developing software can be an art form. While the design can be precisely described in the documentation, the implementation can be subject to the peculiarities of style associated with

---

[148] Heather S. Rosecrans, "Medical Device Regulatory Update," The North Carolina Medical Device Organization Medical Device Forum. Monday, May 16, 2005. Page 61.

[149] "General Principles of Software Validation; Final Guidance for Industry and FDA Staff." U.S. Department of Health and Human Services Food and Drug Administration; Center for Devices and Radiological Health; Center for Biologics Evaluation and Research. January 11th, 2002.

the particular developer or code-writer. Furthermore, software dependencies on third party off-the-shelf (OTS) components cannot be guaranteed in terms of similarities in development style. This extends to the use of software components for which the original intended use was not in a medical setting, but for which the flexibility of the component makes it ideal for such a use relative to a particular software application. For example, software written by a "manufacturer" may employ non-regulated components for which its initial intent was not specifically directed towards developing the medical software "device" itself. Examples such as database engines, off-the-shelf software components, and even development and packaging software may be considered a part of this category. Nonetheless, software may fall within the medical device category. Software which enables or is a component of existing medical hardware is in this category (e.g., software to trace the electrocardiograph waveforms on a telemetry monitor), and software that operates in the role of a device (e.g., collects patient data for use in clinical decision making)[150].

Manufacturing practices for both medical hardware and software is a conformance requirement of the Quality System Regulation (QSR), contained in 21 CFR Part 820. The QSR addresses quality management, device design, purchasing, component handling, production controls, packaging, device labeling, validation and verification, installation, support, and servicing[151]. The CDRH makes clear that "Any software used to automate any part of the device production process or any part of the quality system must be validated for its intended use, as required by 21 CFR § 820.30.[152]" This governance applies to electronic medical records, as well.

Filing 510(k) applications for medical device software follows the standard application process with the concomitant focus on design, validation, and verification. EMR software that receives data from medical devices directly must have demonstrable safety characteristics and must be backed up with test data. All requirements must map to functions and features within the software. One "best practice" I recommend is to map individual requirements to specific test procedure steps, and to then map these to specific design document sections and specific lines or blocks of source code. This provides for

---

[150] "General Principles of Software Validation; Final Guidance for Industry and FDA Staff." U.S. Department of Health and Human Services Food and Drug Administration; Center for Devices and Radiological Health; Center for Biologics Evaluation and Research. January 11th, 2002.

[151] Ibid.

[152] Ibid., Page 3.

unambiguous association between requirements and implementation within the software product itself.

The need to file a 510(k) application must be made relative to the risks to both the patient and the user of the software. An analysis of these risks must be undertaken to quantify them in terms of the likelihood of adverse events and the potential impact of those adverse events on patients. While subjective to a degree, this does assist in determining whether the possible risks are unacceptable (i.e., life threatening) and what mitigation methods can be employed to reduce the likelihood of occurrence, increase patient safety, or both together. However, if a manufacturer is unable to determine for sure whether a proposed product should be classified, it is possible to request a ruling from the FDA. This process involves filing a 513(g) application. The FDA makes a ruling on the basis of predicate devices, substantial equivalence, and details relating to intended use, design, and labeling. If the FDA determines that the proposed product requires no clearance, then the manufacturer may market without requiring labeling. However, if the FDA determines that the device requires clearance, then the manufacturer must abide by their ruling prior to marketing.

Frequently there is a need to update software—improvements in design, or additional design features are required. However, a dilemma results: how to update the code without impacting intended use? After all, if the software is updated, won't that require a re-filing?

The answer is that it is not always necessary to file anew when standard or noninvasive engineering changes to software occur. The FDA has a process for ascertaining whether changes in software (or hardware) merit filing a new 510(k) application. This process contains a series of flow diagrams supported by descriptive text which enables a developer to determine and to document the process for determining whether the amended software falls within the bounds of the indications for use and labeling or whether sufficient changes warrant filing anew[153]. This algorithm is intended for both hardware and software. However, I will omit those portions of the algorithm which apply primarily to hardware devices. These are adapted from the original FDA documentation and are illustrated in Figure 9-2, Figure 9-3, and Figure 9-4. I have excluded the algorithm relating to materials changes as this is not applicable to software.

---

[153] "Deciding When to Submit a 510(k) for a Change to an Existing Device." 510(k) Memorandum #K97-1. U.S. Food and Drug Administration; Center for Devices and Radiological Health. January 10th, 1997.

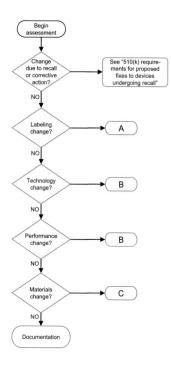

Figure 9-2
Determining whether changes in
software or hardware design merit
filing a new 510(k)-main algorithm
(Used with permission of the Food
and Drug Administration)

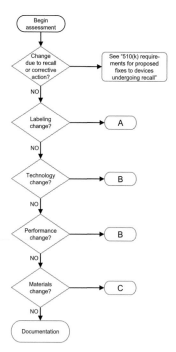

Figure 9-3
Labeling changes algorithm
(Used with permission of the
Food and Drug Administration)

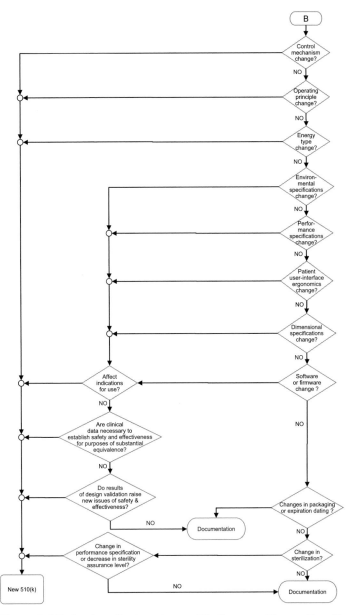

Figure 9-4 Technology, Engineering, and Performance Change Algorithm
(Used with permission of the Food and Drug Administration)

205

9.4 FDA and the EMR

The communication mechanisms between medical devices and the EMR often require transmitting and translating proprietary data from the device to an EMR-acceptable format. Because the application software that communicates with the medical device is performing data translation and the resulting data are used to influence patient decision making, it is most likely that the application software will itself be a medical device. A rule of thumb that I have learned over time is that if I write an application that communicates using proprietary formats with a medical device and provides the primary communication mechanism between the device and an external system, such as an EMR, then my software is most probably a medical device. Since other systems will be listening for data from my application, then my application is a critical linkage point, and its performance and the accuracy with which it communicates to a recipient system is paramount. Hence, the application software used to bridge the gap between the proprietary device communication protocols and an EMR is substantially equivalent to other communication software that performs similar functions. The key elements that determine whether clearance is necessary include risk to the patient, intended use, and predicate devices or systems.

As of publication, the FDA is floating for comment a new regulation (21 CFR § 880) for reclassification of Medical Device Data Systems (MDDS) to a Class-I medical device (i.e., general controls as opposed to pre-market notification or approval requirements)[154].

Per this draft, the definition of the MDDS is as follows:

A medical device data system (MDDS) is a device intended to provide one or more of the following uses:

1) electronic transfer or exchange of medical device data from a medical device, without altering the function or parameters of any connected devices;

2) electronic storage and retrieval of medical device data, without altering the function or parameters of connected devices; or

3) electronic display of medical device data, without altering the function or parameters of connected devices.

---

[154] Daniel G. Schultz, Director, Center for Devices and Radiological Health; Department of Health and Human Services Food and Drug Administration. Docket No. 2007N-0484. 21 CFR Part 880. 25-Jan-2008. Page 5

In particular, an MDDS cannot provide real-time data such as alarms or be used as a substitute for in-room patient monitors. They can be used to record the occurrence of events such as alarms but they cannot be used to make diagnostic or clinical decisions as a substitute for a live clinician.

An important takeaway for medical device data and the EMR is that only general controls would be necessary to manage such systems. However, this does not mean that good manufacturing practices or quality system regulations should not be followed—this only removes the need for pre-market notification of such interfaces and integration.

9.5 Summary

Medical device data provide critical information from which clinical assessment, physician orders, and interventions stem. Thus, the level of risk to patient safety must be assessed when considering any interface into the EMR. Highly reliable, available, and performing health information software and systems may be noteworthy accomplishments in and of themselves. In a clinical environment at the point-of-care, reliability and availability are expected and assumed. These performance characteristics, considered salient selling points in other industries, must be common characteristics in the healthcare environment to ensure clinical usability. Inasmuch as performance and reliability are fundamental to any health information system in clinical practice, the mandate to "do no harm" must be observed. Developing and fielding a clinical information system involves risk and hazard assessment and mitigation as well as regulatory evaluation to establish the potential likelihood of adverse events. Hazard analysis ranks potential adverse events from the incredible to the likely, and the potential degree of harm that can be caused from the negligible to the catastrophic. The span of the hazard mitigation envelope in these two dimensions is represented by the risk assessment graphic as follows in Figure 9-5. [155, 156]

---

[155] Krishna Govindarajan, "Risk management for Product Safety." 3-Dec-08. Revision 0903. Siemens Medical Solutions USA, Inc. Health Services Division.

[156] James T. Luxhoj, "Probabilistic Causal Analysis for System Safety Risk Assessments in Commercial Air Transport." Department of Industrial and System Engineering, Rutgers University, 2003. Page 4.

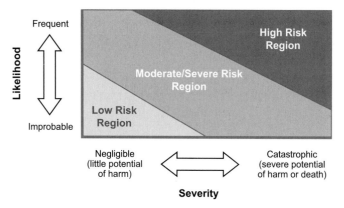

Figure 9-5 Likelihood-Severity Matrix: a tool with which to define and
calibrate regions of risk when evaluating medical devices
and their impact on patient safety

The lower left of the figure identifies regions of acceptable risk, either
from the perspective of incredibility of occurrence or negligibility of
effect. The upper right identifies intolerable regions. The center must
be evaluated individually to assess overall impact. As software contin-
ues to be developed and deployed throughout the healthcare enterprise it becomes exceedingly important to adhere to standards that
ensure its safe use and application in patient care.

10 The Future of Medical Device Integration, Including Device Command & Control

10.1 Introduction

As discussed in Chapter 1, medical device plug-and-play architectures will become the norm over time. This plug-and-play interoperability will extend not only to the integration with the EMR but among medical devices which will be able to communicate and exchange data among one another as part of the standard of care. Beyond this, automatic control of medical devices will also become the norm, although this may take a while longer to implement in clinical environments. In this chapter I will discuss, by way of example, a method for controlling a medical device (mechanical ventilator) using an automatic feedback control mechanism.

Controlling or changing the settings or operation of a medical device can be a risky business. Devices that sustain life (e.g., infusion pumps, mechanical ventilators, intra-arterial balloon pumps, etc.) must be under the supervision of trained clinical staff. Manufacturers of such devices must engage in careful study with live patients to ensure there are sufficient safety and back-up systems in place to mitigate hazards and risks as much as possible. Trusting the process of sustaining life to a computer algorithm and hardware that lacks perspective and longitudinal knowledge on a patient assumes that all relevant information has been identified, measured, and processed to ensure safe and proper operation. While this can be achieved to a degree in a highly controlled environment, relationships among many variables and their impact both individually and collectively on predicting patient system response is dubious at best—for now. This is not to say that such systems cannot be implemented. Studies relating to such activities as controlling mechanical ventilation have been researched through clinical trials. However, generally available products and systems do not presently exist for managing such devices automatically throughout the hospital enterprise. Exceptions in terms of devices that provide features and functionality for limited control do exist (certain ad hoc vitals monitors, mechanical ventilators). But by and large, the ability for a clinician to remotely control a device through a secure hospital network does not presently exist.

Nevertheless, the objective here is to ask and answer the often-asked question "what if...?" Therefore, I will approach this topic from the perspective of how one might accomplish device control for a single specific system and how this can be generalized to other systems.

10.2 Automatic Control Systems

The use of automated methods for controlling medical equipment is not a new concept. Ideas and methodologies related to this are reported in the literature and have been thought about for years, especially in the area of weaning patients from mechanical ventilation[157, 158]. Other applications have included automated infusion pump medication administration and cardiac pacemakers.

Automatic control of patient systems is a developing capability but may have a long way to go in terms of commercial viability and acceptability. The standardized plug-and-play of medical devices will certainly assist in the process of defining a standardized communication process, including language and syntax for communicating among devices. But, other items will be required; specifically, a standardized interface, whereby a medical device can communicate directly to an EMR without requiring a specialized communication transport method for transmitting, processing, and reducing these data.

The benefits of automatic control of medical devices are many in theory, but would need to be proven in practice. One obvious benefit is in the increase in uniformity that automatic control brings to patient care management. Continuous monitoring and responsiveness to changes in patient condition as measured through medical devices can ensure speed and homogeneity in terms of medical device response—something that is difficult for humans to match. Automatic control of medical devices is also a logical extension of clinical decision support whereby resulting clinical actions can be taken as a result of specific conditions or criteria in comparison with measured

---

[157] David A. Tong, "Weaning patients from mechanical ventilation, A knowledge-based system approach." Computer Methods and Programs in Biomedicine, 35 (1991) 267-278.

[158] Carlos Hernandez-Sande, Vicente Moret-Bonillo, Amparo Alonso-Betanzos, "ESTER: An Expert System for Management of Respiratory Weaning Therapy." IEEE Transactions on Biomedical Engineering, Vol. 36, No. 5, May 1989.

values. The use of automatic control theory is limited only by the accuracy and precision with which the system being controlled can be modeled and measured. The human body and physiology in general are fairly well understood in terms of their basic mechanics. Still, no perfect model of the human body exists, and trusting in the "judgment" of a machine to make human-like decisions is chancy. We must remind ourselves that medicine is artful practice. Nonetheless, the breadth and depth of human experience cannot be matched—at least not presently. The ability of a human being to draw upon education and experience from years past in the practice of medicine is invaluable and cannot be programmed into any automatic control system. Some day this may be possible, especially with advances in processing speed, memory, etc. We tend to reflect on the capabilities of automation in accomplishing astonishing tasks, such as playing chess. Yet, the complexities of medicine require drawing upon more than just possible chess moves in a game. Medicine is multi-dimensional, as are many functions in life. The training of automatic control mechanisms has been tested and instantiated in practical applications such as driving subway trains. However, the use of these same types of expert systems for controlling and predicting behavior belies a very rich and dense assemblage of data from which to interpolate multi-dimensional output from multi-dimensional input. The database of necessary information simply does not exist.

Some functions can be modeled, measured, and controlled within the confines of the systems they represent. Respiratory weaning may be one of those areas. The evidence of this is supported by the existence of algorithms (protocols) that provide step-by-step instruction on the weaning of patients from post-operative mechanical ventilation. Yet, many systems (including those related to clinical decision support) tend to fall into the advisory capacity, having no direct control over the apparatus or appliance in direct contact with the patient but rather, provide advice to an intervening care giver. In this role, the method suggests actions that can be easily over-ruled or ignored by the clinician. This is the safest use of these automated methods. While, as referred to above, some manufacturers are enabling semi-automated methods for controlling equipment (for example, methods to assist in respiratory support reduction), these do not supplant human intervention, nor will they in the foreseeable future. Shortliffe and Cimino perhaps sum this up best[159]:

---

[159] Edward H. Shortliffe, Ed. and James J. Cimino, Assoc. Ed. Biomedical Informatics Computer Applications in Health Care and Biomedicine, 3rd Edition. Springer Science & Business Media, LLC: 2006; Pages 619-620.

"The natural outcome ... would seem to be closed-loop control of physiological processes. It can be argued that pacemakers and implantable defibrillators are such devices. In the ICU, however, precisely controlled intravenous pumps are available for drug infusions... The major impediments include the difficulty of creating closed-loop systems with tolerance for the kind of artifacts and measurement errors...and the difficult medicolegal environment..."

Several key factors bear repeating and underscoring: 1) impediments due to tolerance with respect to artifacts and (2) a difficult medicolegal environment. I would go further: the ability to truly represent the control system (i.e., the actual state model of the human body) is a necessary aspect of automatic control system theory and is an important future direction for medical device development. While experimental methods for automatic device control, conducted under clinical trials, have been investigated, commercially available and widely-distributed automatic control of medical devices is still down the road. While the basic physiological and mechanical systems are reasonably well understood, knowledge of neurological processes and brain function in general have barely been touched by comparison. An example of what I mean is the modeling of the sympathetic nervous system. Suggested approaches include the use of expert systems in which patient responses to known inputs are used to "train" system behavior, thereby providing a representation of the human state model. Those grounded in expert systems and neural networks are all too familiar with the limitations of these methods which typically require enormous quantities of data and usually only provide a limited range of accurate performance. Oftentimes, the temptation by users has been to misapply said methods beyond the scope and capacity for accurate responses. This is both reckless and dangerous.

In the process of describing these methods I will discuss in some detail a method which I developed for weaning patients from postoperative mechanical ventilation. I do this to illustrate a very limited application of automatic control system theory. I will add the obvious disclaimer that this method has not been directly applied to patients but is validated against real patient data subject to the influence and control of licensed physicians and respiratory therapists. I will then generalize to other devices.

10.3 Mathematical Development and Application

Weaning from post-operative mechanical ventilation involves the manual reduction of ventilator support by a respiratory therapist under physician supervision. This manual process is labor intensive and inexact: the gradual reduction in respiratory support is performed by the respiratory therapist in finite steps during rounds within the surgical intensive care unit (SICU). Variations in the patient revisit time and errors in judging the patient's spontaneous respiratory capabilities may prolong the duration of mechanical ventilation.

Automating the respiratory weaning process requires near-real-time knowledge of the patient physiological, cardiovascular, and respiratory states. Patient height and weight correlate with the size of the pulmonary cavity, and are used to set inspired volume and breathing frequency.

Respiratory parameters, such as the arterial Oxygen saturation (S_aO_2), mixed venous oxygen saturation (S_vO_2), spontaneous respiratory rate (RR_{sp}) and spontaneous or patient minute ventilation (MV_{sp}) are all indicators of the physiologic stability of the patient. Each of these parameters must remain within normal limits as a patient is weaned from post-operative mechanical ventilation. The importance of spontaneous respiratory rate and tidal volume to the success of weaning has been described in the literature[160], especially through the work of Tobin *et al.*

One such parameter identified as a threshold for successful weaning of patients undergoing continuous positive airway pressure (CPAP) trials is the rapid-shallow breathing index, or RSBI. The RSBI is the ratio RR_{sp}/TV_{sp}. Tobin showed in a retrospective study of 36 patients that RSBI values below 105 liters/breath/minute resulted in highly successful weans from post-operative mechanical ventilation, then tested prospectively on 64 mechanically-ventilated patients.

Traditional approaches to weaning from mechanical ventilation have depended on clinical assessment and laboratory tests such as the arterial blood gas (ABG). Weaning is typically accomplished by reducing the mandatory respiratory rate (RR_m) in fixed stages[161, 162]. However, this approach is performed via the intervention of a physician

---

[160] Tobin M.J., Alex C.G.: Discontinuation of Mechanical Ventilation. In: Tobin M.J., Ed. Principles and Practice of Mechanical Ventilation. New York: McGraw-Hill, 1994, 1194.

[161] Ibid.

and respiratory therapist. I have shown[163] that patients within the Fast-Track weaning protocol experienced predictable changes in minute ventilation. This finding suggested a means for automating the weaning process by monitoring spontaneous minute ventilation from its initial value upon patient arrival following surgery to its final value upon extubation[164]. Actually, it is precisely because of such protocols (essentially, algorithms) that support and suggest the notion that automating the weaning process is plausible. In many institutions, the CABG patient is weaned according to a manual algorithm or protocol in which respiratory support is reduced in direct proportion to the amount of support assumed by the patient over time.

Hypothesize that spontaneous minute ventilation (i.e., the patient-initiated component of minute ventilation) can be used to automate the respiratory weaning of mechanically-ventilated patients. This method differs from traditional approaches that involve manual reduction in respiratory support and use arterial blood gas measurements as a measure of respiratory sufficiency[165] in that patient spontaneous minute volume is employed as the key parameter guiding reduction in respiratory support. The method itself serves to illustrate an approach for using an automatic control based algorithm, and is not intended for actual use in its current form. Strict clinical trials and close oversight of the methodology as well as careful monitoring would need to be conducted before this method could be employed for actual clinical use on live patients.

10.4 Automatic Control System Theory

In developing the mathematical model it is important to define nomenclature. A glossary of variables, subscripts, and superscripts used in the model is summarized in Table 10-1 and Table 10-2.

Automatic Control Systems (ACS) theory is normally applied to mechanical systems to both understand their stability and controlla-

---

[162] J.R. Zaleski: Modeling Post-Operative Respiratory State in Coronary Artery Bypass Graft Patients: A Methodology for Weaning Patients from Mechanical Ventilation, Ph.D. Dissertation, The University of Pennsylvania, 1996, 64-128

[163] Ibid., pages 128-152

[164] J.R. Zaleski: Modeling Spontaneous Minute Volume in Coronary Artery Bypass Graft Patients. Engineering in Medicine and Biology 1998, 17:122-127.

[165] J.R. Zaleski: Modeling Post-Operative Respiratory State in Coronary Artery Bypass Graft Patients: A Methodology for Weaning Patients from Mechanical Ventilation, Ph.D. Dissertation, The University of Pennsylvania, 1996, page 164.

Table 10-1 Glossary of Mathematical Subscripts

Subscript	Definition
0	Initial value at the time respiratory weaning begins
c	Controller-related
d	Delay
e	Event
obs	Observed value
r	Reaction
sp	Spontaneous, or patient value
m	Mandatory, or controlled value
t	Total, or sum of spontaneous and mandatory components
v	Mechanical ventilator related

Table 10-2 Glossary of Mathematical Terms

Variables	Definition
CABG	Coronary Artery Bypass Grafting
IMV	Intermittent Mandatory Ventilation
K	Control gain
L	Laplace Transform
MV	Minute Ventilation, liters per minute
RR	Respiratory Rate, breaths per minute
RSBI	Rapid Shallow Breathing Index, liters per breath per minute
S	Frequency, or S-plane, domain variable
t	Time in weaning process, seconds
τ	Time offset from some initial value, t_0
TV	Tidal Volume, liters per breath

bility in the presence of specific environmental or external input or influences. Renderings of such systems are normally represented in the form of a block diagram. A typical block diagram associated with a feedback control system is depicted in Figure 10-1.

The figure defines all input and output in the time domain. The input to the control system is the variable $r(t)$. This input operates on the transfer function, $g(t)$, to produce the output, $c(t)$. Input $r(t)$ is the desired time-dependent control applied to the system. The transfer

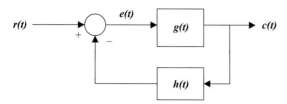

Figure 10-1 Automatic feedback control system block diagram

function, $g(t)$, is the model of system behavior that responds to the applied input, $r(t)$. This input could either be a manual adjustment to a medical device (e.g., a mandatory setting change on a mechanical ventilator) or a measured input from a patient (e.g., change in spontaneous breathing rate, heart rate, etc.)

Error term $e(t)$ is the difference between the desired value, $r(t)$, and the output value, $c(t)$. Feedback to the system is modeled through a feedback block, $h(t)$, which transforms the output into a form and state compatible for comparison with the applied input, $r(t)$.

The transfer function $g(t)$ operates on $e(t)$ to produce an output $c(t)$. The output is fed back to the controller via $h(t)$. The output signal $c(t)$ is fed back through the function $h(t)$ and subtracted from the input signal $r(t)$ to produce an estimate of the error, $e(t)$. The input signal, in comparison with the feedback signal, provides a means for driving the value of the error to zero, resulting in a controllable and stable system. The independent variable t represents time. The variables r, g, e, c, and h are all understood to be functions of time. The stable response, $c(t)$, of the system to an applied input, $r(t)$, is dependent on the form of the system model, $g(t)$, and the feedback model, $h(t)$. Oftentimes the feedback through $h(t)$ does not occur immediately, implying the $h(t)$ can include a model of time delay. Such influences serve to destabilize the system, as overcompensation for behavior anticipated by the system to an applied input can only be gauged on the basis of the measured feedback. For example, if input values such as respiratory rate are adjusted too quickly and in too large a magnitude, an under-damped (that is, highly sensitive) controller would respond by attempting to negate the input rather wildly, potentially resulting in a dangerous situation for the patient. A specific example could be a situation in which a patient, breathing normally during surgical recovery, suddenly deviates from normal respiratory patterns by sighing or yawning. This could be interpreted as cessation of breathing. So, if a patient were breathing at, say, 15 breaths per minute and then the controller interprets the patient as suddenly not breathing at all (patient sighs, breathing pattern is interrupted), then the automatic controller might respond with a large mandatory respiratory rate and an overcompensated tidal volume in order to achieve the correct breathing value. If this is done suddenly then lung injury can result, not to mention the discomfort felt by the patient.

If a comparative output signal is not available immediately, the response of the system to the applied input may result in unstable or widely varying responses, $c(t)$, to known input $r(t)$.

While the block diagram is presented in the time domain, analysis usually proceeds in the frequency domain, or S-plane. For this reason the Laplace transform[166] of the temporal variables is computed. The S-plane representation of the aforementioned variables is as follows:

$$L[r(t)] = R(S) \tag{10.1}$$

$$L[g(t)] = G(S) \tag{10.2}$$

$$L[e(t)] = E(S) \tag{10.3}$$

$$L[c(t)] = C(S) \tag{10.4}$$

$$L[h(t)] = H(S) \tag{10.5}$$

In the S-plane the relationship between the error, the input, and the output signals are as follows:

$$E(S) = R(S) - H(S)C(S) \tag{10.6}$$

The output signal is given by:

$$C(S) = E(S)G(S) \tag{10.7}$$

Substituting (10.6) into (10.7) yields:

$$C(S) = [R(S) - H(S)C(S)]G(S) \tag{10.8}$$

Solving (10.8) for $C(S)$ in terms of the remaining variables yields:

---

[166] Laplace transform $f(S) = L\{F(t)\} = \int_0^\infty e^{-st} F(t)dt$

$$C(S) = R(S)G(S) - G(S)H(S)C(S) \qquad (10.9)$$

Collecting terms:

$$R(S)G(S) = C(S) + G(S)H(S)C(S) \qquad (10.10)$$

$$R(S)G(S) = C(S)[1 + G(S)H(S)] \qquad (10.11)$$

Dividing through by the term in brackets, and bringing the input $R(s)$ to the left side yields:

$$\frac{C(S)}{R(S)} = \frac{G(S)}{1 + G(S)H(S)} \qquad (10.12)$$

This ratio given in the right side of (10.12) is defined so long as $1 + G(S)H(S) \neq 0$. Furthermore, the functions $G(S)$ and $H(S)$ must be continuous.

The application of feedback control to managing ventilator-dependent patients during post-operative weaning is hypothesized assuming the following conditions are true:

1) the patient is in a technologically-dependent state, which is highly-monitored and controlled, leaving relatively little room for variability in patient response outside of known behavior;

2) the patient is at the beginning of the process and is unable to sustain spontaneous respiratory function; and,

3) tidal and minute volume, *TV* and *MV*, correlate to patient weight and height. As weight and height are known, a relatively straightforward relationship exists between the patient's state upon arrival from surgery and the patient's respiratory state at extubation time.

Statement (3) can be visualized with the aid of Figure 10-2, which plots the average patient spontaneous minute ventilation MV_{sp}, as a function of time. The trend shows spontaneous minute ventilation at zero and increasing over time to the final value at extubation. Final value is dependent on the size of the pulmonary cavity. Therefore, final value of MV_{sp} varies for each patient.

The patient's spontaneous respiratory rate and minute ventilation both vary with time (generally from zero, due to the administration of anesthetic and paralyzing drugs during surgery), and the patient's system requires a constant flow of oxygen. Hence, the total minute

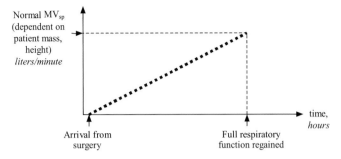

Figure 10-2 Example of a normal evolving trend in spontaneous minute
ventilation, MV_{sp}

ventilation must remain fairly constant over time. This is shown in
Figure 10-3. Total minute ventilation is the sum of the mandatory and
spontaneous minute ventilation components. Total minute ventilation must remain relatively constant during weaning (unless a
change is ordered by a physician) so that the patient receives adequate respiratory support.

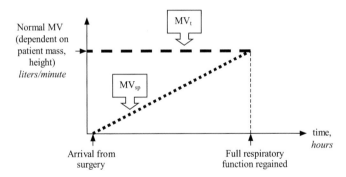

Figure 10-3 Plot showing a notional comparison between total minute
ventilation (MV_t) and spontaneous minute ventilation

However, achieving constant minute ventilation requires altering the
mandatory minute ventilation support to the patient over time. The
respiratory therapist, or nurse, who periodically reviews the patient's
spontaneous minute ventilation, reduces the mandatory minute ventilation proportionally with the increase in patient spontaneous respiratory function. This effect is shown notionally in Figure 10-4. During weaning, the objective of the physician and respiratory therapist
is to decrease the mandatory component of minute ventilation (MV_m)

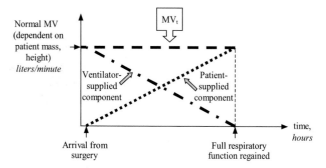

Figure 10-4 Plot showing notional depiction of total minute ventilation with spontaneous and mandatory components overlaid

in direct proportion to an increasing spontaneous component of minute ventilation. The net result will be constant total minute ventilation.

While the total minute ventilation, MV_t, must remain constant throughout the weaning process, both the mandatory and spontaneous components of minute ventilation can vary. The total minute ventilation can be represented as a linear superposition of the patient's spontaneous component, MV_{sp}, and the mandatory component, MV_m. Thus, the total minute ventilation as a function of time can be written as:

$$MV_t(t) = MV_{sp}(t) + MV_m(t) = const \tag{10.13}$$

To illustrate this simple model of respiratory function, we can approximate the functions $MV_{sp}(t)$ and $MV_m(t)$ as follows:

$$MV_{sp}(t) = K_{sp}(t - t_0) \tag{10.14}$$

and

$$MV_m(t) = K_m(t - t_0) \tag{10.15}$$

where $(t - t_0)$ defines the time between arrival from surgery and extubation, and K_{sp} & K_m are constants.

To facilitate further analysis we can re-express the time-based block diagram of Figure 10-1 in the frequency domain (i.e., the S-plane) shown in Figure 10-5.

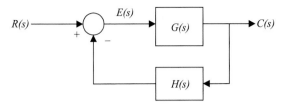

Figure 10-5 Figure depicting the S-plane representation of the automatic feedback control system block diagram

The S-plane is determined by computing the Laplace transform of the time domain signals. This process facilitates mathematical evaluation of the controller and the input & output signals to determine regions of stable operation. The input, $R(S)$, is the desired or "commanded" signal to the ventilator, defined by:

$$R(S) = MV_t(S) - MV_{sp}(S) \qquad (10.16)$$

$R(S)$ behavior is modeled on the basis of typical respiratory support reduction over time. The transfer function, $G(S)$, must allow for altering the input to the ventilator as well as the time lag between the application of the commanded input to the ventilator, $R(S)$, and the realization of the signal at the output, $C(S)$. The output $C(S)$ is simply $MV_m(S)$. Let's now turn to the operation of the ACS.

Changes in spontaneous minute ventilation can result in changes in total minute ventilation unless compensated by changes in the mandatory component of minute ventilation. I'll describe the modeling of this event-response relationship with the aid of Figure 10-6.

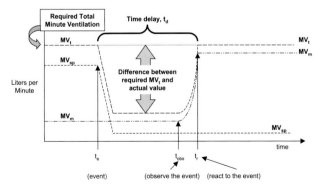

Figure 10-6 Overview of minute ventilation controller response

A change in spontaneous minute ventilation occurs at time t_e (event time). The spontaneous minute ventilation decreases to some new value. However, this change remains unknown until a later time, t_{obs} (observation time). Once spontaneous minute ventilation has been observed to change, a correction can be issued to the ventilator. This correction is executed by time t_r (reaction time). The corrective action raises total minute ventilation to its pre-event value. However, during the delay between event and the end of the reaction time, t_r, the patient has received less respiratory support than prescribed. This is illustrated by the dip in total minute ventilation between event and reaction times, as per (10.13).

Before the mandatory minute ventilation can change, the change in spontaneous minute ventilation must be observed. This is illustrated as an event at time t_{obs} (observation time). Once it is observed that the spontaneous minute ventilation has changed, its impact on total minute ventilation must be assessed, and the mandatory minute ventilation must be adjusted. Because the controller and ventilator are components of a physical system, a delay occurs between when the observation is made and when the ventilator reacts with the correct respiratory support level. This reaction is shown to occur by time t_r (reaction time). Once the mandatory minute ventilation is adjusted to its new value, the required total minute ventilation is once again achieved.

The time period between when an observation is made and when the ventilator is caused to react to the observation involves understanding the physical delays of the ventilator itself. The desire is to minimize the delay time such that:

$$\frac{t_r - t_{obs}}{t_r - t_e} \ll 1 \tag{10.17}$$

Naturally, reducing the time delay between when the event occurs and when the observation is made must also be minimized. The dependency here is on how regularly the observations are made (i.e., the observation frequency).

Simply stated, the reaction time of the mechanical ventilator must be smaller (as small as physically possible). This implies that the dwell time between when spontaneous minute ventilation changes and when this event is observed is much longer than it takes to cause the ventilator to react to the event. In practice, this is a true statement. In effect, we will represent the ventilator's reaction as a step function: an immediate response to the change in spontaneous minute ventilation event, once observed.

The block diagram illustrating this simple controller is visualized in Figure 10-7.

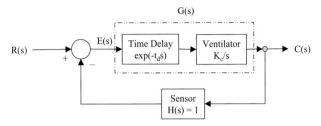

Figure 10-7 Figure illustrating simplified ventilator controller

To represent the delay and ventilator reaction times described in the previous illustration, a delay modeled in the controller as $e^{-t_d s}$ is included[167]. The controller is modeled as a simple step function. The transfer function, $G(S)$, is approximated as follows:

$$G(S) = \frac{K_c \exp(-t_d s)}{s},$$

(10.18)

where t_d is the ventilator time delay and K_c is the gain of the controller, to be determined as part of the controller design process. The controller gain is a mathematical model of a mechanical function: an increase in minute ventilation as manifested through increased respiratory rate, tidal volume, or both. The feedback function, $H(s)$, is assumed to be the actual ventilator mandatory minute ventilation. Hence, $H(s)$ is approximated as having a value equal to 1. The exponential term is a delay. It is represented as a *Padé* approximation as follows:

$$\exp(-t_d s) = \frac{1 - \dfrac{t_d s}{2}}{1 + \dfrac{t_d s}{2}}$$

(10.19)

---

[167] Sometimes referred to as a Padé Approximant, which is a model for a delay in the feedback from the output signal, C(S), through H(S) in automatic control systems theory.

Substituting into (10.18):

$$G(S) = \frac{K_c(1 - t_d S/2)}{S(1 + t_d S/2)} \tag{10.20}$$

We can now develop the equations describing the system transfer function. The error, $E(S)$, is given by the difference between the specified (or commanded) and the mandatory minute ventilation

$$E(S) = R(S) - MV_m(S) \tag{10.21}$$

and,

$$MV_m(S) = E(S)G(S) \tag{10.22}$$

Substituting (10.21) into (10.22) yields:

$$MV_m(S) = [R(S) - MV_m(S)]G(S) \tag{10.23}$$

Multiplying through:

$$MV_m(S) = R(S)G(S) - MV_m(S)G(S) \tag{10.24}$$

Collecting like terms:

$$MV_m(S)[1 + G(S)] = R(S)G(S) \tag{10.25}$$

Rearranging and defining a new variable, $M(S)$:

$$M(S) = \frac{MV_m(S)}{R(S)} = \frac{G(S)}{1 + G(S)} \tag{10.26}$$

Substituting (10.20) into (10.26) yields:

$$M(S) = \frac{K_c(1 - t_d S/2)}{S + t_d S^2/2 + K_c(1 - t_d S/2)} \tag{10.27}$$

Simplifying:

$$M(S) = \frac{K_c(1 - t_d S/2)}{t_d S^2/2 + (1 - K_c t_d/2)S + K_c} \tag{10.28}$$

Normalize by multiplying through numerator and denominator by $2/t_d$:

$$M(S) = \frac{2K_c/t_d(1-t_dS/2)}{S^2 + (2/t_d - K_c)S + 2K_c/t_d} \tag{10.29}$$

Rewrite (10.29) as two equations:

$$M(S) = \frac{2K_c/t_d}{S^2 + (2/t_d - K_c)S + 2K_c/t_d} - \frac{K_cS}{S^2 + (2/t_d - K_c)S + 2K_c/t_d} \tag{10.30}$$

Substitute $R(S) = MV_t(S) - MV_{sp}(S)$ into (10.26):

$$M(S) = \frac{MV_m(S)}{MV_t(S) - MV_{sp}(S)} \tag{10.31}$$

Multiply across by $MV_t(S) - MV_{sp}(S)$:

$$MV_m(S) = \left[MV_t(S) - MV_{sp}(S) \right] M(S) \tag{10.32}$$

Let's approximate MV_{sp} as a step function. This is consistent with the approach of reducing MV support in steps over time:

$$MV_{sp}(S) = K_{sp}(t - \tau), \tag{10.33}$$

in which τ is a reference time indicative of the absolute time at which the control reaction is initiated. Setting $\tau = 0$ and taking the Laplace transform:

$$L[MV_{sp}(t)] = \frac{K_{sp}}{S^2}, \tag{10.34}$$

the total minute volume is approximated as a constant, $MV_t(t) = K_t$. Taking the Laplace transform:

$$L[MV_t(t)] = \frac{K_t}{S} \tag{10.35}$$

substitute (10.34) and (10.35) into (10.32):

$$MV_m(S) = \left\{ \frac{K_t}{S} - \frac{K_{sp}}{S^2} \right\} M(S) \tag{10.36}$$

The time domain solution is realized by taking the inverse Laplace transform of both sides of (10.36).

Each term will be derived separately. Before proceeding, it is useful to recognize that the transfer function, $M(S)$, together with $MV_m(S)$ and $MV_{sp}(S)$, has a form similar to the following three known inverse transforms:

$$L^{-1}\left\{\frac{\omega_n^2}{S(S^2 + 2\zeta\omega_n S + \omega_n^2)}\right\} = 1 - \frac{1}{\sqrt{1-\zeta^2}} e^{-\zeta\omega_n t} \sin\left(\omega_n\sqrt{1-\zeta^2}\, t + \cos^{-1}\zeta\right) \quad (10.37)$$

$$L^{-1}\left\{\frac{\omega_n^2}{S^2(S^2 + 2\zeta\omega_n S + \omega_n^2)}\right\} = t - \frac{2\zeta}{\omega_n} - \frac{1}{\omega_n^2\sqrt{1-\zeta^2}} e^{-\zeta\omega_n t} \sin\left(\omega_n\sqrt{1-\zeta^2}\, t + \cos^{-1}(2\zeta^2 - 1)\right) \quad (10.38)$$

and

$$L^{-1}\left\{\frac{\omega_n^2}{s^2 + 2\zeta\omega_n s + \omega_n^2}\right\} = \frac{\omega_n}{\sqrt{1-\zeta^2}} \exp(-\zeta\omega_n)t \times \sin(\omega_n\sqrt{1-\zeta^2}\, t) \quad (10.39)$$

From the model in (10.39), a comparison with the denominator in (10.30) results in:

$$\zeta = \sqrt{t_d/(2K_c)}(1/t_d - K_c/2) \quad (10.40)$$

and,

$$\omega_n = \sqrt{2K_c/t_d}. \quad (10.41)$$

The expression given by (10.32) is now analyzed by reviewing each of its component parts. Let's begin with the MV_t:

$$L^{-1}\left[MV_t(S) = \frac{K_t}{S}\left\{\frac{2K_c/t_d}{S^2 + (2/t_d - K_c)S + 2K_c/t_d} - \frac{t_s S}{2}\frac{2K_c/t_d}{S^2 + (2/t_d - K_c)S + 2K_c/t_d}\right\}\right] = \quad (10.42)$$

$$MV_t(t) = K_t\left(1 - \frac{1}{\sqrt{1-\zeta^2}}\exp(-\zeta\omega_n t)\times\sin(\omega_n\sqrt{1-\zeta^2}\, t + \cos^{-1}\zeta\right) - \frac{K_t t_d}{2}\left(\frac{\omega_n}{\sqrt{1-\zeta^2}}\exp(-\zeta\omega_n t)\times\sin(\omega_n\sqrt{1-\zeta^2}\, t)\right)$$

$$L^{-1}\left[MV_{sp}(S) = \frac{K_{sp}}{s^2}\left\{\frac{2K_c/t_d}{s^2 + (2/t_d - K_c)s + 2K_c/t_d} - \frac{t_d s}{2}\frac{2K_c/t_d}{s^2 + (2/t_d - K_c)s + 2K_c/t_d}\right\}\right] = \quad (10.43)$$

$$MV_{sp}(t) = K_{sp}\left(t - \frac{2\zeta}{\omega_n} + \frac{1}{\omega_n^2\sqrt{1-\zeta^2}}\exp(-\zeta\omega_n t)\times\sin(\omega_n\sqrt{1-\zeta^2}\, t + \cos^{-1}[2\zeta^2 - 1]\right) - \frac{K_{sp}t_d}{2}\left(1 - \frac{1}{\sqrt{1-\zeta^2}}\exp(-\zeta\omega_n t)\times\sin(\omega_n\sqrt{1-\zeta^2}\, t + \cos^{-1}\zeta)\right)$$

The significance of the controller gain K_c and the time delay t_d are as follows. The controller gain defines the strength or forcefulness of controller response experienced in relation to a deviation between the input and output signal. The theoretical range on controller gain is $0 \leq K_c \leq \infty$.

However, the practical limit is dependent on the nature of the controller. For example, if the mechanism for changing ventilator support is a motor, which increases speed as a function of decreased spontaneous support, then the controller gain defines the amount of voltage applied to the motor to implement the change. Applying too high a gain (e.g., too high a voltage) could have the effect of burning out the motor. On the other hand, too small a controller gain will result in sluggish system response. The time delay defines the interval between when a measurement was taken that deviated with the desired input to the ventilator and when a corrective response is issued to the ventilator motor. Long dwell times can result in non-linear responses in motor voltage, ultimately producing an unstable response in the mechanical ventilator. Typically, we wish the time delay to be small (< 1 minute) and the controller gain to be moderate.

One approach for selecting these two parameters is to perform a root-locus analysis on the ventilator controller transfer function. Then, a value for controller gain is selected which results in stable performance of the ventilator (i.e., poles in the left plane of the root-locus diagram) with sufficient agility to permit rapid ventilator response. Such a condition often occurs when the region of critical damping is selected, based on the roots of the denominator of the controller transfer function, given in (10.44). This condition occurs when

$$K_c = \frac{6}{t_d} + \frac{\sqrt{128}}{2t_d}. \tag{10.44}$$

Values of t_d and K_c satisfying equation (10.44) are shown in Figure 10-8. Gain increases with decreasing delay to accommodate more rapid changes in controller input signal. This plot illustrates the conditions required on K_c and t_d to achieve a critically-damped controller. In practice, it is anticipated that normal time delays will be less than approximately 1 minute. Hence, for critical damping, K_c must be ≥ 10.

In practice, the time delay between measurement of spontaneous minute ventilation and controller reaction is quite short—less than a minute. Therefore, we can expect that just about any value of controller gain will result in an active controller (since gain must be greater

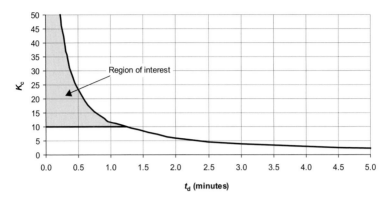

Figure 10-8 Figure illustrating the controller gain as a function of the time delay, t_d

than zero). We will assume $t_d = 10$ seconds (0.167 minutes). This value of delay ensures that data are collected rapidly and changes can be made quickly. A modest controller gain of $K_c = 10$ will be assumed. This is a reasonable value and implies that the controller's response is fast, but not immediate. Once the gain and delay have been determined, we can then demonstrate the operation of the controller.

The controller minute ventilation is computed by substituting (10.42) and (10.43) into (10.45):

$$MV_m(t) = MV_t(t) - MV_{sp}(t). \qquad (10.45)$$

A plot of (10.45) for specific values of K_t, K_{sp}, t_d, and K_c is shown in Figure 10-9.

This plot shows total minute, spontaneous, and mandatory minute ventilation as a function of time. Note that as the sample spontaneous minute ventilation increases, the automatic controller decreases to maintain constant total minute ventilation. (Sample assumptions: $K_t = 10$ liters per minute, $K_{sp} = 1$ liter per minute per minute, $t_d = 0.167$ minutes.)

It is apparent from this plot that the mandatory component of minute ventilation follows the spontaneous component—that is, as the spontaneous component increases, the mandatory component decreases, resulting in (relatively) constant total minute ventilation. This model and approach need to be verified against actual patient spontaneous minute ventilation and the concomitant mandatory component set by the respiratory therapist.

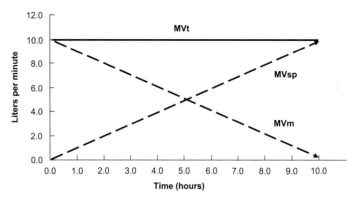

Figure 10-9 Figure illustrating a sample problem demonstrating the performance of automatic controller

This methodology was originally tested during a study involving 24 CABG patients.[168] Analysis of these 24 patients confirmed the hypothesis that spontaneous minute ventilation provides sufficient information required for effectively reducing mandatory support to the patient.

Figure 10-10, plots (a) through (d), show the comparison between spontaneous and mandatory data for one patient from the study. Plot (a) shows patient spontaneous minute ventilation in comparison with manual decrease in mandatory minute ventilation as a function of time. The spontaneous component of minute ventilation is compared with the manually-controlled mandatory component of minute ventilation as set by the respiratory therapist. One can see from (a) the dynamic change in minute ventilation as the patient regains respiratory ability. Plot (c) illustrates the total minute ventilation for this case. Note the variability in total minute ventilation: total minute ventilation begins varying greatly at around 280 minutes. As can be seen, the total minute ventilation varies widely and, at one point during the weaning process, actually drops to approximately 50% of its baseline value (approximately 10 liters per minute). Patient spontaneous minute ventilation in comparison with automatically-controlled mandatory minute ventilation as a function of time is shown in plot (b). Total minute ventilation for this case is shown in plot (d). Note the variability is essentially gone. However, the controller permits the

---

[168] Based on an IRB-approved study of 25 mechanically-ventilated patients within the Surgical Intensive Care Unit (SICU) of the Hospital of the University of Pennsylvania (HUP) during the Spring of 1996. Data collected under Human Studies Protocol #570-0.

patient to breathe spontaneously, sometimes in excess of baseline (beginning at around 280 minutes). Controller assumptions: $K_c = 10$, $t_d = 0.17$ minutes. Hence, our objective is achieved: as the patient regains spontaneous respiratory ability, the ventilator controller response decreases in proportion to maintain constant (physician-defined) total minute ventilation.

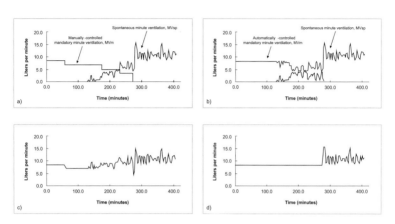

Figure 10-10 Comparison between manual and automatic controllers for a single patient

There are no decreases in total minute ventilation below the physician-prescribed total minute ventilation level. Since the automatic controller imposes no restriction on spontaneous breathing ability, once the patient begins to breathe spontaneously, the patient is free to breathe at whatever level is comfortable. This is illustrated near $t = 280$ minutes, at which time this patient was breathing spontaneously. Therefore, there was no need for the controller to exert any respiratory control over the patient. It is interesting to note the correlation between the mandatory ventilator setting defined by the respiratory therapist and the ventilator controller. In comparing plots (a) and (b) it is observed that the rate of decrease in mandatory support for both the manual and automatic case coincides in time reasonably well. This comparison was performed for all patients, and the results are presented in Table 10-3 which shows the average deviation between mandatory and automatic controller support levels to be within 2 liters per minute in the vast majority of patients. This implies reasonable agreement between the automatic controller and the setting prescribed by the respiratory therapist.

Table 10-3 Average deviation between controller and manual minute ventilation setting

Patient	Deviation (l/min)	Patient	Deviation (l/min)
1	0.36	13	2.42
2	0.66	14	1.03
3	1.17	15	0.81
4	0.70	16	0.86
5	1.68	17	0.83
6	0.96	18	0.52
7	0.64	19	1.07
8	0.58	20	0.93
9	1.24	21	0.87
10	0.58	22	0.94
11	1.40	23	1.61
12	2.27	24	1.23

It must further be noted that some differences do exist between the ventilator controller setting and the desired intermittent mandatory ventilation (IMV) setting prescribed by the physician. This occurs as a result of the chosen value of the controller gain in conjunction with the time delay. The controller gain was set at 10 and the time delay to 0.17 minutes (about 10 seconds). Selecting appropriate gain values to minimize delay without overcompensating in responsiveness is somewhat of an art and must be undertaken during the design of the controller for a particular medical device. No two transfer functions, $G(S)$, will likely be similar for any two different medical devices for which automatic control is desired. The sensitivity of the controller is dependent on the value of this gain. If the gain is too small, the response of the controller will be sluggish. If the gain is set too high, the controller will respond to random noise events, and could also result in mechanical problems to the ventilator (such as the burning out of motors and power supplies). The selection of the controller value for optimum support, while important, is also dependent on the specifics of the mechanical interface between the ventilator and the automatic control system.

The median deviation between the automatic and manual control settings of the mechanical ventilator in this rudimentary example is less than 1 liter per minute. At the 80th percentile, this deviation is less than 2 liters per minute, as determined by accumulating individual deviations from measurements taken from the ventilators and sorting these data by minute ventilation bin. The total quantity of measurements per bin, divided by the total quantity, defines the fraction of data points within the bounds of the bin. When accumulated over all patients, a measure of this fraction is determined for the entire patient population.

Tobin[169] described an approach for reducing mechanically ventilated support to patients. Tobin's approach involved reducing respiratory support in increments of 1 to 3 breaths per minute. Arterial blood gas (ABG) measurements were taken at intervals of approximately 30 minutes after the change in mandatory respiratory rate, RR_m. In Tobin's approach, if the patient's pH remained above approximately 7.3, then the RR_m level was further reduced until the patient was breathing totally on his or her own ($RR_m = 0$). In this way, weaning was guided based on pH. This approach, albeit feasible, requires an ABG measurement. In my experience, ABG measurements are normally taken only 3-5 times during the normal weaning trial[170]. Tobin recognized the importance of the spontaneous MV, RR, and TV to the weaning process. Tobin's measure—the ratio RR/TV—reliably established the patient's viability to wean. Patients at extubation whose RR/TV ratio fell below 105 were deemed ready to wean. Patients with RR/TV ratios above 105 were probably not ready. The RR/TV ratio was determined at the time of desired extubation.

As a confirmation of Tobin's method, RR and TV were measured during the final 30 seconds just prior to extubation on aforementioned patients. This resulted in the acquisition of up to 40 individual measurements of RR and TV for each patient. A scatter plot of RR versus TV was generated incorporating each measurement from each patient. Thus, this related data tends to support the correlation between successful weaning and the importance of the MV, RR, and TV as indicators of respiratory sufficiency as a model for respiratory support reduction. Similar models need to be developed for other types of medical devices and must be validated against live data to establish their efficacy as viable approaches for automatic control.

---

[169] M.J. Tobin, C.G. Alex: Discontinuation of Mechanical Ventilation. In: Tobin M.J., Ed. Principles and Practice of Mechanical Ventilation. New York: McGraw-Hill, 1994, 1194.

[170] Fast-Track Weaning Protocol, published by The Hospital of the University of Pennsylvania, provided as appendix.

10.5 Discussion

Automatic control of medical devices is in its infancy. Manufacturers of devices are beginning to include algorithms to automate simple functions and tasks (such as weaning protocols) into their devices. These methods can be augmented by taking live data into account and building new transfer functions based upon larger sets of data. Such methods fall in the category of neural control or expert systems, in which the transfer functions, $G(S)$, are modeled on patient data. These transfer functions "evolve" over time as the automatic control systems "learn" from more and more patient data, thereby categorizing the type of response based on specific input provided on a particular type of patient. For example, the need to take into account the height and weight of a patient to provide insight into body surface area for titration of infusion or for estimating the nominal size of the pulmonary cavity.

In the proposed method I have described relative to one very important area of mechanical ventilation (a major activity in critical care units), I employ only respiratory parameters for guiding reduction in respiratory support. This method could be applied to any patient who is ventilator-dependent and who needs to be weaned. Furthermore, the proposed controller could be modified with the addition of in-line arterial blood-gas measurements. It is necessary to add to the complexity of automatic control systems to generalize and improve the modeling of the patient system in order to establish confidence that the proposed control system will take into account variability that may be encountered during the standard course of treatment. For example, by incorporating arterial blood-gas measurements the model of the patient system, through $G(S)$, would enhance the utility of the methodology by making it applicable to more patients. Furthermore, broader variations in treatment can be supported by adding to the complexity of the methodology and improving the fidelity of the model of the patient. By increasing the level of complexity of the modeling it becomes possible to apply the same control mechanism to a broader range of functions. The method I described is useful for patients who are weaned from IMV modes down to CPAP. Pressure support ventilator assistance is in no way affected by the automatic controller. Pressure support modes can be accommodated without altering the methodology and with no effect on the patient. This latter statement is supported since the patient, breathing spontaneously, would be monitored on a non-interference basis by the controller. In effect, such a controller could perform a safety role in the event a patient lost the ability to sustain spontaneous respiratory control. The controller would accomplish this by automatically sensing the patient's inability to sustain support. As a result of such an event, the controller would provide the necessary support level, based on a pre-set limit specified in accordance with the patient's physiology (weight and height).

Because delays exist between when minute ventilation is measured and when the controller responds, a slight time lag will result between the spontaneous response and the controller's response. As delays are reduced to zero, differences between spontaneous response and controller response diminish. Therefore, minimizing the time difference between when measurements are taken and when the controller responds is imperative to the utility of the controller. Even time delays on the order of 10 seconds can result in significant differences between spontaneous and controller response. This is the reason why manual control of the ventilator can cause patients to experience insufficient respiratory support. The net result of this time lag was shown in Table 10-3, in which the average difference between the respiratory therapist's manual setting and the automatic controller is greater than zero.

Moreover, selection of the controller gain can affect the precision with which the controller follows the patient spontaneous minute ventilation. It was shown that by increasing the controller gain, a more accurate controller response could be obtained. I also pointed out that the proper controller gain setting is dependent on the interface hardware between the controller and the ventilator, and that setting this gain too high or too low could result in performance which is too sensitive to changes or too sluggish in response. However, this potential for less than adequate performance can be compensated for using feed-forward gain in the controller. In this way, the anticipated response of the patient can be used to cause the controller to respond more quickly initially. Implementing this, however, still requires details of the physical hardware interface between the controller and ventilator.

Because automatic controllers remain continuously attentive to changes in the patient's spontaneous minute ventilation progress, whether the application is mechanical ventilation or infusion, the level of control will always remain at the correct level for the patient. In the case of manual control, changes are made only as often as a patient is visited within intensive care. Hence, the controller responds more quickly and actively to changes in respiratory support levels, whereas the manual level is changed much more slowly. The manual support tends to lag behind the patient spontaneous respiratory support, implying that the manual settings tend to be sub-optimal for the patient.

11 Example Methods and Software

11.1 Implementation Overview

This chapter provides some examples of computer code and methods to retrieve data from several devices, as well as to illustrate methods described in Chapter 7 and Chapter 8 relating to data analysis and user interfaces. The methods provided here are not exhaustive and are not intended to be used in medical devices as-is. The development of medical-grade software must be undertaken in accord with the Quality System Regulations (QSR) of the Food and Drug Administration, to include Good Manufacturing Practices (GMP). I provide these examples to impact an understanding of some of the medical device communication methods.

In most cases the methods for data communication are straightforward in that they involve transmission of standard, manufacturer-provided commands over serial Ethernet or USB communication ports to retrieve data. Still, to the uninitiated, until one gains some experience actually doing this, these methods can provide a valuable head start so that questions such as "how does he do that?" are answered.

One of the reasons I cannot provide all these methods is that their communication mechanisms are proprietary or require special software development kits that must be procured under special arrangement with manufacturers. I provide the communication methods for those devices that are typically published and available from the manufacturer for custom development purposes. A best practice is to always obtain the official device communication or connectivity specifications for a given medical device. Aside from the legal requirements, there are safety and hazard implications associated with not having official documentation.

The reasons are important. If one is not using official specifications then the possibility exists that the developer may not have access or knowledge of commands, limitations, or communication requirements that are necessary to accurately communicate with the medical devices. Another is that in the event the manufacturer should change a command or update the interface, then the developer will not have these updates should a new model of the device be procured. Having stale information on device communication can result in incorrect or no data being retrieved from the device—an obvious hazard.

It is also useful to employ serial and USB port communication analysis tools to validate the data communication between a computer and a medical device in order to see the actual handshaking and validate that the data retrieved are true and accurate. I recommend two software tools which I have found invaluable in such endeavors, both available for purchase from AGG Software, Inc. These are the *Advanced Serial Port Monitor* and the *Advanced USB Port Monitor*. Presently both retail for approximately $60 (US). One of the benefits of experimenting with these tools is that a user can employ standard manufacturer communication software to transmit commands to the medical devices and then view, or sniff, the serial or USB packets. This provides the user with a clear understanding of the handshaking mechanism, so that when using a manufacturer supplied standard communicate command, it is possible to implement techniques such as error checking to determine when communication is established and successful between the computer and the device.

All of the programs are written in Java and can be compiled with a Sun Java Software Development Kit[171]. I recommend downloading and installing the latest version of the Sun Java SDK. In addition, you will need either Sun's or IBM's version of the Java Communication API. In the newest versions of the Java Platform the communications API, or javax.comm, is a standard extension. The communications API is also available for download (upon registration) from the Sun Web site.

As a final note, none of the following programs were designed to follow specific programming standards. I have no doubt that these may be re-written more succinctly and elegantly by more able individuals. That was not the purpose expressed here. I encourage the interested reader to do so.

11.2 Serial Port Communications

Serial communications using Java are rather straitghtforward. There are several class libraries that enable communicating with serial USB and Ethernet ports. The class library I prefer is the Java Communications Application Programming Interface (API).

---

[171] Available for download at http://java.sun.com/javase/downloads/index.jsp

The specific serial port communication handshake depends on the medical device. Typical settings for serial ports are as follows:

Baud rate: 9600

Parity: None

Data bits: 8

Stop bits: 1

Of course, exceptions abound. Yet, given the various medical devices that support only serial communication, the mechanism for opening and closing communication ports is the same. The differences involve the specific proprietary commands required by the medical device, the associated data response and its content, and the communications settings. The Java Communications API library provides examples of serial port communication that include some error handling. In the examples below I have developed my own methods that accomplish the task and are straightforward. I will demonstrate serial port communication with respect to the LifeScan ONE TOUCH, SureStep, and Ultra brand of glucometer, a simple handheld device to be used in the home.

The ONE TOUCH brand of glucometers by LifeScan provide a series of specifications[172] that may be used to communicate between a computer and the glucometers via a proprietary (i.e., manufacturer-supplied) serial cable. The glucometers also can be used with a software application that is available for sale from the manufacturer. The listing in Table 11-1 is a self-contained program featuring a user interface that allows the user to retrieve data from the glucometer using a standard command. This program will work with the Ultra and SureStep models of glucometers, per the manufacturers communication specification as of 2005.

Command line compilation proceeds as follows:

```
Javac glucose.java
```

Command line execution is as follows:

```
Java glucose
```

---

[172] Examples: "ONE TOUCH Ultra Meter RS-232 Communication Specification." "SureStep Meter RS-232 Communication Specification." LifeScan, Inc. 1000 Gibralter Drive, Milpitas, CA 95035-6312.

Table 11-1 glucose.java

```
import java.awt.*;
import java.awt.event.*;
import java.io.*;
import java.io.BufferedInputStream;
import javax.swing.border.*;
import javax.comm.*;
import javax.swing.*;
import javax.swing.event.*;
import javax.swing.JFrame;
import javax.swing.event.ChangeEvent;
import javax.swing.event.ChangeListener;


//
//*********************************************************************
//
// glucose.java
//
// Retrieve data from SureStep(r) or OneTouch(r) glucometer
//
// Commands: DMF -- Send date and time from meter on-board clock
//           DM@ -- Send meter serial number
//           DMP -- Dump meter data
//
// Recompile with new Baud Rate, COM port setting.
// Default settings: 9600, COM1
//
// Author: John Zaleski
//
//
//*********************************************************************

public class glucose extends JPanel implements SerialPortEventListener
{
    private JButton DMF;
    private JButton DMa;
    private JButton DMP;
    private JButton exitB;
    public static int baudRate = 9600;
    public static String comPort = „COM1";
    public static int  maxWidth = 800;
    public static int  maxHeight = 400;
    JTextArea jta;
    static CommPortIdentifier portId;
    InputStream inputStream;
    OutputStream outputStream;
    SerialPort serialPort;
    char chr[] = new char[30];

    public void serialEvent(SerialPortEvent event)
    {
        switch(event.getEventType())
        {
            case SerialPortEvent.BI:
            case SerialPortEvent.OE:
            case SerialPortEvent.FE:
            case SerialPortEvent.PE:
            case SerialPortEvent.CD:
            case SerialPortEvent.CTS:
            case SerialPortEvent.DSR:
            case SerialPortEvent.RI:
            case SerialPortEvent.OUTPUT_BUFFER_EMPTY:
            jta.append( „\n Output buffer empty „ );
          break;
        }
    }
```

Table 11-1 glucose.java *(continued)*

```
//-----------------------------------------------------------
// Main method
//-----------------------------------------------------------
public static void main(String[] args)
{
    try {
        glucose gl = new glucose();
        JFrame jf = new JFrame( „Glucose");
        jf.setContentPane( gl );
        jf.setSize( maxWidth, maxHeight );
        jf.setVisible( true );
        jf.setLocation( 10,10);
        jf.addWindowListener( new WindowAdapter() {
            public void windowClosing(WindowEvent e ) {
                System.exit( 0 );
            }
        });
    } catch (Exception e) {
    }
} // end main

//
// Converts command sent as String into character array
// and appends a Hexadecimal <CR> to the end of the array.
//
public int convertToCharArray( char array[], String s )
{
    int cmdLength = s.length();
    for ( int k = 0; k < cmdLength; k++ )
    {
        array[k] = s.charAt(k);
    }
    array[cmdLength] = 0x0D;
    return (cmdLength+1);
} // end convertToCharArray


//
// Closes serial port and I&O streams
//
public void closestreams()
{
    try {
        inputStream.close();
        outputStream.close();
        serialPort.close();
    } catch ( Exception e ) {}
}


//
// Constructor.
//
public glucose()
{
    buildUI();
}

//
// Create a rudimentary user interface.
//
public void buildUI()
{
    //
    // Text area layout
```

Table 11-1 glucose.java *(continued)*

```
        //
        int rows = 15;
        int cols = 105;
        jta = new JTextArea( „", rows, cols );
        Font font = new Font(„Courier", Font.BOLD, 12 );
        Font font2= new Font(„Tahoma", Font.BOLD, 12 );
        jta.setFont( font );
        jta.setForeground( Color.yellow );
        jta.setBackground( Color.blue );
        jta.append(„Starting...\n\n" );

        //
        // Scroll message pane
        //
        final boolean autoscroll = true;
        JScrollPane messagePane = new JScrollPane( jta,
                                         JScroll-
Pane.VERTICAL_SCROLLBAR_ALWAYS,

                                         JScroll-
Pane.HORIZONTAL_SCROLLBAR_NEVER
                                         );
        //
        // Included for autoscrolling to always show the latest data in
pane
        //
        final JScrollBar vsb = messagePane.getVerticalScrollBar();
            vsb.addAdjustmentListener(new AdjustmentListener() {
                public void adjustmentValueChanged(AdjustmentEvent e) {
                    if ( autoscroll && !e.getValueIsAdjusting())
                    {
                        vsb.setValue(vsb.getMaximum());
                    }
                }
            });

        //
        // Panel for the textarea
        //
        JPanel jtaPanel = new JPanel();
        jtaPanel.setLayout( new FlowLayout() );
        jtaPanel.add( messagePane );

        //
        // Button panel
        //
        JPanel buttonP = new JPanel( new FlowLayout() );

        //
        // Author's Note:
        //

        DMF = new JButton( „Get DMF" );
        DMF.addActionListener( new ActionListener() {
            public void actionPerformed(ActionEvent ev1 ){
                communicate( „DMF" );
            }
        });
        DMa = new JButton( „Get DMa" );
        DMa.addActionListener( new ActionListener() {
            public void actionPerformed(ActionEvent ev2 ){
                communicate( „DM@" );
            }
        });
        DMP = new JButton( „Get DMP" );
        DMP.addActionListener( new ActionListener() {
```

Table 11-1 glucose.java *(continued)*

```
            public void actionPerformed(ActionEvent ev3 ){
                communicate( „DMP" );
            }
        });
        exitB = new JButton(„Exit");
        exitB.addActionListener( new ActionListener() {
            public void actionPerformed(ActionEvent ev4 ) {
                System.exit(0);
            }
        });
        buttonP.add( DMF );
        buttonP.add( DMa );
        buttonP.add( DMP );
        buttonP.add( exitB );
        this.setLayout( new FlowLayout() );
        this.setBorder(new EmptyBorder(20,20,20,20));
        this.add(buttonP);
        this.add(jtaPanel);
    }


    //
    // Communication method that opens serial port and sends each
    // command to device
    //
    public void communicate( String Command )
    {
      closestreams();
        try {
            portId = CommPortIdentifier.getPortIdentifier( comPort );
            serialPort = (SerialPort) portId.open(„glucose", 1234);
            jta.append( „\n" + portId.getName() + „ opened for output");
        } catch (Exception e) {
          jta.append( „\n Exception thrown in Communicate opening serial
port: „ + e
                            + „\n");
        }
        try {
            serialPort.setSerialPortParams( baudRate,
                                            SerialPort.DATABITS_8,
                                            SerialPort.STOPBITS_1,
                                            SerialPort.PARITY_NONE);
            serialPort.enableReceiveTimeout(1000); // 0.5 seconds

            inputStream = serialPort.getInputStream();
            outputStream = serialPort.getOutputStream();
            int nChars = 0;
            StringBuffer readBuffer = new StringBuffer();
            int c = 0;

            //
            // Send DM? command first. This causes meter
            // to send all options settings
            //
            nChars = convertToCharArray( chr, „DM?" );

            jta.append („\n Command length: „ + nChars );

            //
            // Write DMS characters to serial port
            //
            for (int i = 0; i < nChars; i++ )
            {
                outputStream.write(chr[i]);
                System.out.println(„chr[„ + i + „] = „ + chr[i] );
            }
```

Table 11-1 glucose.java *(continued)*

```
              //
              // Read response characters from serial port
              //

              while ((c=inputStream.read()) != 04)
                                              // Decimal <10> = Ascii
<LF> = Hex <0x0A>
                      {                             // Can also try:
                                              // Decimal <13> = Ascii
<CR> = Hex <0x0D>
                      System.out.println( „c = („ + c + „)" );
                      jta.append(„\n" + c );
                      if ( c == -1 ) break;
                      }

              //
              // Now, send command passed in through Command String
              //

              for ( int i = 0; i < 10; i++ ) chr[i] = , ,;

              jta.append( „\n Command Sent: [„ + Command + „]");
              nChars = convertToCharArray( chr, Command );


              //
              // Write Command characters to serial port
              //
              for (int i = 0; i < nChars; i++ )
              {
                  outputStream.write(chr[i]);
                  System.out.println(„chr[„ + i + „] = „ + chr[i] );
              }

              jta.append( „\n Raw input received: „ );

              //
              // Read response to Command from serial port
              //
              while ((c=inputStream.read()) != 04)
                            // Decimal <10> = Ascii <LF> = Hex <0x0A>
                      {                     // Can also try:
                            // Decimal <13> = Ascii <CR> = Hex <0x0D>
                      System.out.println( „c = („ + c + „)" );
                      if ( c == -1 ) break;
                      jta.append( „ „ + c );
                      if(c!=13)  readBuffer.append((char) c);
                      }

              String receivedInput = readBuffer.toString();
              jta.append(„\n Input received: [„ + receivedInput + „]");

              closestreams();
          } catch (Exception e) {
              jta.append(„\n Exception thrown in Communicate: „ + e );
          }
      } // end communicate()

} // end glucose
```

11.3 Mechanical Ventilator

By now I think I've conveyed the point that proprietary interfaces exist requiring custom tailoring. I will now illustrate a more sophisticated program that communicates with a device normally used in the intensive care unit: a mechanical ventilator. In the following implementation I employ a client-server method to retrieve data from a Servo^j mechanical ventilator. The client transmits proprietary commands synchronously to the server over a standard TCP/IP network interface. As the commands are received by the server they are communicated via serial port via commands specified in the Computer Interface Emulator (CIE) Reference Manual.[173]

The user interface client ("Client"), ServoClient.java, creates a user interface in which the user selects desired data channels to be displayed. This, in turn communicates with the proxy server ("Proxy Server"), ServoProxy.java. The proxy server is a class that is event-triggered either on cyclic thread awakening or on transmission of a user request. Either case results in a ventilator command being sent from the Client to the Proxy Server. The Proxy Server extracts the content of the command and formats the data using binary coding (together with a checksum calculation, as required by the particular brand of mechanical ventilator) and transmits the binary command through a particular COM port to which the mechanical ventilator is attached. Note that a serial cable may be ordered from the manufacturer to make this physical connection. A cable can also be fabricated.

When using a Serial-to-Ethernet interface server (such as the Moxa Technologies DE-211 or DE-311, for instance) the fact that the data are physically transmitted over Ethernet LAN to the serial server is of no consequence to the design of the serial interface connection between the Proxy Server and the particular mechanical ventilator: to the Proxy Server, this is transparent. The interface server enables up to 255 virtual COM ports to be opened, thereby implying that up to 255 simultaneous ventilators can be managed by the Proxy Server and associated software if appropriately modified. A code snippet of the Proxy Server serial communication method is provided below. This particular code segment opens a particular serial port, retrieves the data using ServoProxy.java, transmits the command to the ventilator, awaits a response from the ventilator, packages the response in the form of a string, and sends the response to the Client via TCP/IP port.

---

[173] Siemens Servo^j Computer Interface Emulator Reference Manual. E382 E407E 119010102. Siemens-Elema AB, Electromedical Systems Division (c) 2001.

Table 11-2 Servo^i Basic Channels Example

ID	ChNo	TrendNo	ParmName	ScaleF	Label	ParmUnits	Units
1	01	20	Insp. Tidal vol. (breath)	5000	mib Tvi	l	mV/l
2	03	21	Exp. Tidal vol. (breath)	5000	mib Tve	l	mV/l
3	04	0	O2-concen-tration (breath)	50	iO2	%	mV/%
4	08	2	Resp. rate calc (breath)	50	mib RRc	breaths/min	mV/breaths/min
5	10	4	Exp. Minute vol. (breath)	200	mib Mve	l/min	mV/l/min

An example of the existing database structure for basic channels of the Servo^i ventilator is shown in Table 11-2. These tables are available from the Computer Interface Manual that accompanies the Servo^i mechanical ventilator[174].

The Basic Channels table lists a small sampling of the parameters that are normally accessible from the Servo^i brand of mechanical ventilator, accessed through the Channel Number, or ChNo, field within the table. Each valid parameter channel contains a parameter name, a scale factor, a unit label, and, where applicable, a standard label. The textual descriptive fields are those normally presented to the user within the user interface. The client, upon user selection of desired fields, automatically extracts the associated channel number and creates a command from the one or more selected user fields.

Table 11-3 Basic Commands table contents for Servo^i ventilator

ID	commandname	description
1	HO	Hello
2	RB	Read Breath
3	RT	Read Time
4	DB	Define Breath

174 Siemens Servo^i, Computer Interface Emulator Reference Manual. E382 E407E 119010102, Siemens-Elema AB.

The Client directs the Proxy Server to request results based on one of the standard commands it issues from the Basic Commands, Table 11-3. In the case of the Servo^i, standard syntax requires that a breath be defined according to the types of parameters the user requests. Therefore, the Client issues a "Define Breath", or DB, command together with the channel numbers associated with the specific user-selected data to the ventilator. The Command Server then follows this command with a "Read Breath", or RB, command, which causes the ventilator to issue the specified data result via the Proxy Server.

However, the types of data are not limited to these basic channels. A set of extended channel data are also available from the Servo^i, and these are accessed using a combination of Extended Commands, Table 11-4, together with a complex set of data extraction methods.

Table 11-4 Subset of Extended Commands Table for Servo^i ventilator

ID	commandname	description
1	RADA	Read Acquired Data
2	RPAI	Read Patient Information

The Extended Commands shown in Table 11-5 are extracted from the table via the Command Name column and sent to the Proxy Server together with a specific set of commands. An example of the sample commands for the 200-level (i.e., measured breath data) channels is provided.

The proprietary command structure that each ventilator requires is one reason for employing a database approach for storing commands. In this way, commands can be appended or even swapped out, and new tables can be added which will not affect the functioning of the computer program. Table 11-5 is supplemented by the Units Table, Table 11-6.

Table 11-5 Subset of Extended Channels for measured breath data on the Servo^i ventilator

ID	ChNo	ParmName	gain	offset	gain_x	gain_y	offset_x	offset_y	unit	type
1	200	Measured breath frequency	+1000E -004	+0000E +000	4	3	4	3	06	BT
2	201	Exp. Tidal volume	+1000E -003	+0000E +000	5	4	5	4	01	BT
3	202	Insp. Tidal volume	+1000E -003	+0000E +000	5	4	5	4	01	BT

Table 11-6 Units for data values associated with extended Servo[i] ventilator commands

ID	code	description
1	01	ml
2	02	ml/s
3	03	ml/min
4	04	cmH2O
5	05	ml/cmH2O
6	06	breaths/min
7	07	%
8	08	l/min
9	09	cmH2O/l/s
10	10	mmHg
11	11	kPa
12	12	mbar
13	13	mV

As the Proxy Server returns data to the Client, the Client writes these data to the database tables. The entire Client-Server communication process is visualized in the event trace diagram of Figure 11-1.

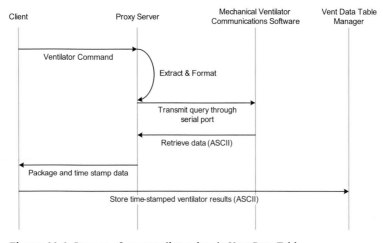

Figure 11-1 Storage of raw ventilator data in Vent Data Table

Table 11-7 contains a sampling of data retrieved from the Servo[i] ventilator. This table holds both the basic and extended channel results.

Table 11-7 Sample Vent Data table contents collected from Servo[i] ventilator

ID	cmdsent1	cmdrcvd1	cmdsent2	cmdrcvd2	vtime
663	DB0103081011	*	RB	2558 2554 2161 2271 2145	031218 112855

The shading is used to help illustrate the example for calculating a breath parameter from the raw results. Begin by reviewing the contents of the Basic Channels table. A subset of these table cells are reprinted in Table 11-8 below.

Table 11-8 Re-print of a subset of cells from the Basic Channel table

ID	ChNo	TrendNo	ParmName	ScaleF	Label	ParmUnits	Units
2	01	20	Insp. Tidal vol. (breath)	5000	mib Tvi	l	mV/l
4	03	21	Exp. Tidal vol. (breath)	5000	mib Tve	l	mV/l
9	08	2	Resp. rate calc (breath)	50	mib RRc	breaths/ min	mV/breaths/ min
11	10	4	Exp. Minute vol. (breath)	200	mib Mve	l/min	mV/l/min
12	11	23	Mean airway pressure (breath)	50	mib MAP	cm H2O	mV/cm H2O

The shading in Table 11-7 and Table 11-8 serves to link specific integer values associated with parameters and data between the two tables. Note the table entry for item 663 in Table 11-9 Examples of transmitted and received data.

Table 11-9 Examples of transmitted and received data

ID	cmdsent1	cmdrcvd1	cmdsent2	cmdrcvd2	vtime
663	DB0103081011	*	RB	2558 2554 2161 2271 2145	031218 112855

In this row, the Client has sent a command containing text DB0103081011♦ to the Proxy Server (the final diamond shape is the command line terminator in ASCII—in Hexadecimal this is the number string '0x04' followed by a carriage return '0x0D' and a line feed '0x0A').

The line terminator is not shown in the table, but is required as a terminus for each command string transmitted to the ventilator to signify the end of the command. For the Servo^j, this command defines a breath containing five parameters in integer-coded form. Table 11-8 shows these parameters to be "Inspiratory Tidal Volume", "Expiratory Tidal Volume", "Respiratory Rate (calculated)", "Expiratory Minute Volume", and "Mean Airway Pressure," respectively. The Proxy Server responds with an "*"—indicating acceptance of the command with no syntax errors. The response sent back to the Proxy Server from the ventilator is the integer string "25582554216122712145." Finally, a time stamp, also retrieved from the ventilator in similar fashion, is written to the table, establishing a time-stamp for the recorded result. This time stamp is "031218112855."

The table cell shading serves to segment the individual strings into associated queries and responses. Thus, in the case of the defined breath code "01" (i.e., inspiratory tidal volume), the response is "2558." In the case of the defined breath code "03" (i.e., expiratory tidal volume), the response is "2554," and so on.

These coded results are translated into physical readings using a computational method. For the basic channels associated with the Servo^j ventilator, this method is:

$$BasicValue = \frac{(BasicValueCode - 2048) \times 4.883}{ScaleF}$$

The BasicValueCode for "Inspiratory Tidal Volume" is (at this instant) 2558 and the scale factor (ScaleF) is found in column 5 of the Basic Channels table. For "Inspiratory Tidal Volume" this happens to be 5000. Proceeding with the calculation:

$$BasicValue = \frac{(2558 - 2048) \times 4.883}{5000} = 0.498$$

The parameter units associated with this value are taken from column 7 of the same table: "liters" or the symbol "l".

The time stamp is:

03 12 18 11 28 55

This text translates as follows:

03—Year

12—Month

18—Day

11—Hour

28—Minute

55—Second

This same process can be repeated for the other basic channel parameters.

For the extended channels associated with the Servo[i], the process is somewhat more complicated, and I will proceed with an example calculation. As in the Basic Channel case, a breath is defined in which one or more breath parameters are queried from the ventilator. The Client transmits a define breath ("DB") command to the Proxy Server. Note that the line termination character is omitted from the end of the line to enable the reader to focus on the message content itself.

A valid example is:

SDADB200201202203204

Appended to this command is a checksum[175], computed according to the following algorithm, Table 11-10:

Table 11-10 Checksum algorithm

```
public static String checksum(String cmd)
{
    int chk=0;
    for (int i=0; i<cmd.length(); i++)
        chk = chk ^ cmd.getBytes()[i];
    return Integer.toHexString(chk).toUpperCase();
}
```

---

[175] Ibid. Page 45

In the case of the command issued above, the checksum, when appended to the original command string, causes the string to be modified as follows:

SDADB200201202203204 66

The last two characters constitute the check sum for this string. The terminator characters are appended to this string prior to transmission to the ventilator. This is appended to all commands, as in the basic channel cases. In hexadecimal, the above string is given by:

5344414442323030323031323032323303332303404

A result is obtained using the extended channel equivalent of read breath (i.e., "RADAB"). The exact syntax of extended channel read breath, in which the command literally appears as follows, with checksum and line terminator appended, is:

RADAB54

An actual response to this command appears below:

0111 0500 0501 0055 0055

The subset of the extended channels table associated with the 200 series of *Servo*[i] from the CIE document is shown in Table 11-11.

Table 11-11 Extended Channel table for 200-series commands (breath data)

ID	ChNo	ParmName	gain	offset	gain_x	gain_y	offset_x	offset_y	unit	type
1	200	Measured breath frequency	+1000E -004	+0000E +000	4	3	4	3	06	BT
2	201	Exp. Tidal volume	+1000E -003	+0000E +000	5	4	5	4	01	BT
3	202	Insp. Tidal volume	+1000E -003	+0000E +000	5	4	5	4	01	BT
4	203	Insp. Minute volume	+1000E -004	+0000E +000	5	4	5	4	08	BT
5	204	Exp. Minute volume	+1000E -004	+0000E +000	5	4	5	4	08	BT

We can again employ cell shading to help illustrate the parameter value calculation process. From the command, let us segment the individual parameter codes, as follows:

SDADB `200` `201` `202` `203` `204` 66

For example, from Table 11-11 the channel number "202" corresponds to "Inspiratory Tidal Volume." Also, note the columns headed "gain_x...offset_y." The values contained in these columns are necessary for computing the parameter values. First, we must compute a gain and an offset:

$Gain = +1000\text{E-}003 = 1$

$Offset = +0000\text{E}+000 = 0$

The parameter value is then computed as:

$$ExtendedValue = Gain \times ExtendedValueCode - Offset \qquad (11.1)$$

$$ExtendedValue = 1 \times 501 - 0 = 501$$

Also, note the unit code for this parameter is "01" and, from Table 11-6, this corresponds to units of milliliters, ml. Thus, the inspiratory tidal volume is 501 ml, or 0.501 liters.

The programs are compiled as follows:

```
Client: javac ServoClient.java
Server: javac ServoProxy.java
```

The Programs must be run concurrently from two separate command shells (i.e., cmd.exe). The proxy server is run as follows:

```
Java ServoProxy COMx
```

Here, COMx refers to the serial communications port to which the computer on which ServoProxy is run and is connected to the mechanical ventilator via a serial cable. Client execution is as follows:

```
Java ServoClient
```

Both the client and server may be run on the same computer. Figure 11-2 shows the client user interface with some sample data populated to illustrate how it appears during normal operation. Table 11-12 and Table 11-13 are listings of the client and server code, respectively.

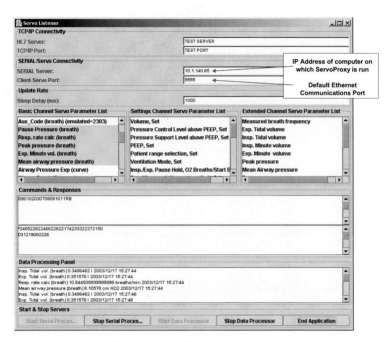

Figure 11-2 ServoClient User Interface

Table 11-12 Listing: ServoClient.java

```
// ***************************************************************
// ServoClient.java
//
// Reads channels from DB, fetches data from ServoProxy.
//
// Author (original): John Zaleski
// ***************************************************************

import java.io.*;
import java.awt.*;
import java.net.*;
import java.sql.*;
import java.sql.Connection;
import java.sql.DriverManager;
import java.sql.SQLException;
import java.lang.*;
import java.util.*;
import java.lang.Math;
import java.text.*;
import java.awt.event.*;
import javax.swing.*;
import javax.swing.event.*;
import javax.swing.border.*;
import java.lang.Thread;
import java.lang.*;


public class ServoClient extends JFrame implements AdjustmentListener,
ActionListener, ListSelectionListener
{
```

Table 11-12 Listing: ServoClient.java *(continued)*

```
public static String TCPIPsrvrText = "TEST SERVER";
public static String TCPIPportText = "TEST PORT";
public static String url = "jdbc:odbc:Servo";
public boolean KEEP_RUNNING = true;
public boolean KEEP_RUNNING2 = true;
public String SERIALportText = "5555";
public String SERIALsrvrText = "stet: 10.1.140.165";
public String basicChannels[][] = new String[50][9];
public String extndChannels[][] = new String[50][15];
public String settsChannels[][] = new String[50][15];
public String unitsChannels[][] = new String[50][4];
public String selectedBasicChannels[] = new String[50];
public String selectedExtndChannels[] = new String[50];
public String selectedSettsChannels[] = new String[50];
public String sBasicFactors[] = new String[50];
public String sExtndFactors[][] = new String[50][15];
public String sSettsFactors[][] = new String[50][15];
public int basicchannelCounter = 0;
public int extndchannelCounter = 0;
public int settschannelCounter = 0;
JList basicChannelList = null;
JList extndChannelList = null;
JList settsChannelList = null;
public int maxBasicChannels = 0;
public int maxExtndChannels = 0;
public int maxSettsChannels = 0;
public int maxUnitsChannels = 0;
DefaultListModel basicChannelListModel;
DefaultListModel extndChannelListModel;
DefaultListModel settsChannelListModel;
public String basicconcatChannels = null;
public String extndconcatChannels = null;
public String settsconcatChannels = null;
public int basicchanNum[] = new int[50];
public int extndchanNum[] = new int[50];
public int settschanNum[] = new int[50];
public String basicchannelResults = null;
public String extndchannelResults = null;
public String settschannelResults= null;
public String timeResults = null;
public TextField TCPIPsrvrField;
public TextField TCPIPportField;
public TextField SERIALsrvrField;
public TextField SERIALportField;
public TextField mshField;
public TextField pidField;
public TextField pv1Field;
public TextField obrField;
public TextField sleepDelayField;
public JTextArea rawCmdsArea;
public JTextArea rawDataArea;
public JTextArea prcDataArea;
public int frameWidth = 788;
public int frameHeight = 700;
public int TCPIP_PORT = 0;
public int SLEEP_DELAY = 1000;
public int SLEEP_DELAY2 = 2000;
public int SERIAL_PORT = 5555;
public double realventResults[] = new double[150];
SERIALListener listen;
DATAListener data;
JButton SPstartButton;
JButton SPstopButton;
JButton DPstartButton;
JButton DPstopButton;
JButton endButton;
```

Table 11-12 Listing: ServoClient.java *(continued)*

```java
Connection dbConn = null;
Connection dbConn2 = null;
Connection dbConn3 = null;
Statement st = null;
Statement st2 = null;
Statement st3 = null;
ResultSet RS1 = null;
ResultSet RS2 = null;

//===============================================================
//:::::
//::::: adjustmenValueChanged method to detect adjustments in
//::::: windows.
//:::::
public void adjustmentValueChanged ( AdjustmentEvent event )
{
    this.update();
} // End actionPerformed()

//===============================================================
//:::::
//::::: update method updates the user interface window
//:::::
protected void update() {}

//:::::
//::::: ServoClient constructor
//:::::
public ServoClient() { super ( "Servo Listener" ); }

//:::::
//::::: Main
//:::::
public static void main(String[] args)
{
    ServoClient sc = new ServoClient();
    sc.makeDBConnection( url );
    sc.queryDBBasic();
    sc.queryDBExtnd();
    sc.queryDBSetts();
    sc.queryUnits();
    sc.closeDBConnection();
    sc.buildUI();
} // main()

//:::::
//::::: Action listener for buttons
//:::::
public void actionPerformed ( java.awt.event.ActionEvent event )
{
    if ( event.getActionCommand().equals( "start" ) )
    {
        listen = new SERIALListener( this );
        KEEP_RUNNING = true;
        listen.start();
        SPstartButton.setEnabled( false );
        SPstopButton.setEnabled( true );
    }
    if ( event.getActionCommand().equals( "start1" ) )
    {
        data = new DATAListener( this );
        KEEP_RUNNING2 = true;
        data.start();
        DPstartButton.setEnabled( false );
```

Table 11-12 Listing: ServoClient.java *(continued)*

```
            DPstopButton.setEnabled( true );
        }
        if ( event.getActionCommand().equals( "stop" ) )
        {
            KEEP_RUNNING = false;
            SPstartButton.setEnabled( true );
            SPstopButton.setEnabled( false );
        }
        if ( event.getActionCommand().equals( "stop1" ) )
        {
            KEEP_RUNNING2 = false;
            DPstartButton.setEnabled( true );
            DPstopButton.setEnabled( false );
        }
        if ( event.getActionCommand().equals( "end" ) )
        {
            KEEP_RUNNING = false;
            KEEP_RUNNING2= false;
            System.exit( 0 );
        }
    } // End actionPerformed()


//::::
//:::: This method is required by ListSelectionListener.
//::::
    public void valueChanged( ListSelectionEvent e )
    {
        if ( e.getValueIsAdjusting() == false )
        {
            //::::
            //:::: Basic Channels
            //::::
            if ( basicChannelList.getSelectedIndex() == -1 )
            {
            } else {
                // Selection, enable the launch button.
                // Get the index of all the selected items
               int[] selectedIx = basicChannelList.getSelectedIndices();
                // Get all the selected items using the indices
                for (int i=0; i<selectedIx.length; i++)
                {
                  Object sel = basicChannelList.getModel().getElementAt
                      (selectedIx[i]);
                }
                basicconcatChannels = "";
                basicchannelCounter = 0;
                for (int j=0; j < maxBasicChannels; j++ )
                {
                  boolean isSel = basicChannelList.isSelectedIndex(j);
                    if ( isSel == true )
                    {
                        selectedBasicChannels[basicchannelCounter] =
                                basicChannels[j][2];
                        sBasicFactors[basicchannelCounter] =
                                basicChannels[j][5];
                        basicchanNum[basicchannelCounter] = j;
                        basicconcatChannels += basicChannels[j][2];
                        basicchannelCounter += 1;
                    }
                }
                System.out.println( " BASIC concatenated channels: " +
                        basicconcatChannels );
            } // end basic channel selection
            //::::
            //:::: Extended Channels
```

Table 11-12 Listing: ServoClient.java *(continued)*

```
//:::
if ( extndChannelList.getSelectedIndex() == -1 )
{
} else {
    // Selection, enable the launch button.
    // Get the index of all the selected items
    int[] selectedIx = extndChannelList.getSelectedIndices();
    // Get all the selected items using the indices
    for (int i=0; i<selectedIx.length; i++)
    {
        Object sel = extndChannelList.getModel().getElementAt
            (selectedIx[i]);
    }
    extndconcatChannels = "";
    extndchannelCounter = 0;
    for (int j=0; j < maxExtndChannels; j++ )
    {
        boolean isSel = extndChannelList.isSelectedIndex(j);
        if ( isSel == true )
        {
            selectedExtndChannels[extndchannelCounter] =
                extndChannels[j][2];
            for ( int k = 0; k < 15; k++ )
sExtndFactors[extndchannelCounter][k] = extndChannels[j][k];
            extndchanNum[extndchannelCounter] = j;
            extndconcatChannels += extndChannels[j][2];
            extndchannelCounter += 1;
        }
    }
    System.out.println( " EXTENDED concatenated channels: "
        + extndconcatChannels );
} // end extended channel selection


//:::
//::: Settings Channels
//:::
if ( settsChannelList.getSelectedIndex() == -1 )
{
} else {
    // Selection, enable the launch button.
    // Get the index of all the selected items
    int[] selectedIx = settsChannelList.getSelectedIndices();
    // Get all the selected items using the indices
    for (int i=0; i<selectedIx.length; i++)
    {
        Object sel = settsChannelList.getModel().getElementAt
            (selectedIx[i]);
    }
    settsconcatChannels = "";
    settschannelCounter = 0;
    for (int j=0; j < maxSettsChannels; j++ )
    {
        boolean isSel = settsChannelList.isSelectedIndex(j);
        if ( isSel == true )
        {
            selectedSettsChannels[settschannelCounter] =
                settsChannels[j][2];
            for ( int k = 0; k < 15; k++ )
sSettsFactors[settschannelCounter][k] = settsChannels[j][k];
            settschanNum[settschannelCounter] = j;
            settsconcatChannels += settsChannels[j][2];
            settschannelCounter += 1;
        }
    }
    System.out.println( " SETTINGS concatenated channels: "
```

Table 11-12 Listing: ServoClient.java *(continued)*

```
                        + settsconcatChannels );
             } // End settings channel selection
        }
    } // End valueChanged


    //::::
    //:::: buildUI()
    //::::
    public void buildUI()
    {
        //
        // Set fonts
        //
        String fontName = "Arial";
        int type = Font.BOLD;
        int size = 10;
        Font font;
        FontMetrics fm;
        font = new Font( fontName, type, size );
        //::::
        //:::: TCP/IP Server
        //::::
        JLabel TCPIPsrvrFieldLabel = new JLabel("<HTML><CENTER> <FONT
FACE=arial STYLE=bold SIZE=3 " + "COLOR=BLUE>HL7 Server:</FONT></CEN-
TER></HTML>");
        TCPIPsrvrField = new TextField( TCPIPsrvrText );
        TCPIPsrvrField.setFont( font );
        TCPIPsrvrField.addActionListener( new ActionListener() {
        public void actionPerformed( ActionEvent event )
        {
            TCPIPsrvrText = TCPIPsrvrField.getText();
        }
        });
        TCPIPsrvrField.addTextListener( new TextListener() {
        public void textValueChanged( TextEvent event )
        {
            TCPIPsrvrText = TCPIPsrvrField.getText();
        }
        });
        JPanel TCPIPserverPanel = new JPanel();
        TCPIPserverPanel.setLayout( new GridLayout(0,2) );
        TCPIPserverPanel.add( TCPIPsrvrFieldLabel );
        TCPIPserverPanel.add( TCPIPsrvrField );
        //::::
        //:::: TCP/IP Port
        //::::
        JLabel TCPIPportFieldLabel = new JLabel("<HTML><CENTER><FONT
FACE=arial STYLE=bold SIZE=3 " + "COLOR=BLUE>TCP/IP Port:</FONT></CEN-
TER></HTML>");
        TCPIPportField = new TextField( TCPIPportText );
        TCPIPportField.setFont( font );
        TCPIPportField.addActionListener( new ActionListener() {
        public void actionPerformed( ActionEvent event )
        {
            TCPIP_PORT = Integer.valueOf( TCPIPportField.getText()
).intValue();
        }
        });
        TCPIPportField.addTextListener( new TextListener() {
        public void textValueChanged( TextEvent event )
        {
            TCPIP_PORT = Integer.valueOf( TCPIPportField.getText()
).intValue();
        }
        });
```

Table 11-12 Listing: ServoClient.java *(continued)*

```
        JPanel TCPIPportPanel = new JPanel();
        TCPIPportPanel.setLayout( new GridLayout(0,2) );
        TCPIPportPanel.add( TCPIPportFieldLabel );
        TCPIPportPanel.add( TCPIPportField );
        JPanel TCPIPPanel = new JPanel();
        TCPIPPanel.setLayout( new GridLayout(2,0) );
        Border TCPIPPanelBorder = BorderFactory.createTitledBorder( "TCP/
IP Connectivity" );
        TCPIPPanel.setBorder( TCPIPPanelBorder );
        TCPIPPanel.add( TCPIPserverPanel );
        TCPIPPanel.add( TCPIPportPanel );
        //::::
        //:::: SERIAL Server
        //::::
        JLabel SERIALsrvrFieldLabel = new JLabel("<HTML><CENTER><FONT
FACE=arial STYLE=bold SIZE=3 " + "COLOR=BLUE>SERIAL Server:</FONT></
CENTER></HTML>");
        SERIALsrvrField = new TextField( SERIALsrvrText );
        SERIALsrvrField.setFont( font );
        SERIALsrvrField.addActionListener( new ActionListener() {
        public void actionPerformed( ActionEvent event )
        {
            SERIALsrvrText = SERIALsrvrField.getText();
        }
        });
        SERIALsrvrField.addTextListener( new TextListener() {
        public void textValueChanged( TextEvent event )
        {
            SERIALsrvrText = SERIALsrvrField.getText();
        }
        });
        JPanel SERIALserverPanel = new JPanel();
        SERIALserverPanel.setLayout( new GridLayout(0,2) );
        SERIALserverPanel.add( SERIALsrvrFieldLabel );
        SERIALserverPanel.add( SERIALsrvrField );
        //::::
        //:::: SERIAL Port
        //::::
        JLabel SERIALportFieldLabel = new JLabel("<HTML><CENTER><FONT
FACE=arial STYLE=bold SIZE=3 " + "COLOR=BLUE>Client-Servo Port:</FONT></
CENTER></HTML>");
        SERIALportField = new TextField( SERIALportText );
        SERIALportField.setFont( font );
        SERIALportField.addActionListener( new ActionListener() {
        public void actionPerformed( ActionEvent event )
        {
            SERIAL_PORT = Integer.valueOf( SERIALportField.getText()
).intValue();
        }
        });
        SERIALportField.addTextListener( new TextListener() {
        public void textValueChanged( TextEvent event )
        {
            SERIAL_PORT = Integer.valueOf( SERIALportField.getText()
).intValue();
        }
        });
        JPanel SERIALportPanel = new JPanel();
        SERIALportPanel.setLayout( new GridLayout(0, 2) );
        SERIALportPanel.add( SERIALportFieldLabel );
        SERIALportPanel.add( SERIALportField );
        JPanel SERIALPanel = new JPanel();
        SERIALPanel.setLayout( new GridLayout(2,0) );
        Border SERIALPanelBorder = BorderFactory.createTitledBorder(
"SERIAL/Servo Connectivity" );
        SERIALPanel.setBorder( SERIALPanelBorder );
```

Table 11-12 Listing: ServoClient.java *(continued)*

```
        SERIALPanel.add( SERIALserverPanel );
        SERIALPanel.add( SERIALportPanel );
        //::::
        //:::: Sleep delay field label
        //::::
        JLabel sleepDelayFieldLabel = new JLabel("<HTML><FONT FACE=arial
STYLE=bold SIZE=3 " + "COLOR=BLUE>Sleep Delay (ms):</FONT></HTML>");
        sleepDelayField = new TextField( ""+SLEEP_DELAY );
        sleepDelayField.setFont( font );
        sleepDelayField.addActionListener( new ActionListener() {
        public void actionPerformed( ActionEvent event )
        {
            SLEEP_DELAY = Integer.valueOf( sleepDelayField.getText()
).intValue();
        }
        });
        sleepDelayField.addTextListener( new TextListener() {
        public void textValueChanged( TextEvent event )
        {
            SLEEP_DELAY = Integer.valueOf( sleepDelayField.getText()
).intValue();
        }
        });
        JPanel sleepPanel = new JPanel();
        sleepPanel.setLayout( new GridLayout(0,2) );
        Border sleepPanelBorder = BorderFactory.createTitledBorder(
"Update Rate" );
        sleepPanel.setBorder( sleepPanelBorder );
        sleepPanel.add( sleepDelayFieldLabel );
        sleepPanel.add( sleepDelayField );
        //::::
        //:::: Build scroll pane lists
        //::::
        JLabel basicFieldLabel = new JLabel("<HTML><CENTER>
            <FONT FACE=arial STYLE=bold SIZE=3 " + "COLOR=BLUE>
              Basic Channels:</FONT></CENTER></HTML>");
        basicChannelListModel = new DefaultListModel();
        for ( int i = 0; i < maxBasicChannels; i++ )
        {
            basicChannelListModel.addElement( basicChannels[i][4] );
        }
        basicChannelList = new JList( basicChannelListModel );
        basicChannelList.setSelectionMode( ListSelection-
Model.MULTIPLE_INTERVAL_SELECTION );
        basicChannelList.setSelectedIndex( -1 );
        basicChannelList.addListSelectionListener( this );
        basicChannelList.setVisibleRowCount( 10 );
        JScrollPane basicChannelListScrollPane = new JScrollPane(
basicChannelList );
        basicChannelListScrollPane.setPreferredSize( new Dimension( 250,
150 ) );
        JPanel basicscrollPanel = new JPanel();
        basicscrollPanel.setLayout( new BorderLayout() );
        Border basicscrollPanelBorder = BorderFactory.createTitledBorder(
"Basic Channel Servo Parameter List" );
        basicscrollPanel.setBorder( basicscrollPanelBorder );
    //      basicscrollPanel.add( basicFieldLabel, BorderLayout.WEST );
        basicscrollPanel.add( basicChannelListScrollPane, BorderLay-
out.EAST );
        //::::
        //:::: Build scroll pane lists
        //::::
        JLabel extFieldLabel = new JLabel("<HTML><CENTER><FONT FACE=arial
STYLE=bold SIZE=3 " + "COLOR=BLUE>Extended Channels:</FONT></CENTER></
HTML>");
        extndChannelListModel = new DefaultListModel();
```

Table 11-12 Listing: ServoClient.java *(continued)*

```
        for ( int i = 0; i < maxExtndChannels; i++ )
        {
            extndChannelListModel.addElement( extndChannels[i][3] );
        }
        extndChannelList = new JList( extndChannelListModel );
        extndChannelList.setSelectionMode( ListSelection-
Model.MULTIPLE_INTERVAL_SELECTION );
        extndChannelList.setSelectedIndex( -1 );
        extndChannelList.addListSelectionListener( this );
        extndChannelList.setVisibleRowCount( 10 );
        JScrollPane extndChannelListScrollPane = new JScrollPane(
extndChannelList );
        extndChannelListScrollPane.setPreferredSize( new Dimension( 250,
150 ) );
        JPanel extscrollPanel = new JPanel();
        extscrollPanel.setLayout( new BorderLayout() );
        Border extscrollPanelBorder = BorderFactory.createTitledBorder(
"Extended Channel Servo Parameter List" );
        extscrollPanel.setBorder( extscrollPanelBorder );
    //      extscrollPanel.add( extFieldLabel, BorderLayout.WEST );
        extscrollPanel.add( extndChannelListScrollPane, BorderLayout.EAST
);
        //::::
        //:::: Build scroll pane lists
        //::::

        JLabel setFieldLabel = new JLabel("<HTML><CENTER><FONT FACE=arial
STYLE=bold SIZE=3 " + "COLOR=BLUE>Settings Channels:</FONT></CENTER></
HTML>");
        settsChannelListModel = new DefaultListModel();
        for ( int i = 0; i < maxSettsChannels; i++ )
        {
            settsChannelListModel.addElement( settsChannels[i][3] );
        }
        settsChannelList = new JList( settsChannelListModel );
        settsChannelList.setSelectionMode( ListSelection-
Model.MULTIPLE_INTERVAL_SELECTION );
        settsChannelList.setSelectedIndex( -1 );
        settsChannelList.addListSelectionListener( this );
        settsChannelList.setVisibleRowCount( 10 );
        JScrollPane settsChannelListScrollPane = new JScrollPane(
settsChannelList );
        settsChannelListScrollPane.setPreferredSize( new Dimension( 250,
150 ) );
        JPanel setscrollPanel = new JPanel();
        setscrollPanel.setLayout( new BorderLayout() );
        Border setscrollPanelBorder = BorderFactory.createTitledBorder(
"Settings Channel Servo Parameter List" );
        setscrollPanel.setBorder( setscrollPanelBorder );
    //      setscrollPanel.add( setFieldLabel, BorderLayout.WEST );
        setscrollPanel.add( settsChannelListScrollPane, BorderLayout.EAST
);
        //::::
        //:::: Cmds and Resp Scrolling Panes
        //::::
        JLabel rawCmdsAreaLabel = new JLabel("<HTML><CENTER><FONT
FACE=arial STYLE=bold SIZE=4 " + "COLOR=BLUE>Commands:</FONT></CEN-
TER></HTML>");
        rawCmdsArea = new JTextArea( "No Segments Yet", 20, 150 );
        rawCmdsArea.setFont( font );
        rawCmdsArea.setEditable( false );
        rawCmdsArea.setLineWrap( true );
        JScrollPane scrollingcmdsArea = new JScrollPane( rawCmdsArea );
        scrollingcmdsArea.setPreferredSize( new Dimension( 100, 150 ) );
        JPanel rawCmdsPanel = new JPanel();
```

Table 11-12 Listing: ServoClient.java *(continued)*

```
      rawCmdsPanel.setLayout( new BorderLayout() );
      rawCmdsPanel.add( scrollingcmdsArea, BorderLayout.CENTER );
      JLabel rawDataAreaLabel = new JLabel("<HTML><CENTER><FONT
FACE=arial STYLE=bold SIZE=4 " + "COLOR=BLUE>Responses:</FONT></CEN-
TER></HTML>");
      rawDataArea = new JTextArea( "No Segments Yet", 20, 150 );
      rawDataArea.setFont( font );
      rawDataArea.setEditable( false );
      rawDataArea.setLineWrap( true );
    JScrollPane scrollingdataArea = new JScrollPane( rawDataArea );
      scrollingdataArea.setPreferredSize( new Dimension( 100, 150 ) );
      JPanel rawDataPanel = new JPanel();
      rawDataPanel.setLayout( new BorderLayout() );
      rawDataPanel.add( scrollingdataArea, BorderLayout.CENTER );
      JPanel CmdsPanel = new JPanel();
      CmdsPanel.setLayout( new GridLayout(2,0) );
      Border CmdsPanelBorder = BorderFactory.createTitledBorder(
"Commands & Responses" );
      CmdsPanel.setBorder( CmdsPanelBorder );
      CmdsPanel.add( rawCmdsPanel );
      CmdsPanel.add( rawDataPanel );
      //:::
      //:::: DataView window
      //:::


      JLabel prcDataAreaLabel = new JLabel("<HTML><CENTER><FONT
FACE=arial STYLE=bold SIZE=4 " + "COLOR=BLUE>Processed Data:</FONT></
CENTER></HTML>");

      prcDataArea = new JTextArea( "No Data Yet", 20, 80 );
      prcDataArea.setFont( font );
      prcDataArea.setEditable( false );
      prcDataArea.setLineWrap( true );
    JScrollPane scrollingDataArea = new JScrollPane( prcDataArea );
      scrollingDataArea.setPreferredSize( new Dimension( 20, 80 ) );
      JPanel prcDataPanel = new JPanel();
      prcDataPanel.setLayout( new BorderLayout() );
      prcDataPanel.add( scrollingDataArea, BorderLayout.CENTER );
      //
      // Now, add this panel to the dataView panel
      //
      JPanel dataViewPanel = new JPanel();
      dataViewPanel.setLayout( new GridLayout(1,0) );
      Border dataViewPanelBorder = BorderFactory.createTitledBorder(
"Data Processing Panel" );
      dataViewPanel.setBorder( dataViewPanelBorder );
      dataViewPanel.add( prcDataPanel );
      //:::
      //:::: Start, Stop buttons
      //:::
      SPstartButton = new JButton( "Start Serial Processor" );
      SPstartButton.setActionCommand( "start" );
      SPstartButton.addActionListener( this );
      SPstartButton.setEnabled( true );
      SPstopButton = new JButton( "Stop Serial Processor" );
      SPstopButton.setActionCommand( "stop" );
      SPstopButton.addActionListener( this );
      SPstopButton.setEnabled( false );
      DPstartButton = new JButton( "Start Data Processor" );
      DPstartButton.setActionCommand( "start1" );
      DPstartButton.addActionListener( this );
      DPstartButton.setEnabled( true );
      DPstopButton = new JButton( "Stop Data Processor" );
      DPstopButton.setActionCommand( "stop1" );
      DPstopButton.addActionListener( this );
```

261

Table 11-12 Listing: ServoClient.java *(continued)*

```
        DPstopButton.setEnabled( false );
        endButton = new JButton( "End Application" );
        endButton.setActionCommand( "end" );
        endButton.addActionListener( this );
        endButton.setEnabled( true );
        JPanel ssPanel = new JPanel( new GridLayout(0,5) );
        ssPanel.setLayout( new GridLayout( 0, 5 ) );
      Border ssPanelBorder = BorderFactory.createTitledBorder( "Start
& Stop Servers" );
        ssPanel.setBorder( ssPanelBorder );
        ssPanel.add( SPstartButton );
        ssPanel.add( SPstopButton );
        ssPanel.add( DPstartButton );
        ssPanel.add( DPstopButton );
        ssPanel.add( endButton );
        JPanel superscrollPanel = new JPanel( new BorderLayout() );
        superscrollPanel.add( basicscrollPanel, BorderLayout.WEST );
        superscrollPanel.add( setscrollPanel, BorderLayout.CENTER );
        superscrollPanel.add( extscrollPanel, BorderLayout.EAST );
        JPanel fieldPanel0 = new JPanel();
        JPanel fieldPanel1 = new JPanel();
        JPanel fieldPanel2 = new JPanel();
        fieldPanel0.setLayout( new BorderLayout() );
        fieldPanel1.setLayout( new BorderLayout() );
        fieldPanel2.setLayout( new BorderLayout() );
        fieldPanel0.add( TCPIPPanel, BorderLayout.NORTH );
        fieldPanel0.add( SERIALPanel,    BorderLayout.CENTER );
        fieldPanel0.add( sleepPanel, BorderLayout.SOUTH );
        fieldPanel1.add( superscrollPanel,    BorderLayout.NORTH );
        fieldPanel1.add( CmdsPanel,      BorderLayout.CENTER );
        fieldPanel2.add( dataViewPanel, BorderLayout.NORTH );
        fieldPanel2.add( ssPanel,     BorderLayout.CENTER );
        Container content = getContentPane();
        content.setLayout ( new BorderLayout() );
        content.setBackground( Color.white );
        content.setForeground( Color.blue );
        content.add( fieldPanel0, BorderLayout.NORTH );
        content.add( fieldPanel1, BorderLayout.CENTER );
        content.add( fieldPanel2, BorderLayout.SOUTH );
        //::::
        //:::: Set frame size
        //::::
        setSize ( frameWidth, frameHeight );
        //::::
        //:::: Set frame window listener
        //::::
        addWindowListener( new WindowAdapter() {
        public void windowIconified( WindowEvent e ) {
            System.out.println( " Window ICONIFIED" );
        }
        public void windowDeiconified( WindowEvent e ) {
            System.out.println( " Window DE_ICONIFIED" );
        }
        public void windowClosing( WindowEvent e ) {
            System.exit( 0 );
        }
        });
        //::::
        //:::: Set frame location
        //::::
        setLocation( 10,10 );
        setVisible( true );
    } // buildUI

    //::::
    //:::: Make the DB connection
```

Table 11-12 Listing: ServoClient.java *(continued)*

```
//:::
public void makeDBConnection( String path )
{
    try {
        Class.forName("sun.jdbc.odbc.JdbcOdbcDriver");
        String uname = "";
        String pword = "";
        dbConn = DriverManager.getConnection( path, uname, pword );
        st = dbConn.createStatement();
    } catch( Exception e ) {
        System.out.println( "***Error making connection***");
        System.out.println( "MakeJDBConnection " + e );
    }
} // End makeDBConnection()


//:::
//::: Close the DB connection
//:::
public void closeDBConnection()
{
    try {
        dbConn.close();
        st.close();
    } catch ( Exception e ) { System.err.println( "***cannot close
JDBC*** " + e );}
} // End closeDBConnection()


//:::
//::: Query the DB for Basic channel data
//:::
public void queryDBBasic( )
{
    ResultSetMetaData rsmd = null;
    try {
        //:::
        //::: Actual query statement containing WHERE clause.
        //:::
        ResultSet rec = st.executeQuery("SELECT * FROM BasicChannels");
        rsmd = rec.getMetaData();
        int numberOfColumns = rsmd.getColumnCount();
        //:::
        //::: Print all instances of these objects out
        //:::
        int i = 0;
        while(rec.next() )
        {
            for (int j = 1; j <= numberOfColumns; j++)
            {
                String columnValue = rec.getString(j);
                basicChannels[i][j] = columnValue;
                System.out.print( " " + basicChannels[i][j] + ", " );
            }
            System.out.println();
            i = i + 1;
        } // End While
        maxBasicChannels = i-1;
    } catch( Exception e ) {
        System.err.println( "***Error in queryDBBasic()*** " + e );
    }
} // End queryDBBasic()


//:::
//::: Query the DB for Extended channel data
```

Table 11-12 Listing: ServoClient.java *(continued)*

```
//:::::
public void queryDBExtnd( )
{
    ResultSetMetaData rsmd = null;
    try {
        //:::::
        //::::: Actual query statement containing WHERE clause.
        //:::::
        ResultSet rec = st.executeQuery("SELECT * FROM
ExtendedChannels200");
        rsmd = rec.getMetaData();
        int numberOfColumns = rsmd.getColumnCount();
        System.out.println( " EXTENDED COMMANDS");
        System.out.println( " Number of columns: " + numberOfColumns );
        //:::::
        //::::: Print all instances of these objects out
        //:::::
        int i = 0;
        while(rec.next() )
        {
            for (int j = 1; j <= numberOfColumns; j++)
            {
                String columnValue = rec.getString(j);
                extndChannels[i][j] = columnValue;
                System.out.print( " " + extndChannels[i][j] + ", " );
            }
            System.out.println();
            i = i + 1;
        } // End While
        maxExtndChannels = i-1;
    } catch( Exception e ) {
        System.err.println( "***Error in queryDBExtnd()*** " + e );
    }
} // End queryDBExtnd()


//:::::
//::::: Query the DB for Settings channel data
//:::::
public void queryDBSetts( )
{
    ResultSetMetaData rsmd = null;
    try {
        //:::::
        //::::: Actual query statement containing WHERE clause.
        //:::::
        ResultSet rec = st.executeQuery("SELECT * FROM
ExtendedChannels300");
        rsmd = rec.getMetaData();
        int numberOfColumns = rsmd.getColumnCount();
        //:::::
        //::::: Print all instances of these objects out
        //:::::
        int i = 0;
        while(rec.next() )
        {
            for (int j = 1; j <= numberOfColumns; j++)
            {
                String columnValue = rec.getString(j);
                settsChannels[i][j] = columnValue;
                System.out.print( " " + settsChannels[i][j] + ", " );
            }
            System.out.println();
            i = i + 1;
        } // End While
        maxSettsChannels = i-1;
```

Table 11-12 Listing: ServoClient.java *(continued)*

```
        } catch( Exception e ) {
    System.err.println( "***Error in queryDBSetts()*** " + e );
        }
    } // End queryDBSetts()


    //:::::
    //::::: Query the Units for channel data
    //:::::
    public void queryUnits( )
    {
        ResultSetMetaData rsmd = null;
        try {
            //:::::
            //::::: Actual query statement containing WHERE clause.
            //:::::
            ResultSet rec = st.executeQuery("SELECT * FROM units");
            rsmd = rec.getMetaData();
            int numberOfColumns = rsmd.getColumnCount();
            //:::::
            //::::: Print all instances of these objects out
            //:::::
            int i = 0;
            while(rec.next() )
            {
                for (int j = 1; j <= numberOfColumns; j++)
                {
                    String columnValue = rec.getString(j);
                    unitsChannels[i][j] = columnValue;
                  System.out.print( " " + unitsChannels[i][j] + ", " );
                }
                System.out.println();
                i = i + 1;
            } // End While
            maxUnitsChannels = i-1;
            System.out.println( " Max units: " + maxUnitsChannels );
        } catch( Exception e ) {
            System.err.println( "***Error in queryUnits()*** " + e );
        }
    } // End queryUnits()
} // ServoClient


//==========================================
//:::::NEW CLASS
//==========================================

class DATAListener extends Thread {

    //:::::
    //::::: Link to the ServoClient
    //:::::
    ServoClientsource;

    DATAListener ( Frame s )
    {
        super();
        source = ( ServoClient ) s;
    }

    //:::::
    //::::: Run method communicates with database
    //:::::
    public void run()
    {
```

Table 11-12 Listing: ServoClient.java *(continued)*

```
        while ( source.KEEP_RUNNING2 )
        {
            ResultSetMetaData rsmd = null;
            try {
                Class.forName("sun.jdbc.odbc.JdbcOdbcDriver");
                String uname = "";
                String pword = "";
            source.dbConn3 = DriverManager.getConnection( source.url,
uname, pword );
                source.st3 = source.dbConn3.createStatement();
                //:::::
                //::::: Actual query statement containing WHERE clause.
                //:::::
                ResultSet rec = source.st3.executeQuery("SELECT * FROM
ventdata");
                rsmd = rec.getMetaData();
                int numberOfColumns = rsmd.getColumnCount();
            System.out.println( " number of columns: " + numberOfColumns
);
                //:::::
                //::::: Print all instances of these objects out
                //:::::
                source.prcDataArea.setText( "" );
                int i = 0;
                while(rec.next() )
                {
                    String cmdsValue = rec.getString(2);
                    String respValue = rec.getString(4);
                    String dataValue = rec.getString(5);
                    String timeValue = rec.getString(6);
                    System.out.println( "------------------");
                    System.out.println( respValue );
                    if ( respValue.equals("RB" ) )
                    {
                        parseBasicResults( cmdsValue,
                                           dataValue,
                                           source.basicChannels,
                                           source.maxBasicChannels,
                                           timeValue );
                    }
                    if ( respValue.equals("RADAB") )
                    {
                        parseExtndResults( cmdsValue,
                                           dataValue,
                                           source.extndChannels,
                                           source.maxExtndChannels,
                                           source.unitsChannels,
                                           source.maxUnitsChannels,
                                           timeValue );
                    }
                } // End While
                source.dbConn3.close();
                source.st3.close();
                Thread.sleep( source.SLEEP_DELAY2 );
            } catch (Exception e ) {
                System.err.println( " Caught in run method of DATAListener
Class: " + e );
            }
        } // End while
    } // End run method


    public void parseBasicResults( String sentCmd,
                                   String result,
                                   String factors[][],
                                   int nVals,
```

Table 11-12 Listing: ServoClient.java *(continued)*

```
                                String time )
    {
        // 2426207122282109 --> 2426 2071 2228 2109
        int nResults = result.length() / 4;
        System.out.println( " sent Cmd = " + sentCmd + " nResults = " +
nResults );
        int k = 2;
        for ( int i = 0; i < nResults; i++ )
        {
            int data = Integer.parseInt(result.substring(i*4, (i*4)+4));
            String cmd = sentCmd.substring(k, k+2);
            System.out.println( " cmd = " + cmd + " data = " + data + "
nVals = " + nVals );
            for ( int j = 0; j < nVals; j++ )
            {
                if ( cmd.equals( factors[j][2] ) )
                {
                    System.out.print( " " + factors[j][4] + " | " +
factors[j][5] + " | " + factors[j][6] + " | " + factors[j][7] + " | " +
factors[j][8] );
                    double sf = Double.valueOf( factors[j][5]
).doubleValue();
                    double Val = (data - 2048) * 4.883 / sf;
                    System.out.println( " Val = " + Val );
                    source.prcDataArea.append( "" + factors[j][4] + " " +
                                            Val + " " +
                                            factors[j][7] + " " );
                    source.prcDataArea.append( parseTime( time ) + "\n" );
                }
            }
            k = k + 2;
        }
    } // End parseBasicResults()


    public String parseTime( String time )
    {
        String dummy = null;
        if ( time.length() > 0 )
        {
            dummy = "20" + time.substring(0,2) + "/";
            dummy += time.substring(2,4) + "/";
            dummy += time.substring(4,6) + " ";
            dummy += time.substring(6,8) + ":";
            dummy += time.substring(8,10)+ ":";
            dummy += time.substring(10,12) + " ";
        }
        System.out.println( " dummy = " + dummy );
        return dummy;
    }


    public void parseExtndResults( String sentCmd,
                                   String result,
                                   String factors[][],
                                   int    nVals,
                                   String units[][],
                                   int    maxUnits,
                                   String time )
    {
        // 2426207122282109 --> 2426 2071 2228 2109
        int nResults = result.length() / 4;
        String selUnit = null;
        int k = 5;
```

267

Table 11-12 Listing: ServoClient.java *(continued)*

```
for ( int i = 0; i < nResults; i++ )
        {
            int data = Integer.parseInt(result.substring(i*4, (i*4)+4));
            String cmd = sentCmd.substring(k, k+3);
            for ( int j = 0; j < nVals; j++ )
            {
                // System.out.println( "   factors = " + factors[j][2] );
                if ( cmd.equals( factors[j][2] ) )
                {
                    int Xg = Integer.parseInt( factors[j][6] );
                    int Yg = Integer.parseInt( factors[j][7] );
                    int Xo = Integer.parseInt( factors[j][8] );
                    int Yo = Integer.parseInt( factors[j][9] );
                    double Gain = Xg * Math.pow(10, Yg );
                    double Offs = Xo * Math.pow(10, Yo );
                    double Val = data*Gain - Offs;
                    for ( int l = 0; l < maxUnits; l++ )
                    {
                        if ( factors[j][10].equals( units[l][2] ) )
                        {
                            selUnit = units[l][3];
                        }
                    }
                    source.prcDataArea.append( "" + factors[j][3] + " "
+ Val + " " + selUnit + "\n" );
                    selUnit = "";
                }
            }
            k = k + 3;
        }
    } // End parseExtndResults()
} // End class dataListener




//===========================================
//:::::NEW CLASS
//===========================================

class SERIALListener extends Thread {
    //:::::
    //::::: Link to the ServoClient
    //:::::
    ServoClientsource;
    String channels[] = new String [30];
    int channelCount = 0;


    SERIALListener ( Frame s )
    {
        super();
        source = ( ServoClient ) s;
    }


    //:::::
    //::::: Run method communicates with ServoProxy
    //:::::
    public void run()
    {
        boolean basicparms = false;
        boolean extndparms = false;
        boolean settsparms = false;

        while (source.KEEP_RUNNING)
```

Table 11-12 Listing: ServoClient.java *(continued)*

```
        {
            try {
                // Create connection with ServoProxy
                Socket talkSock;
                OutputStream netOut = null;
                InputStream netIn = null;
                talkSock = new Socket(source.SERIALsrvrText,
source.SERIAL_PORT);
                System.out.println("Connected with server  " +
talkSock.getInetAddress() + ":" + talkSock.getPort());
                netOut = talkSock.getOutputStream();
                netIn = talkSock.getInputStream();
                String basicData = "DB"    + source.basicconcatChannels;
                String extndData = "SDADB" + source.extndconcatChannels;
                String settsData = "SDADS" + source.settsconcatChannels;
                if ( basicData.indexOf("null") <= 0 ) basicparms = true;
                if ( extndData.indexOf("null") <= 0 ) extndparms = true;
                if ( settsData.indexOf("null") <= 0 ) settsparms = true;
                System.out.println( " basicparms, extndparms, settsparms
" + basicparms + extndparms + settsparms );
                String extString;
                StringTokenizer st = null;
                double data;
                // Make sure we start in BASIC mode
                // send 'set channels', receive 'set OK', send 'receive
data', receive data string for BASIC mode channels
                try {
                    Class.forName("sun.jdbc.odbc.JdbcOdbcDriver");
                    String uname = "";
                    String pword = "";
                    source.dbConn2 = DriverManager.getConnection(
source.url, uname, pword );
                    source.st2 = source.dbConn2.createStatement();
                    sendToVent("HO", netOut);
                    recvFromVent(netIn);
                    sendToVent("RT", netOut);
                    source.timeResults = "" + recvFromVent(netIn);
                    String localTime = source.timeResults.trim();
                    if ( basicparms )
                    {
                    System.out.println( " BAS------------------------
----------");

                        sendToVent(basicData, netOut);
                        String s1 = basicData;
                        String r1 = recvFromVent(netIn);
                        source.rawCmdsArea.setText( "" );
                        source.rawDataArea.setText( "" );
                        source.rawCmdsArea.append( s1 );
                        source.rawDataArea.append( r1 );
                        sendToVent("RB", netOut);
                        source.basicchannelResults = recvFromVent(netIn);
                        String s2 = "RB";
                        String r2 = source.basicchannelResults;
                        String t1 = source.timeResults;
                        source.rawCmdsArea.append( s2 + "\n" );
                        source.rawDataArea.append( r2 + "\n" );
                        source.rawDataArea.append( t1 + "\n" );
                        System.out.println( " t1 = " + t1 );
                        String ins1 = "INSERT INTO [ventdata] (cmdsent1,
cmdrcvd1, cmdsent2, cmdrcvd2, vtime) VALUES ( '" + s1 + "', '" + r1 +
"', '" + s2 + "', '" + r2 + "', '" + localTime + "' );";
                        int i = source.st2.executeUpdate( ins1 );
                    }
                    if ( extndparms )
                    {
```

Table 11-12 Listing: ServoClient.java *(continued)*

```
                     System.out.println( " EXT----------------------
------------");
                     //
                     // transfer into extended mode
                     //
                     sendToVentCHK("RCTY", netOut);
                     sendToVentCHK( extndData, netOut );
                     recvFromVent(netIn);
                     String s3 = extndData;
                     String r3 = recvFromVent(netIn);
                     sendToVentCHK( "RADAB", netOut );
                source.extndchannelResults = recvFromVent( netIn );
                     String s4 = "RADAB";
                     String r4 = source.extndchannelResults;
                     String t4 = "";
                     String ins2 = "INSERT INTO [ventdata] (cmdsent1,
cmdrcvd1, cmdsent2, cmdrcvd2, vtime) VALUES ( '" + s3 + "', '" + r3 +
"', '" + s4 + "', '" + r4 + "', '" + localTime + "' );";
                     int j = source.st2.executeUpdate( ins2 );
                     } // End if extndparms
                     if ( settsparms )
{
                     System.out.println( " SET----------------------
------------");
                     //
                     // transfer into extended mode
                     //
                     sendToVentCHK("RCTY", netOut);
                     System.out.println( " SET----------------------
------------");
                     sendToVentCHK( settsData, netOut );
                     recvFromVent(netIn);
                     sendToVentCHK("RADAS", netOut );
                source.settschannelResults = recvFromVent(netIn);
                     // parseSettsResults( source.settschannelResults,
                     // source.sSettsFactors,
                     // source.timeResults );
                     } // End if settsparms
                     source.dbConn2.close();
                     source.st2.close();
                } catch ( Exception sqle ) {
                     System.out.println( " sql insert error: " + sqle );
                }
                Thread.sleep( source.SLEEP_DELAY );
                talkSock.close();
            }
          catch (UnknownHostException unke) {System.out.print("Unknown
host.");}
            catch (IOException ioe) {System.err.println(ioe);}
            catch (Exception e ) { System.err.println( e ); }
        } // end While
    } // run


    //:::::
    //::::: Takes a string, adds EOT to it, and writes it to the given
outputstream
    //:::::
    public static int sendToVent(String cmdToSend, OutputStream netOut)
    {char eot = (char)0x04;
        try {
            cmdToSend = cmdToSend + " ";
            System.out.print("Sending: " + cmdToSend + "\n");
            netOut.write(cmdToSend.getBytes());
        } catch (IOException ioe) {return -1;}
```

Table 11-12 Listing: ServoClient.java *(continued)*

```
        return 0;
    }

    //:::::
    //::::: Waits for a reply from the given inputstream,
    //::::: strips the EOT, and returns the remaining string
    //:::::
    public static String recvFromVent(InputStream netIn)
    {
        int bytesRead;
        byte []inBytes = new byte[2048];
        byte []inBytesAdjusted = null;
        String stringIn;
        try {
            bytesRead = netIn.read(inBytes);
            inBytesAdjusted = new byte[bytesRead];
            for(int i=0; i<bytesRead; i++)
                inBytesAdjusted[i] = inBytes[i];
            stringIn = new String(inBytesAdjusted);
            System.out.print("Received: " + stringIn + "\n");
        } catch (IOException ioe) {return ("Error: " + ioe); }
        return stringIn.substring(0, stringIn.length()-1);
    }

    //:::::
    //::::: Returns the checksum for a given string
    //:::::
    public static String checksum(String cmd)
    {
        int chk=0;
        for (int i=0; i<cmd.length(); i++)
            chk = chk ^ cmd.getBytes()[i];
        return Integer.toHexString(chk).toUpperCase();
    }

    //:::::
    //::::: Takes a string, adds EOT and a checksum to it,
    //::::: and writes it to the given outputstream
    //:::::
    public static int sendToVentCHK(String cmdToSend, OutputStream
netOut)
    {char eot = (char)0x04;
        cmdToSend = cmdToSend + checksum(cmdToSend) + " ";
        System.out.print("Sending: " + cmdToSend + "\n");
        try {
            netOut.write(cmdToSend.getBytes());
        } catch (IOException ioe) {return -1;}
        return 0;
    }

    //:::::
    //::::: Waits for a reply from the given inputstream,
    //::::: strips the EOT and the checksum, and returns the remaining
string
    //:::::
    public static String recvFromVentCHK(InputStream netIn)
    {
        int bytesRead;
        byte []inBytes = new byte[2048];
        byte []inBytesAdjusted = null;
        String stringIn;
        try {
            bytesRead = netIn.read(inBytes);
            inBytesAdjusted = new byte[bytesRead];
            for(int i=0; i<bytesRead; i++)
                inBytesAdjusted[i] = inBytes[i];
```

Table 11-12 Listing: ServoClient.java *(continued)*

```
            stringIn = new String(inBytesAdjusted);
            System.out.print("Received: " + stringIn + "\n");
        } catch (IOException ioe) {return ("Error: " + ioe); }
        return stringIn.substring(0, stringIn.length()-3);
    }

    public void parseSettsResults( String result,
                                   String factors[][],
                                   String time )
                             {
        // 2426207122282109 --> 2426 2071 2228 2109
        int nResults = result.length() / 4;
        System.out.println( " nResults: " + nResults );
    } // End parseSettsResults()


    public void HL7ORU()
    {
        String myString = null;
        String pString = null;
        int basePort = source.TCPIP_PORT;
        Socket cConn = null;
        PrintWriter otSocket = null;
        try {
            InetAddress IPAddress = InetAddress.getByName(
source.TCPIPsrvrText );
            cConn = new Socket( IPAddress, basePort );
           otSocket = new PrintWriter( cConn.getOutputStream(), true );
            // otSocket.println( msgString ); // Would contain HL7 ORU
            cConn.close();
            otSocket.close();
        } catch ( Exception e ) {
            System.err.println(" Cannot open socket " + e );
            System.exit(0);
        }
    } // End HL7ORU()
} // class SERIALListener()
```

Table 11-13 Listing: ServoProxy.java

```
// **********************************************************************
// ServoProxy
//
// Queries ventilatory and forwards all incoming serialdata on TCP/IP to
// specified COM port and vice-versa
//
// Author: John Zaleski
//
// **********************************************************************


import java.io.*;
import java.util.*;
import javax.comm.*;
import java.net.*;
import java.lang.String;

public class ServoProxy implements Runnable, SerialPortEventListener {
    // Variables for serial communication
    static CommPortIdentifier portId;
    static Enumeration portList;
    static OutputStream outCOMData;
    static InputStream inCOMData;
    static SerialPort serialPort;
```

Table 11-13 Listing: ServoProxy.java *(continued)*

```
// Thread for reading from COM port
static Thread readThread;
// Variables for network communication
static ServerSocket sSock = null;
static Socket talkSock = null;
static InputStream inNetData = null;
static OutputStream outNetData = null;
// Variables used to go between network and COM
static byte []inBytes = new byte[256];
static byte []outBytes = new byte[256];
static int bytesRead;
static String read;

    public static void main(String[] args)
{
        if (args.length != 1)
        {
            System.out.print("usage: java ServoProxy COMx\n");
            System.exit(0);
        }
        portList = CommPortIdentifier.getPortIdentifiers();
        while (portList.hasMoreElements())
        {
            portId = (CommPortIdentifier) portList.nextElement();
            if (portId.getPortType() == CommPortIdentifier.PORT_SERIAL)
            {
                if (portId.getName().equals(args[0]))
                {
                    System.out.print("Listening on serial port " +
portId.getName() + ".\n");
                    // open the port
                    try {
                        serialPort = (SerialPort) portId.open("comPort",
2000);
                    } catch (PortInUseException e) {}
                    // set parameters for serial communcation
                    try {
                        serialPort.setFlowControlMode(seri-
alPort.FLOWCONTROL_XONXOFF_IN + serialPort.FLOWCONTROL_XONXOFF_OUT);
                        serialPort.setSerialPortParams(9600,
serialPort.DATABITS_8, serialPort.STOPBITS_1, serialPort.PARITY_EVEN);
                    } catch (UnsupportedCommOperationException e) {};
                    try {
                        inCOMData = serialPort.getInputStream();
                        outCOMData = serialPort.getOutputStream();
                    } catch (IOException e) {}
                    ServoProxy reader = new ServoProxy();
                }
            }
        }

        int port = 5555;
        // Main loop
        System.out.print("Press Control-C to end.\n");
        while(true)
        {
            try {
                // Create the server socket
                sSock = new ServerSocket(port);
                System.out.print("Listening on TCP/IP port " + port +
".\n");
                // Wait for a connection
                talkSock = sSock.accept();
                System.out.print("Client connected.\n");
                inNetData = talkSock.getInputStream();
                outNetData = talkSock.getOutputStream();
```

Table 11-13 Listing: ServoProxy.java *(continued)*

```
                while (talkSock.isConnected())
                {
                    bytesRead = inNetData.read(inBytes);
                    if (bytesRead < 0)
                        break;
                    outBytes = new byte[bytesRead];
                    for(int i=0; i<bytesRead; i++)
                        outBytes[i] = inBytes[i];
                    String s = new String(outBytes);
                    System.out.print("From Net Port: " + s + "\n");
                    if (talkSock.isConnected())
                        outCOMData.write(outBytes);
                }
                System.out.print("Client disconnected.\n");
            }
        catch (IOException e) { // If there is an error (namely the
client has abruptly ended the connection),
            try {                    // then we close both the server and talk
sockets on this end so that we can
                sSock.close();  // wait again for another connection
                talkSock.close();
            } catch (IOException ioerr) {System.err.println(ioerr);}
            }
        }
    } // end main

    public ServoProxy()
    {
        try {
            serialPort.addEventListener(this);
        } catch (TooManyListenersException e) {}
        serialPort.notifyOnDataAvailable(true);
        readThread = new Thread(this);
        readThread.start();
    }

    public void run() {}

    public void serialEvent(SerialPortEvent event)
    {
        switch(event.getEventType()) {
        case SerialPortEvent.BI:
        case SerialPortEvent.OE:
        case SerialPortEvent.FE:
        case SerialPortEvent.PE:
        case SerialPortEvent.CD:
        case SerialPortEvent.CTS:
        case SerialPortEvent.DSR:
        case SerialPortEvent.RI:
        case SerialPortEvent.OUTPUT_BUFFER_EMPTY:
            break;
        case SerialPortEvent.DATA_AVAILABLE:
            try {
                Thread.sleep(100);   // This is to wait until all data is
buffered on port before   read
            } catch (InterruptedException e) {}
            try {
                bytesRead = inCOMData.read(inBytes);
                if (bytesRead < 0)
                    break;
                outBytes = new byte[bytesRead];
                for(int i=0; i<bytesRead; i++)
                    outBytes[i] = inBytes[i];
                String s = new String(outBytes);
                System.out.print("From COM Port: " + s + "\n");
                outNetData.write(outBytes);
```

Table 11-13 Listing: ServoProxy.java *(continued)*

```
        } catch (IOException e) {System.err.println(e);}
            break;
        }
    }
}
```

In Chapter 7, I focused on analytical and computational methods for reducing and processing data. I will now detail several of these, the first being the chi-square probability distribution function, which is used to establish the likelihood that two data sets are drawn from the same distribution. Next, I will address the Haar Wavelet transform and I will provide details regarding matrix inversion. Finally, I provide the code related to a patented user interface for displaying findings in real time.

11.4 Chi-Square Probability Distribution

As I've already discussed the theory and application of the chi-square distribution function, I will not address it in more detail here, save to discuss the computational schema.

The method involves computing the incomplete Gamma function, $Q(\chi^2, N_{DOF})$, which is computed based on the values of chi-square and the number of degrees of freedom, N_{DOF}.

A method was developed that runs as a macro within Microsoft Excel. The listing is provided in Table 11-14 below.

Table 11-14 Listing: *chi_squared()*

```
Sub chi_squared()
'
'  chi_squared Macro
'  Macro recorded 1/12/2008 by JRZ
'
'  Based on an original method by John P. Pezzulo
'  http://statpages.org/JCPhome.html & http://statpages.org/pdfs.html
'
'  Implemented as a visual basic macro in Miscrosoft Excel
'
'  Based on an approximation presented in equation 26.6.15 of the
'  Handbook of Mathematical Functions by Abramowitz and Stegun.

ndof = Worksheets("FreqDist-Coarse").Cells(2, 25)
chsq = Worksheets("FreqDist-Coarse").Cells(2, 26)
Worksheets("FreqDist-Coarse").Cells(2, 27) = ChiSq(chsq, ndof)

End Sub
```

Table 11-14 Listing: *chi_squared() (continued)*

```
Function ChiSq(ByVal x As Double, ByVal n As Integer) As Double

    Dim pi As Double
    pi = 3.14159265358979
    Dim TINY As Double
    TINY = 0.000000000000001

    If x > 1000 Or n > 1000 Then
        Dim dummy1 As Double
        Dim dummy2 As Double
        Dim dummy3 As Double
        Dim q As Double

        dummy1 = (x / n) ^ (1 / 3) + 2 / (9 * n) - 1
        dummy2 = Sqr(2 / (9 * n))
        dummy3 = dummy1 / dummy2

        q = Norm(dummy3) / 2

        If x > n Then
            ChiSq = q
        End If
        If x <= n Then
            ChiSq = 1 - q
        End If
    Else

        Dim p As Double

        p = 0#
        p = Exp(-0.5 * x)

        If (n Mod 2) = 1 Then
            p = p * Sqr(2 * x / pi)
        End If

        Dim k As Integer

        k = n

        While k >= 2
            p = p * x / k
            k = k - 2
        Wend

        Dim t As Double
        Dim a As Double

        t = p
        a = n

        While t > TINY * p
            a = a + 2
            t = t * x / a
            p = p + t
        Wend

        ChiSq = 1 - p
    End If

End Function

Function Norm(ByVal z As Double) As Double

    Dim pi As Double
    pi = 3.1415926535
```

Table 11-14 Listing: *chi_squared() (continued)*

```
Dim q As Double
q = 0#

q = z * z

If Abs(z) > 7 Then
        Dim c1 As Double
        Dim c2 As Double
        Dim c3 As Double

        c1 = 1 - 1 / q + 3 / (q * q)
        c2 = Exp(-q / 2)
        c3 = Abs(z) * Sqr(pi() / 2)

        Norm = c1 * c2 / c3
    Else
        Norm = ChiSq(q, 1)
    End If

End Function
```

11.5 Matrix Inversion

Utilities for computing the inverse of a matrix are very useful in linear algebra, and especially in least square regression and wavelet transforms. The following method computes the inverse of a matrix. The method is completely self-contained. The function which computes the inverse is named *inverse().*[176]

I created a main calling program that can be used to test the matrix inversion method. The method itself requires two matrices for input and the number of rows (columns). The main program is below. Contained within this program are three methods:

   readDataFile(), inverse(), printMatrix()

The readDataFile method reads a Microsoft Excel .csv (comma separated file) from a local directory. A sample Microsoft Excel input file is shown in Table 11-15.

The data are read and the inverse is computed. Finally, the original matrix and its inverse are printed. Table 11-16 (minv.java) lists the computer program designed to read and compute the inverse of this matrix.

---

[176] Adapted from a method originally developed by Tao Pang, An Introduction to Computational Physics, Cambridge University Press, New York: 1997.

Table 11-15 *data.csv*

15	7	5	2	9
26	23	4	1	8
13	14.5	17.2	19.1	20.9
3.4	7.8	22	24.1	16.4
8.5	5.1	10.7	14.9	5.6

Command line compilation of the program is accomplished as follows:

```
javac minv.java
```

Command line execution is as follows:

```
java minv
```

Table 11-16 Listing: *minv.java*

```java
import java.awt.*;
import java.lang.Math;
import java.io.*;
import java.text.*;
import java.util.*;

public class minv
{
    public void initminv()
    {
        int maxRows = 5;
        double matrix[][] = new double[maxRows][maxRows];
        double matrixInv[][] = new double[maxRows][maxRows];
        int nRows = 0;

        nRows = readDataFile( matrix, maxRows );
        inverse( matrix, matrixInv, nRows );
        printMatrix( matrix, matrixInv, nRows );
    } // initminv

    // ************************************************************
    // readDataFile: read a .csv file containing the matrix
    //
    // parameter      dimension           description
    // -----------------------------------------------------------
    // mat            [nRows][nRows]      matrix
    // maxRows        int                 maximum number of rows
    //                                    and columns
    // ************************************************************

    public int readDataFile( double mat[][], int maxRows )
    {
        String  dataSegment = null;
        String line = null;
        int nRows = 0;
        int row = 0;
```

Table 11-16 Listing: *minv.java (continued)*

```
        int col = 0;

        try {
            File file = new File("data.csv");
            BufferedReader bufRdr  = new BufferedReader(new
FileReader(file));

            // read each line of text file

            while((line = bufRdr.readLine()) != null)
            {
                StringTokenizer st = new StringTokenizer(line,",");
                col = 0;
                while (st.hasMoreTokens())
                {
                    // get next token and store it in the array

                    mat[row][col] = Double.parseDouble(st.nextToken());
                    System.out.print( mat[row][col] + " " );
                    col++;
                }
                System.out.println();
                row++;
            }

            // close file

            bufRdr.close();

            nRows = row;
            System.out.println( "nRows = " + nRows );

        } catch ( Exception ioe ) {
            System.err.println( "All Data Read... " + ioe );
        } // End try
        return nRows;
    }


    // ****************************************************************
    // printMatrix: Print matrix and inverse
    //
    // parameter      dimension              description
    // ----------------------------------------------------------------
    // mat            [nRows][nRows]         original matrix
    // matInv         [nRows][nRows]         matrix inverse
    // nRows          int                    number of rows and columns
    // ****************************************************************
    public void printMatrix( double mat[][], double matinv[][], int nRows
)
    {
        System.out.println( "===============Data=================" );

        //
        // Specify the number formatting parameter to print out
        // numbered axes on plot.
        //

        NumberFormat nf = NumberFormat.getNumberInstance();
        nf.setMinimumFractionDigits(6);
        String NumberString;

        nf.setMinimumFractionDigits(2);

        System.out.println( "Matrix" );
        for ( int i = 0; i < nRows; ++i )
```

Table 11-16 Listing: *minv.java (continued)*

```
        {
            for ( int j = 0; j < nRows; ++j )
            {
                NumberString = nf.format( mat[i][j] );
                System.out.print( NumberString + "    " );
            }
            System.out.println();
        }

        System.out.println( "Inverted Matrix" );
        for ( int i = 0; i < nRows; ++i )
        {
            for ( int j = 0; j < nRows; ++j )
            {
                NumberString = nf.format( matinv[i][j] );
                System.out.print( NumberString + "    " );
            }
            System.out.println();
        }
    }

    //
    ****************************************************************
    // inverse: Print matrix and inverse
    //
    // parameter      dimension              description
    // -----------------------------------------------------------
    // a              [n][n]                 original matrix
    // x              [n][n]                 matrix inverse
    // n              int                    number of rows and columns
    //
    // Based on original version in C written by Tao Pang dated 10/24/
2001.
    //
    // Book Title: An Introduction to Computational Physics
    // Author: Tao Pang
    // Publisher: Cambridge University Press
    // New York.
    // September, 1997
    // ISBN's: 0-521-48143-0 (hardback); 0-521-48592-4 (paperback)
    //
    //
    ****************************************************************
    public void inverse( double a[][], double x[][], int n )
    {
        static int NMAX = 100;
        double b[][] = new double[NMAX][NMAX];
        double c[]   = new double[NMAX];
        int indx[]   = new int[NMAX];
        int i, j, k, itmp;
        double c1, pi, pi1, pj;

        if ( n > NMAX ) n = NMAX;

        for ( i = 0; i < n; ++i )
        {
            for ( j = 0; j < n; ++j )
            {
                b[i][j] = 0;
            }
        }

        for ( i = 0; i < n; ++i )
        {
            b[i][i] = 1;
        }
```

Table 11-16 Listing: *minv.java (continued)*

```
// Initialize the index

for ( i = 0; i < n; ++i )
{
    indx[i] = i;
}

// Find the rescaling factors, one from each row

for ( i = 0; i < n; ++i )
{
    c1 = 0;
    for ( j = 0; j < n; ++j )
    {
        if ( Math.abs(a[i][j]) > c1 ) c1 = Math.abs(a[i][j]);
    }
    c[i] = c1;
}

// Search the pivoting (largest) element from each column

for ( j = 0; j < n-1; ++j )
{
    pi1 = 0;
    k = 0; // Added by me to address initialization error
    for ( i = j; i < n; ++i )
    {
        pi = Math.abs(a[indx[i]][j])/c[indx[i]];
        if (pi > pi1)
        {
            pi1 = pi;
            k = i;
        }
    }

    // Interchange the rows via indx[] to record pivoting order

    itmp = indx[j];
    indx[j] = indx[k];
    indx[k] = itmp;

    for ( i = j+1; i < n; ++i )
    {
        pj = a[indx[i]][j]/a[indx[j]][j];

        // Record pivoting ratios below diagonal

        a[indx[i]][j] = pj;

        // Modify other elements accordingly

        for ( k = j+1; k < n; ++k )
        {
            a[indx[i]][k] = a[indx[i]][k] - pj*a[indx[j]][k];
        } // end for k
    } // end for i
} // end for j

// Completed.

for ( i = 0; i < n-1; ++i )
{
    for ( j = i+1; j < n; ++j )
    {
        for ( k = 0; k < n; ++k )
```

Table 11-16 Listing: *minv.java (continued)*

```
                {
                    b[indx[j]][k] = b[indx[j]][k] -
                                    a[indx[j]][i]*b[indx[i]][k];
                }
            }
        }

        for ( i = 0; i < n; ++i )
        {
            x[n-1][i] = b[indx[n-1]][i]/a[indx[n-1]][n-1];
            for ( j = n-2; j >= 0; j = j - 1)
            {
                x[j][i] = b[indx[j]][i];
                for ( k = j+1; k < n; ++k )
                {
                    x[j][i] = x[j][i] - a[indx[j]][k]*x[k][i];
                }
                x[j][i] = x[j][i] / a[indx[j]][j];
            }
        }
    } // End Inverse

    public static void main( String args[] )
    {
        minv m = new minv();
        m.initminv();
    } // End main
} // End minv()
```

11.6 Haar Wavelet Transform

The program now discussed performs a Haar wavelet transform on one-dimensional data. The one-dimensional transform can be used in such applications as time-series analysis. This differs from image-type analysis primarily in that wavelet transforms of images require two dimensions. A simple program that computes the two-dimensional Haar matrix is listed in Table 11-17. The method that computes the coefficients is labeled WTrans2D. This program creates a Haar matrix and prints to screen.

Table 11-17 Listing: *WTrans2D.java*

```
import java.awt.*;
import java.lang.Math;
import java.io.*;
import java.text.*;
import java.util.*;

public class WTrans2D
{
//----------------------------------------------------------------
--------
    // ****************************************************************
    // computeHaar: Call method to make and print Haar matrix
```

Table 11-17 Listing: *WTrans2D.java (continued)*

```
    //
    // parameter     dimension          description
    // --------------------------------------------------------------
    // mat           [nRows][nRows]     matrix to be printed
    // nRows         int                number of rows
    // nCols         int                number of columns
    // **************************************************************
  public void computeHaar()
  {
      int maxRows = 8;
      int maxCols = 8;
      double[][] HaarMatrix = new double[maxRows][maxCols];
      HaarMatrix = Make2DHaar( maxRows, maxCols );
      printMatrix( HaarMatrix, maxRows, maxCols );
  } // end computeHaar

//-----------------------------------------------------------------------
--------
    // **************************************************************
    // Make2DHaar: Compute Haar transform matrix
    //
    // Based originally on a method by R.G. Baldwin, Copyright 2004
    // Modified by J. Zaleski, April 2008.
    //
    // parameter           dimension        description
    // --------------------------------------------------------------
    // DummyMatrix         [nRows][nRows]   Working matrix
    // HaarMatrixTranspose [nRows][nCols]   Haar matrix-transposed
    // nRows               int              number of matrix rows
    // nCols               int              number of matrix columns
    // halfnRows           int              nRows / 2
    // halfnCols           int              nCols / 2
    // fillColumn          int              defines columns to be
    //                                      written
    // **************************************************************
  public double[][] Make2DHaar( int nRows, int nCols )
  {
      double[][] DummyMatrix = new double[nRows][nCols];
      double[][] HaarMatrixTranspose = new double[nRows][nCols];
      double[][] HaarMatrix = new double[nRows][nCols];

      //**************************************************
      // Fill first half of columns in DummyMatrix
      //**************************************************

  int halfnRows = nRows/2;
  int halfnCols = nCols/2;
  int fillColumn = 0;

      for ( int i = 0; i < nRows; i+=2 ) {
      for ( int j = 0; j < halfnCols; j++ ) {
      if ( j == fillColumn ) {
          DummyMatrix[i][j] = 1.0;
          DummyMatrix[i+1][j] = 1.0;
  } else
      {
  DummyMatrix[i][j] = 0.0;
}
  // end for j (column)
  fillColumn = fillColumn + 1;
  // end for i (row)

      //**************************************************
      // Fill remaining half of columns in DummyMatrix
      //**************************************************
```

283

Table 11-17 Listing: *WTrans2D.java (continued)*

```
            fillColumn = halfnCols;

            for ( int i = 0; i < nRows; i+=2 ) {
                for ( int j = halfnCols; j < nCols; j++ ) {
                    if ( j == fillColumn ) {
                        DummyMatrix[i][j] = -1.0;
                        DummyMatrix[i+1][j] = 1.0;
            } else
{

        DummyMatrix[i][j] = 0.0;
        }
        // end for j (column)
        fillColumn = fillColumn + 1;
        // end for i (row)

        //**************************************************
        // Scale by sqrt(2)/2 in order to make the
        // W-transpose matrix orthogonal
        //**************************************************

        double scaleFactor = Math.sqrt(2.0) / 2.0;
        for ( int i = 0; i < nRows; i++ )
        {
            for ( int j = 0; j < nCols; j++ )
            {
                HaarMatrixTranspose[i][j] = scaleFactor * DummyMa-
trix[i][j];
            }
        }

        //**************************************************
        // Transpose
        //**************************************************

        for ( int i = 0; i < nRows; i++ )
        {
            for ( int j = 0; j < nCols; j++ )
            {
                HaarMatrix[i][j] = HaarMatrixTranspose[j][i];
            }
        }
        return HaarMatrix;
        //end Make2DHaar
    //----------------------------------------------------------------
    // ************************************************************
    // printMatrix: Print matrix
    //
    // parameter      dimension            description
    // ----------------------------------------------------------------
    // mat            [nRows][nRows]       matrix to be printed
    // nRows          int                  number of rows
    // nCols          int                  number of columns
    // ************************************************************
    public void printMatrix( double mat[][], int nRows, int nCols )
    {
      System.out.println( "=================Data==================" );

        //
        // Specify the number formatting parameter to print out
        // numbered axes on plot.
        //

        NumberFormat nf = NumberFormat.getNumberInstance();
        nf.setMinimumFractionDigits(9);
        String NumberString;
```

Table 11-17 Listing: *WTrans2D.java (continued)*

```
        nf.setMinimumFractionDigits(3);

        System.out.println( "Matrix" );
        for ( int i = 0; i < nRows; ++i )
        {
            for ( int j = 0; j < nCols; ++j )
            {
                NumberString = nf.format( mat[i][j] );
                System.out.print( NumberString + "   " );
            }
            System.out.println();
        }
    } // end printMatrix

//------------------------------------------------------------------------
--------
    public static void main( String args[] )
        {
        WTrans2D wt = new WTrans2D();
        wt.computeHaar();
    }
} // End WTrans2D
```

The Haar transform method reads a Microsoft Access database. A sample screen snapshot of this is provided in Table 11-18:

Table 11-18 HaarXform.mdb

data

ID	MRN	Hour	Minute	Second	Data
1	400490	11	9	0	2
2	400490	11	11	0	5
3	400490	11	13	0	8
4	400490	11	15	0	9
5	400490	11	17	0	7
6	400490	11	19	0	4
7	400490	11	21	0	-1
8	400490	11	23	0	1

The table contains several columns, the most important of these is the Data column. The medical record number column (MRN) and those corresponding to Hour, Minute, and Second can be consolidated or eliminated altogether by the user upon redesign or alteration of the method.

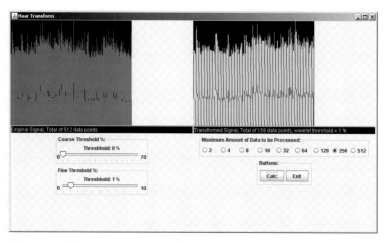

Figure 11-3 HaarXform user interface

A screen snapshot of the user interface is provided in Figure 11-3. The user can specify the number of coefficients to be used in signal reconstruction using two sliders (a coarse and fine selection). These are used to define the threshold—in percentage of the maximum coefficient value—below which the Haar coefficients are not used for reconstruction. The plot on the left of the figure represents the original data. The plot on the right is the reconstructed set. The user can select the amount of data to be used in reconstruction up to 512 data points. Note that the Haar transform operates in even incremental factors of two. This is the reason why buttons are supplied with which to select multiples of two.

The program consists of three separate java files, listed in Table 11-19 (HaarXform.java—main program), Table 11-20 (DataPlotter.java), and Table 11-21 (ReconPlotter.java). DataPlotter.java plots or graphs the original data. ReconPlotter.java plots or graphs the reconstructed data after wavelet coefficient amplitude coefficients are applied to the transformed data and then re-transformed back to the time domain.

Command line compilation is as follows:

```
javac HaarXform.java DataPlotter.java
    ReconPlotter.java
```

Command line execution is as follows:

```
java HaarXform
```

286

Table 11-19 Listing: *HaarXform.java*

```
import javax.comm.*;
import javax.imageio.ImageIO;
import javax.swing.*;
import javax.swing.AbstractButton;
import javax.swing.border.*;
import javax.swing.ButtonModel;
import javax.swing.JCheckBox;
import javax.swing.JFrame;
import javax.swing.event.*;
import javax.swing.event.ChangeEvent;
import javax.swing.event.ChangeListener;
import javax.swing.plaf.*;
import javax.swing.text.NumberFormatter;
import javax.swing.Timer;

import java.sql.*;
import java.sql.Connection;
import java.sql.DriverManager;
import java.sql.SQLException;


import java.applet.*;
import java.awt.*;
import java.awt.BorderLayout;
import java.awt.Color;
import java.awt.Container;
import java.awt.event.*;
import java.awt.event.ActionEvent;
import java.awt.event.ActionListener;
import java.awt.event.ItemEvent;
import java.awt.event.ItemListener;
import java.awt.event.KeyEvent;
import java.awt.Graphics;
import java.awt.Image;
import java.awt.List;
import java.awt.Scrollbar;
import java.awt.Toolkit;
import java.io.*;
import java.io.BufferedInputStream;
import java.lang.*;
import java.lang.Math;
import java.lang.Thread;
import java.net.*;
import java.net.URL;
import java.text.*;
import java.text.DecimalFormat;
import java.util.Date;
import java.util.GregorianCalendar;
import java.util.Properties;
import java.util.Vector;

import javax.swing.border.*;
import javax.swing.event.*;
import javax.swing.JInternalFrame;
import javax.swing.JDesktopPane;
import javax.swing.JMenu;
import javax.swing.JMenuItem;
import javax.swing.JMenuBar;
import javax.swing.JFrame;
import javax.swing.KeyStroke;

import java.util.Hashtable;

// ****************************************************************
// HaarXform.java
//
```

Table 11-19 Listing: *HaarXform.java (continued)*

```
// Author: J. Zaleski
//
// Computes the 1-D Haar transform of time series data.
//

public class HaarXform extends JPanel
{
    String url = "jdbc:odbc:HaarXform";
    Connection conn = null;
    Statement st = null;
    ResultSet rec = null;
    private DefaultListModel listModel1;
    private DefaultListModel listModel2;
    JButton exitB;
    JButton startB;
    JButton stopB;
    JButton calcB;
    double[] rawData = new double[ 1600 ];
    int rawDataCount;
    double[] reconData = new double[ 1600 ];
    int reconDataCount;
    JRadioButton rad2;
    JRadioButton rad4;
    JRadioButton rad8;
    JRadioButton rad16;
    JRadioButton rad32;
    JRadioButton rad64;
    JRadioButton rad128;
    JRadioButton rad256;
    JRadioButton rad512;
    public static int panelWidth = 915;
    public static int panelHeight = 480;
    public static int plotWidth = 300;
    public static int plotHeight = 300;
    public int DEFAULT_SLEEP_TIME = 10;
    public int DEFAULT_DATA_COUNT = 256;
    public TextField outputFileTF;
    public TextField coeffsFileTF;
    public TextField sliderTF;
    public String DEFAULT_OUTPUT_FILE = "..\\output\\haaroutput.txt";
    public String DEFAULT_COEFFS_FILE = "..\\output\\haarcoeffs.txt";
    JTextField originalSignalField;
    JTextField transformedSignalField;
    public int totalSignalThreshold;
    public int totalSignalCoefficients;
    public DataPlotter dataPlotter;
    public ReconPlotter reconPlotter;
    JDesktopPane desktop;

    /* Width of the window */

    public static int maxWidth = 915;
    public static int maxHeight = 530;

    /* Window location */

    public static int    xLocation = 20;
    public static int    yLocation = 0;
    public JSlider        pSlider_fine;
    public int            DEFAULT_PCT_fine = 0;
    public int            minValue_fine = 0;
    public int            maxValue_fine = 10;
    public int            majorStep_fine = 5;
    public int            minorStep_fine = 1;
    public JLabel         vLabel_fine;
    public JSlider        pSlider_coarse;
```

Table 11-19 Listing: *HaarXform.java (continued)*

```
    public int          DEFAULT_PCT_coarse = 0;
    public int          minValue_coarse = 0;
    public int          maxValue_coarse = 70;
    public intmajorStep_coarse = 10;
    public int          minorStep_coarse = 5;
    public JLabel        vLabel_coarse;


    // ************************************************
    // HaarXform
    //
    // Creates UI, reads data, etc.
    //
    // ************************************************
    public HaarXform()
    {
        MakeJDBConnection( url );
        rawDataCount = getParms( rawData );
        CloseJDBConnection();

        System.out.println( " Amount of raw data: " + rawDataCount );
        dataPlotter = new DataPlotter( plotWidth, plotHeight, rawData-
Count, rawData );
        initHaarXform( rawData, rawDataCount );
        reconPlotter = new ReconPlotter( plotWidth, plotHeight, recon-
DataCount, reconData );

        originalSignalField = new JTextField();
        originalSignalField.setBackground( Color.black );
        originalSignalField.setForeground( Color.cyan );
        originalSignalField.setText("Original Signal, Total of " +
rawDataCount + " data points" );

        transformedSignalField = new JTextField();
        transformedSignalField.setBackground( Color.black );
        transformedSignalField.setForeground( Color.green );
        transformedSignalField.setText(" Transformed Signal, Total of "
+ totalSignalCoefficients +
                                " data points, wavelet threshold
= " + totalSignalThreshold + " %" );

        //
        // Calc, Exit buttons
        //

        calcB = new JButton("Calc");
        startB = new JButton("Start");
        stopB = new JButton("Stop");
        exitB  = new JButton("Exit");

        //
        // Actionlisteners for buttons
        //

        startB.addActionListener( new ActionListener() {
            public void actionPerformed( ActionEvent e1 ) {
                Thread originalThread = new Thread( dataPlotter, "Signal
Plotter");
                originalThread.start();
            }
        });

        stopB.addActionListener( new ActionListener() {
            public void actionPerformed( ActionEvent e2 ) {
                dataPlotter.stopClock();
                reconPlotter.stopClock();
```

Table 11-19 Listing: *HaarXform.java (continued)*

```
            }
        });

        exitB.addActionListener( new ActionListener() {
            public void actionPerformed( ActionEvent e3 ) {
                System.exit(0);
            }
        });

        calcB.addActionListener( new ActionListener() {
            public void actionPerformed( ActionEvent e3 ) {
                Thread reconThread = new Thread( reconPlotter,
"Reconstructed Signal");
                reconThread.start();
                initHaarXform( rawData, rawDataCount );
                reconPlotter.updatePlot( reconDataCount, reconData );
                transformedSignalField.setText(" Transformed Signal,
Total of " +
                            totalSignalCoefficients +
                            " data points, wavelet threshold = " +
                            totalSignalThreshold + " %" );
            }
        });

        //--------------------
        // Font metrics
        //--------------------

        String fontName = "Arial";
        int type = Font.BOLD;
        int size = 10;
        Font font;
        FontMetrics fm;
        font = new Font( fontName, type, size );

        //-----------------------------------------------------
        // Build percentage change slider -- fine adjustment
        //-----------------------------------------------------

        pSlider_fine = new JSlider(minValue_fine,
                            maxValue_fine,
                            DEFAULT_PCT_fine );

        pSlider_fine.setMajorTickSpacing( majorStep_fine );
        pSlider_fine.setMinorTickSpacing( minorStep_fine );
        pSlider_fine.setSnapToTicks( true );
        pSlider_fine.setPaintTicks( true );
        pSlider_fine.addChangeListener( new ChangeListener() {
            public void stateChanged( ChangeEvent evt ) {
                int value_fine = 0;
                value_fine = pSlider_fine.getValue();
                vLabel_fine.setText( "Threshhold: " + value_fine + " %" );
                DEFAULT_PCT_fine = pSlider_fine.getValue();
            }
        });

        JLabel minLabel_fine = new JLabel( ""+minValue_fine );
        JLabel maxLabel_fine = new JLabel( ""+maxValue_fine );
        vLabel_fine = new JLabel( "Threshhold: "+DEFAULT_PCT_fine + " %"
);
        vLabel_fine.setHorizontalAlignment( JLabel.CENTER );

        //-----------------------------------------------------
        // Build percentage change slider -- coarse adjustment
        //-----------------------------------------------------
```

Table 11-19 Listing: *HaarXform.java (continued)*

```
        pSlider_coarse = new JSlider( minValue_coarse,
                                      maxValue_coarse,
                                      DEFAULT_PCT_coarse );

        pSlider_coarse.setMajorTickSpacing( majorStep_coarse );
        pSlider_coarse.setMinorTickSpacing( minorStep_coarse );
        pSlider_coarse.setSnapToTicks( true );
        pSlider_coarse.setPaintTicks( true );
        pSlider_coarse.addChangeListener( new ChangeListener() {
        public void stateChanged( ChangeEvent evt ) {
            int value_coarse = 0;
            value_coarse = pSlider_coarse.getValue();
          vLabel_coarse.setText( "Threshhold: " + value_coarse + " %" );
            DEFAULT_PCT_coarse = pSlider_coarse.getValue();
        }
        });

        JLabel minLabel_coarse = new JLabel( ""+minValue_coarse );
        JLabel maxLabel_coarse = new JLabel( ""+maxValue_coarse );
        vLabel_coarse = new JLabel( "Threshhold: "+DEFAULT_PCT_coarse +
" %" );
        vLabel_coarse.setHorizontalAlignment( JLabel.CENTER );

        // FINE SLIDER PANEL

        JPanel sliderPanel_fine = new JPanel( new BorderLayout() );
        Border finesliderPanelBorder = BorderFactory.createTitledBorder(
"Fine Threshold %:" );
        sliderPanel_fine.setBorder( finesliderPanelBorder );
        sliderPanel_fine.add( minLabel_fine, BorderLayout.WEST );
        sliderPanel_fine.add( maxLabel_fine, BorderLayout.EAST );
        sliderPanel_fine.add( pSlider_fine, BorderLayout.CENTER);
        sliderPanel_fine.add( vLabel_fine, BorderLayout.NORTH );

        // COARSE SLIDER PANEL

        JPanel sliderPanel_coarse = new JPanel( new BorderLayout() );
        Border coarsesliderPanelBorder = BorderFactory.createTitledBor-
der( "Coarse Threshold %:" );
        sliderPanel_coarse.setBorder( coarsesliderPanelBorder );
        sliderPanel_coarse.add( minLabel_coarse, BorderLayout.WEST );
        sliderPanel_coarse.add( maxLabel_coarse, BorderLayout.EAST );
        sliderPanel_coarse.add( pSlider_coarse, BorderLayout.CENTER);
        sliderPanel_coarse.add( vLabel_coarse, BorderLayout.NORTH );


        // Button Panel

        JPanel buttonP = new JPanel();
        buttonP.setLayout( new FlowLayout() );
        Border buttonPanelBorder = BorderFactory.createTitledBorder(
"Buttons:" );
        buttonP.setBorder( buttonPanelBorder );
        buttonP.add( calcB );
        buttonP.add( exitB );

        //--------------------------------------
        // Coefficient Selection Radio Buttons
        //--------------------------------------

        rad2 = new JRadioButton("2");
        rad2.setMnemonic(KeyEvent.VK_A);
        rad2.setActionCommand("2");
        rad2.setSelected(false);
```

Table 11-19 Listing: *HaarXform.java (continued)*

```
rad4 = new JRadioButton("4");
rad4.setMnemonic(KeyEvent.VK_B);
rad4.setActionCommand("4");
rad4.setSelected(false);

rad8 = new JRadioButton("8");
rad8.setMnemonic(KeyEvent.VK_C);
rad8.setActionCommand("8");
rad8.setSelected(false);

rad16 = new JRadioButton("16");
rad16.setMnemonic(KeyEvent.VK_D);
rad16.setActionCommand("16");
rad16.setSelected(false);

rad32 = new JRadioButton("32");
rad32.setMnemonic(KeyEvent.VK_E);
rad32.setActionCommand("32");
rad32.setSelected(false);

rad64 = new JRadioButton("64");
rad64.setMnemonic(KeyEvent.VK_F);
rad64.setActionCommand("64");
rad64.setSelected(false);

rad128 = new JRadioButton("128");
rad128.setMnemonic(KeyEvent.VK_G);
rad128.setActionCommand("128");
rad128.setSelected(false);

rad256 = new JRadioButton("256");
rad256.setMnemonic(KeyEvent.VK_G);
rad256.setActionCommand("256");
rad256.setSelected(true);

rad512 = new JRadioButton("512");
rad512.setMnemonic(KeyEvent.VK_H);
rad512.setActionCommand("512");
rad512.setSelected(false);

// Group the radio buttons

ButtonGroup radioGroup = new ButtonGroup();
radioGroup.add(rad2);
radioGroup.add(rad4);
radioGroup.add(rad8);
radioGroup.add(rad16);
radioGroup.add(rad32);
radioGroup.add(rad64);
radioGroup.add(rad128);
radioGroup.add(rad256);
radioGroup.add(rad512);

// Register action listeners

rad2.addActionListener( new ActionListener() {
    public void actionPerformed( ActionEvent e ) {
        String dummy = e.getActionCommand();
        DEFAULT_DATA_COUNT = Integer.valueOf( dummy ).intValue();
    }
});

rad4.addActionListener( new ActionListener() {
    public void actionPerformed( ActionEvent e ) {
        String dummy = e.getActionCommand();
        DEFAULT_DATA_COUNT = Integer.valueOf( dummy ).intValue();
```

Table 11-19 Listing: *HaarXform.java (continued)*

```
            }
    });

    rad8.addActionListener( new ActionListener() {
        public void actionPerformed( ActionEvent e ) {
            String dummy = e.getActionCommand();
            DEFAULT_DATA_COUNT = Integer.valueOf( dummy ).intValue();
        }
    });

    rad16.addActionListener( new ActionListener() {
        public void actionPerformed( ActionEvent e ) {
            String dummy = e.getActionCommand();
            DEFAULT_DATA_COUNT = Integer.valueOf( dummy ).intValue();
        }
    });

    rad32.addActionListener( new ActionListener() {
        public void actionPerformed( ActionEvent e ) {
            String dummy = e.getActionCommand();
            DEFAULT_DATA_COUNT = Integer.valueOf( dummy ).intValue();
        }
    });

    rad64.addActionListener( new ActionListener() {
        public void actionPerformed( ActionEvent e ) {
            String dummy = e.getActionCommand();
            DEFAULT_DATA_COUNT = Integer.valueOf( dummy ).intValue();
        }
    });

    rad128.addActionListener( new ActionListener() {
        public void actionPerformed( ActionEvent e ) {
            String dummy = e.getActionCommand();
            DEFAULT_DATA_COUNT = Integer.valueOf( dummy ).intValue();
        }
    });

    rad256.addActionListener( new ActionListener() {
        public void actionPerformed( ActionEvent e ) {
            String dummy = e.getActionCommand();
            DEFAULT_DATA_COUNT = Integer.valueOf( dummy ).intValue();
        }
    });

    rad512.addActionListener( new ActionListener() {
        public void actionPerformed( ActionEvent e ) {
            String dummy = e.getActionCommand();
            DEFAULT_DATA_COUNT = Integer.valueOf( dummy ).intValue();
        }
    });

    //----------------------------------------
    // Radio Group pane
    //----------------------------------------

    JPanel radioPanel = new JPanel();
    radioPanel.setLayout( new GridLayout(1,9) );
    Border radioPanelBorder = BorderFactory.createTitledBorder(
"Maximum Amount of Data to be Processed:" );
    radioPanel.setBorder( radioPanelBorder );
    radioPanel.add(rad2);
    radioPanel.add(rad4);
    radioPanel.add(rad8);
    radioPanel.add(rad16);
    radioPanel.add(rad32);
```

293

Table 11-19 Listing: *HaarXform.java (continued)*

```
      radioPanel.add(rad64);
      radioPanel.add(rad128);
      radioPanel.add(rad256);
      radioPanel.add(rad512);

      //-------------------------------------------
      // Content pane
      //-------------------------------------------

      this.setLayout( new GridLayout(2,2) );

      JPanel leftPanel = new JPanel();
      leftPanel.setLayout( new FlowLayout() );
      leftPanel.add( sliderPanel_coarse );
      leftPanel.add( sliderPanel_fine );

      JPanel rightPanel = new JPanel();
      rightPanel.setLayout( new FlowLayout() );
      rightPanel.add( radioPanel );
      rightPanel.add( buttonP );

      dataPlotter.setSize( plotWidth, plotHeight );
      reconPlotter.setSize( plotWidth, plotHeight );

      this.add( dataPlotter );
      this.add( reconPlotter );

      JPanel leftField = new JPanel();
      leftField.setLayout( new BorderLayout() );
      leftField.add( originalSignalField, BorderLayout.NORTH );
      leftField.add( leftPanel, BorderLayout.CENTER );

      this.add( leftField );

      JPanel rightField = new JPanel();
      rightField.setLayout( new BorderLayout() );
      rightField.add( transformedSignalField, BorderLayout.NORTH );
      rightField.add( rightPanel, BorderLayout.CENTER );

      this.add( rightField );

  } // End go()

// ****************************************************************
//
// adjustmenValueChanged method to detect adjustments in
// windows.
//
// ****************************************************************
public void adjustmentValueChanged ( AdjustmentEvent event )
{
    this.update();
} // End actionPerformed()

// ****************************************************************
//
// update method updates the user interface window
//
// ****************************************************************
protected void update() {}

// ****************************************************************
//
// initialize public method for accomplishing tasks
// that need to be done once at the beginning of
// execution.
```

Table 11-19 Listing: *HaarXform.java (continued)*

```
//
// ****************************************************************
public void Initialize() throws IOException {}

// ****************************************************************
//
// Make a database connection
//
// ****************************************************************
public void MakeJDBConnection( String path )
{
try {
Class.forName("sun.jdbc.odbc.JdbcOdbcDriver");
String uname = "";
String pword = "";
conn = DriverManager.getConnection( path, uname, pword );
            st = conn.createStatement();
        } catch( Exception e ) {
        //   System.out.println( "***Error making connection***" );
        //   System.out.println( "MakeJDBConnection " + e );
        }
    } // End MakeJDBConnection()

    // ****************************************************************
    // Close a database connection
    // ****************************************************************
    public void CloseJDBConnection()
    {
        try {
            conn.close();
            st.close();
        } catch ( Exception e ) { System.err.println( "***cannot close
JDBC*** " + e );}
    }

    // ****************************************************************
    //
    // Retrieve time-series data from database
    //
    // ****************************************************************
    public int getParms( double [] rd )
    {
        int dataCounter = 0;
        ResultSetMetaData rsmd = null;
        int numberOfColumns = 0;
        String[] colNames;
        double columnValue;

        try
        {
            rec = st.executeQuery( "SELECT * FROM data" );
            rsmd = rec.getMetaData();
            numberOfColumns = rsmd.getColumnCount();
            colNames = new String[ rsmd.getColumnCount() ];

            for ( int col = 0; col < colNames.length; col++ )
            {
                colNames[col] = rsmd.getColumnName(col + 1);
            }

            while(rec.next())
            {
                for (int i = 0; i < numberOfColumns; i++)
                {
                    if ( colNames[i].equals("Data") == true )
                    {
```

295

Table 11-19 Listing: *HaarXform.java (continued)*

```
                        columnValue = rec.getDouble(i+1);
                        rd[dataCounter] = columnValue;
                        dataCounter++;
                  } // End if
             } // End for
        } // End While
    } catch( Exception e ) {
        System.err.println( "***Error in getParms()*** " + e );
    }

    return dataCounter;

} // End getParms()


// ****************************************************************
//
// Initialize and process the Haar DWT
//
// ****************************************************************
public void initHaarxform( double[] f, int nRawRows )
{
    double H[][] = new double[600][600];
    double Hraw[][] = new double[600][600];
    double Hinv[][] = new double[600][600];
    double f1[] = new double[600];
    double b[] = new double[600];
    boolean used[] = new boolean[600];
    String dataSegment = null;
    int index0;
    int index1;
    int indexComma;
    int indexSpace;
    int nRows = 0;
    int nCols = 0;
    int Ncoeffs = DEFAULT_DATA_COUNT;
    int maxExpPower = 15;

    //
    // Set number of rows/columns
    //

    nRows = nRawRows;

    if ( nRows > DEFAULT_DATA_COUNT )
    {
        nRows = DEFAULT_DATA_COUNT;
    }
    nCols = nRows;

    for ( int expPower = 0; expPower < maxExpPower; expPower++ )
    {
        if ( nRows >= Math.pow(2, expPower) & nRows < Math.pow(2,
expPower+1) )
        {
            nRows = (int) Math.pow(2,expPower);
        }
    }

    //
    // Specify the number formatting parameter to print out
    // numbered axes on plot.
    //

    NumberFormat nf = NumberFormat.getNumberInstance();
    nf.setMinimumFractionDigits(6);
```

Table 11-19 Listing: *HaarXform.java (continued)*

```
        String NumberString;
        nf.setMinimumFractionDigits(2);

        //
        // Create the Haar matrix
        //

        makeHaar(H, nRows );

        //
        // Before inverting, copy H to Hraw. H is destroyed during
        // inversion process.
        //

        matcopy( H, Hraw, nRows, nCols );

        //
        // Now invert the H matrix; Hinv contains the inverse, and H
        // is destroyed in the process.
        //

        inverse( H, Hinv, nRows );

        //
        // b = H^(-1)f, where f = vector of signal data;
        //
        // H is Haar matrix;
        //
        // b = vector of wavelet coefficients
        //

        for ( int k = 0; k < nRows; k++ ) used[k] = true;

        mult( b, Hinv, f, nRows, nCols, used );

        //
        // Filter the coefficients...
        //
        // Any coefficient that is > (DEFAULT_PCT_fine +
DEFAULT_PCT_coarse) * bmax / 100, assign to zero.
        //

        filter( b, used, nRows );

        //============================================================
        // Recreate and print the data from the DWT coefficients
        //============================================================

        try {
            PrintWriter out1 = new PrintWriter(new FileOutput-
Stream(DEFAULT_OUTPUT_FILE));
            PrintWriter out2 = new PrintWriter(new FileOutput-
Stream(DEFAULT_COEFFS_FILE));

            mult( f1, Hraw, b, nRows, Ncoeffs, used );

            int useableCoeffs = 0;
            for ( int k = 0; k < nRows; k++ )
            {
              if ( used[k] == true ) useableCoeffs = useableCoeffs + 1;
            }

            int total_threshold = DEFAULT_PCT_fine + DEFAULT_PCT_coarse;

            totalSignalThreshold = total_threshold;
            totalSignalCoefficients = useableCoeffs;
```

Table 11-19 Listing: *HaarXform.java (continued)*

```
          out1.println( "Reconstructed Signal, " + useableCoeffs + "
Data Points, " + total_threshold + "% DWT Threshhold" );
          reconDataCount = nRows;
          for ( int k = 0; k < nRows; ++k )
          {
              NumberString = nf.format( f1[k] );
              reconData[k] = f1[k];
              out1.println( NumberString );
          }

          out2.println( "Wavelet Coefficients " + total_threshold +
"% Threshhold" );
          for ( int k = 0; k < nRows; ++k )
          {
          if ( used[k] == true )
              {
                  NumberString = nf.format( b[k] );
                  out2.println( NumberString );
              }
              else
              {
                  NumberString = "0.0";
                  out2.println( NumberString );
              }
          }

          out1.close(); out2.close();

      } catch ( IOException ioe ) {
          System.err.println( "***Error writing to file: " + ioe );
      } // End try-catch block
  } // initHaarXform


    //
************************************************************************
    //
    // filter
    //
    // Removes coefficients from calculation based on coarse & fine
    // threshold settings.
    //
    //
************************************************************************
    public void filter( double b[], boolean used[], int Nr )
    {
        double zero = 0.0;
        double bmax = 0.0;
        double rlpct = 0.0;

        for ( int i = 0; i < Nr; i++ )
        {
            if ( b[i] > bmax ) bmax = b[i];
        }

      if ( bmax > 0.0 ) rlpct = (DEFAULT_PCT_fine + DEFAULT_PCT_coarse)
* bmax / 100.0;

        for ( int j = 0; j < Nr; j++ )
        {
            double value = Math.abs(b[j]);
            if ( value >= zero && value < rlpct )
            {
                used[j] = false;
```

Table 11-19 Listing: *HaarXform.java (continued)*

```
        }
      }
    } // End filter()


    //
    //*********************************************************************
    //
    // matcopy
    //
    // Copies a matrix from one array variable to another.
    //
    //
    //*********************************************************************
    public void matcopy( double a[][], double b[][], int Nr, int Nc )
    {
        for ( int i = 0; i < Nr; ++i )
        {
            for ( int j = 0; j < Nc; ++j )
            {
                b[i][j] = a[i][j];
            }
        }
    } // end matcopy()


    //
    //*********************************************************************
    //
    // transpose
    //
    // Transpose matrix
    //
    //
    //*********************************************************************
    public void transpose( double aT[][], double bT[][], int Nr, int Nc)
    {
        double dummy[][] = new double[600][600];
        for ( int i = 0; i < Nr; ++i )
        {
            for ( int j = 0; j < Nc; ++j )
            {
                dummy[i][j] = bT[j][i];
            }
        }
        for ( int i = 0; i < Nr; ++i )
        {
            for ( int j = 0; j < Nc; ++j )
            {
                aT[i][j] = dummy[i][j];
            }
        }
    } // end transpose()


    //
    //*********************************************************************
    //
    // mult
    //
    // Multiplies a matrix by a vector, producing a vector.
    //
    //
    //*********************************************************************
    public void mult( double c[],
                      double A[][],
```

Table 11-19 Listing: *HaarXform.java (continued)*

```java
                    double b[],
                    int Nr,
                    int Nc,
                    boolean used[] )
{
    //
    // f[i] = a[i][j] x b[j]
    //
    double sum;
    for ( int i = 0; i < Nr; ++i )
    {
        sum = 0.0;
        for ( int j = 0; j < Nc; ++j )
        {
            if ( used[j] == true ) sum += A[i][j] * b[j];
        }
        c[i] = sum;
    } // end for
} // end mult()


// *****************************************************************
//
// makeHaar
//
// Compute the 1-D Haar matrix.
//
// *****************************************************************
public void makeHaar( double a[][], int n )
{
    double h[][] = new double[600][600];
    int power = 0;
    int CRows = 0;
    int rowSum = 0;
    int startCol = 0;
    int stopCol = 0;
    int startRow = 0;
    int stopRow = 0;

    // How many rows
    //
    try {
        for ( int k = 0; k < 10; ++k )
        {
            if ( (n < Math.pow(2, k+1)) & (n >= Math.pow(2,k)) )
power = k;
        } // end for
    } catch ( Exception AE ) {
        System.err.println( "*** Arithmetic Exception *** " + AE );
        System.err.println( "*** power = " + power );
    } // end try

    //
    // Identify the number rows and columns
    //

    CRows = (int) Math.pow(2,power);

    //
    // Zero h[][]
    //

    for ( int row = 1; row <= CRows; row++ )
        for ( int col = 1; col <= CRows; col++ )
            h[row][col] = 0.0;
```

Table 11-19 Listing: *HaarXform.java (continued)*

```
//
// First column
//
for ( int row = 1; row <= CRows; row++ ) h[row][1] = 1.0;
rowSum = 2;
for ( int pow = power; pow > 0; pow-- )
{
    startCol = (int) Math.pow(2, pow-1)+1;
    stopCol = (int) Math.pow(2, pow);
    startRow = 1;
    for ( int col = startCol; col <= stopCol; col++ )
    {
        for ( int row = startRow; row < startRow+rowSum; row++ )
        {
            if ( (row-startRow) < rowSum/2 ) h[row][col] = 1.0;
            if ( (row-startRow) >= rowSum/2 ) h[row][col] =-1.0;
        } // for row
        startRow += rowSum;
    } // for col
    rowSum *= 2;
} // for pow

//
// Print out.
//

for ( int row = 1; row <= CRows; row++ )
{
    for ( int col = 1; col <= CRows; col++ )
    {
        a[row-1][col-1] = h[row][col];
    } // end for col
} // end for row
} // END makeHaar


// *****************************************************************
// inverse: Compute matrix inverse
//
// parameter      dimension            description
// -------------------------------------------------------------
// a              [n][n]               original matrix
// x              [n][n]               matrix inverse
// n              int                  number of rows and columns
//
// Based on original version in C written by Tao Pang dated 10/24/
2001.
//
// Book Title: An Introduction to Computational Physics
// Author: Tao Pang
// Publisher: Cambridge University Press
// New York.
// September, 1997
// ISBN's: 0-521-48143-0 (hardback); 0-521-48592-4 (paperback)
//
// *****************************************************************
public void inverse( double a[][], double x[][], int n )
{
    double b[][] = new double[n][n];
    double c[]   = new double[n];
    int indx[]   = new int[n];
    int i, j, k, itmp;
    double c1, pi, pi1, pj;

    for ( i = 0; i < n; ++i )
    {
```

Table 11-19 Listing: *HaarXform.java (continued)*

```
        for ( j = 0; j < n; ++j )
        {
            b[i][j] = 0;
        }
    }

    for ( i = 0; i < n; ++i )
    {
        b[i][i] = 1;
    }

    // Initialize the index

    for ( i = 0; i < n; ++i )
    {
        indx[i] = i;
    }

    // Find the rescaling factors, one from each row

    for ( i = 0; i < n; ++i )
    {
        c1 = 0;
        for ( j = 0; j < n; ++j )
        {
            if ( Math.abs(a[i][j]) > c1 ) c1 = Math.abs(a[i][j]);
        }
        c[i] = c1;
    }

    // Search the pivoting (largest) element from each column

    for ( j = 0; j < n-1; ++j )
    {
        pi1 = 0;
        k = 0; // Added by me to address initialization error
        for ( i = j; i < n; ++i )
        {
            pi = Math.abs(a[indx[i]][j])/c[indx[i]];
            if (pi > pi1)
            {
                pi1 = pi;
                k = i;
            }
        }

        // Interchange the rows via indx[] to record pivoting order

        itmp = indx[j];
        indx[j] = indx[k];
        indx[k] = itmp;

        for ( i = j+1; i < n; ++i )
        {
            pj = a[indx[i]][j]/a[indx[j]][j];

            // Record pivoting ratios below diagonal

            a[indx[i]][j] = pj;

            // Modify other elements accordingly

            for ( k = j+1; k < n; ++k )
            {
                a[indx[i]][k] = a[indx[i]][k] - pj*a[indx[j]][k];
            } // end for k
```

Table 11-19 Listing: *HaarXform.java (continued)*

```
        } // end for i
    } // end for j

    // Completed.

    for ( i = 0; i < n-1; ++i )
    {
        for ( j = i+1; j < n; ++j )
        {
            for ( k = 0; k < n; ++k )
            {
                b[indx[j]][k] = b[indx[j]][k] -
a[indx[j]][i]*b[indx[i]][k];
            }
        }
    }

    for ( i = 0; i < n; ++i )
    {
        x[n-1][i] = b[indx[n-1]][i]/a[indx[n-1]][n-1];
        for ( j = n-2; j >= 0; j = j - 1)
        {
            x[j][i] = b[indx[j]][i];
            for ( k = j+1; k < n; ++k )
            {
                x[j][i] = x[j][i] - a[indx[j]][k]*x[k][i];
            }
            x[j][i] = x[j][i] / a[indx[j]][j];
        }
    }
} // End Inverse


public static void main( String args[] )
{
    HaarXform hrxfm = new HaarXform();
    JFrame jf = new JFrame("Haar Transform");
    jf.setContentPane( hrxfm );
    jf.setSize( maxWidth, maxHeight );
    jf.setVisible( true );
    jf.setLocation( xLocation, yLocation );
    jf.addWindowListener( new WindowAdapter() {
        public void windowClosing(WindowEvent e ) {
            System.exit( 0 );
        }
    });
} // End main
} // End HaarXform()
```

Table 11-20 Listing: *DataPlotter.java*

```
import javax.comm.*;
import javax.imageio.ImageIO;
import javax.swing.*;
import javax.swing.AbstractButton;
import javax.swing.border.*;
import javax.swing.ButtonModel;
import javax.swing.JCheckBox;
import javax.swing.JFrame;
import javax.swing.event.*;
import javax.swing.event.ChangeEvent;
import javax.swing.event.ChangeListener;
import javax.swing.plaf.*;
```

303

Table 11-20 Listing: *DataPlotter.java (continued)*

```java
import javax.swing.SwingUtilities;
import javax.swing.text.NumberFormatter;
import javax.swing.Timer;

import java.applet.*;
import java.awt.*;
import java.awt.BorderLayout;
import java.awt.Color;
import java.awt.Container;
import java.awt.event.*;
import java.awt.event.ActionEvent;
import java.awt.event.ActionListener;
import java.awt.event.ItemEvent;
import java.awt.event.ItemListener;
import java.awt.event.KeyEvent;
import java.awt.Graphics;
import java.awt.Graphics2D;
import java.awt.color.ColorSpace;
import java.awt.geom.AffineTransform;
import java.awt.image.AffineTransformOp;
import java.awt.image.BufferedImage;
import java.awt.image.BufferedImageOp;
import java.awt.image.ByteLookupTable;
import java.awt.image.ColorConvertOp;
import java.awt.image.ConvolveOp;
import java.awt.image.Kernel;
import java.awt.image.LookupOp;
import java.awt.image.RescaleOp;

import java.awt.Image;
import java.awt.image.*;

import java.awt.List;
import java.awt.Scrollbar;
import java.awt.Toolkit;
import java.io.*;
import java.io.BufferedInputStream;
import java.lang.*;
import java.lang.Math;
import java.lang.Thread;
import java.net.*;
import java.net.URL;
import java.text.*;
import java.text.DecimalFormat;
import java.util.Date;
import java.util.GregorianCalendar;
import java.util.Properties;
import java.util.Vector;

import javax.swing.border.*;
import javax.swing.event.*;
import javax.swing.JInternalFrame;
import javax.swing.JDesktopPane;
import javax.swing.JMenu;
import javax.swing.JMenuItem;
import javax.swing.JMenuBar;
import javax.swing.JFrame;
import javax.swing.KeyStroke;
import java.util.Random;


public class DataPlotter extends JComponent implements Runnable
{
    static int plotWidth;
    static int plotHeight;
    static int maxValues = 1600;
```

Table 11-20 Listing: *DataPlotter.java (continued)*

```
static int rawValueCount = 0;
static double [] rawValues = new double [maxValues];
public long normalSleepTime = 2000; // milliseconds
private volatile boolean keepRunning;
public volatile String timeMsg;

public DataPlotter( int pWidth, int pHeight, int rawDataCount, double
[] rawData )
    {
        plotWidth = pWidth;
        plotHeight = pHeight;
        rawValueCount = rawDataCount;
        for ( int i = 0; i < rawValueCount; i++ )
        {
            rawValues[i] = rawData[i];
        }
    }

public void run()
    {
        runClock();
    }

public void runClock()
    {
        DecimalFormat dfmt = new DecimalFormat("0.00");
        keepRunning = true;
        long nextSleepTime = normalSleepTime;
        int counter = 0;
        long startTime = System.currentTimeMillis();
        try {
            Thread.sleep( nextSleepTime );
        }
        catch ( InterruptedException iex )
        {
         System.err.println( " *** Thread Interrupted: " + iex + " ***");
        }

        counter++;

        double counterSeconds = counter / 10.0;
        double elapsedSeconds = ( System.currentTimeMillis() - startTime
) / 1000.0;
        double diffSeconds = counterSeconds - elapsedSeconds;

      nextSleepTime = normalSleepTime + ( (long) (diffSeconds * 1000.0)
);

        if ( nextSleepTime < 0 )
        {
            nextSleepTime = 0;
        }

        timeMsg = dfmt.format(counterSeconds) + " - " +
                  dfmt.format(elapsedSeconds) + " = " +
                  dfmt.format(diffSeconds);

        repaint();
    } // end runClock()

public void stopClock()
    {
        keepRunning = false;
    }

public void paint( Graphics g )
```

305

Table 11-20 Listing: *DataPlotter.java (continued)*

```
    {
            Graphics2D g2d = (Graphics2D)g;
            AffineTransform originalTransform = g2d.getTransform();

            // Find maximum plotting value

            double max = 0;
            for ( int i = 0; i < rawValueCount; i++ )
                if ( rawValues[i] > max ) max = rawValues[i];
            if ( ((int) max) > plotHeight ) plotHeight = (int) max;

            // We are constrained to a rectangle plotWidth x plotHeight in
area. // Let's first rotate the area and then begin plotting.

            g2d.setColor( Color.black );
            g2d.fillRect(0,0,plotWidth,plotHeight);
            g2d.setColor( Color.red );
            for ( int i = 0; i < rawValueCount-1; i++ )
            {
                int x0 = (int) ((i+0) * plotWidth/rawValueCount);
                int x1 = (int) ((i+1) * plotWidth/rawValueCount);
                int y0 = plotHeight - (int) (rawValues[i] * 1/plotHeight );
              int y1 = plotHeight - (int) (rawValues[i+1] * plotHeight/max );
                g2d.drawLine( x0, y0, x1, y1 );
            }
        } // end paint
    }
```

Table 11-21 Listing: *ReconPlotter.java*

```
import javax.comm.*;
import javax.imageio.ImageIO;
import javax.swing.*;
import javax.swing.AbstractButton;
import javax.swing.border.*;
import javax.swing.ButtonModel;
import javax.swing.JCheckBox;
import javax.swing.JFrame;
import javax.swing.event.*;
import javax.swing.event.ChangeEvent;
import javax.swing.event.ChangeListener;
import javax.swing.plaf.*;
import javax.swing.SwingUtilities;
import javax.swing.text.NumberFormatter;
import javax.swing.Timer;

import java.applet.*;
import java.awt.BorderLayout;
import java.awt.Color;
import java.awt.Container;
import java.awt.event.*;
import java.awt.event.ActionEvent;
import java.awt.event.ActionListener;
import java.awt.event.ItemEvent;
import java.awt.event.ItemListener;
import java.awt.event.KeyEvent;
import java.awt.Graphics;
import java.awt.Graphics2D;
import java.awt.color.ColorSpace;
import java.awt.geom.AffineTransform;
import java.awt.image.AffineTransformOp;
import java.awt.image.BufferedImage;
```

Table 11-21 Listing: *ReconPlotter.java (continued)*

```java
import java.awt.image.BufferedImageOp;
import java.awt.image.ByteLookupTable;
import java.awt.image.ColorConvertOp;
import java.awt.image.ConvolveOp;
import java.awt.image.Kernel;
import java.awt.image.LookupOp;
import java.awt.image.RescaleOp;

import java.awt.Image;
import java.awt.image.*;

import java.awt.List;
import java.awt.Scrollbar;
import java.awt.Toolkit;
import java.io.*;
import java.io.BufferedInputStream;
import java.lang.*;
import java.lang.Math;
import java.lang.Thread;
import java.net.*;
import java.net.URL;
import java.text.*;
import java.text.DecimalFormat;
import java.util.Date;
import java.util.GregorianCalendar;
import java.util.Properties;
import java.util.Vector;

import javax.swing.border.*;
import javax.swing.event.*;
import javax.swing.JInternalFrame;
import javax.swing.JDesktopPane;
import javax.swing.JMenu;
import javax.swing.JMenuItem;
import javax.swing.JMenuBar;
import javax.swing.JFrame;
import javax.swing.KeyStroke;
import java.util.Random;


public class ReconPlotter extends JComponent implements Runnable
{
    static int plotWidth;
    static int plotHeight;
    static int maxValues = 1600;
    static int rawValueCount = 0;
    static double [] rawValues = new double [maxValues];
    public long normalSleepTime = 1500; // milliseconds
    private volatile boolean keepRunning;
    public volatile String timeMsg;

    public ReconPlotter( int pWidth, int pHeight, int rawDataCount,
    double [] rawData )
    {
        plotWidth = pWidth;
        plotHeight = pHeight;
        rawValueCount = rawDataCount;
        for ( int i = 0; i < rawValueCount; i++ )
        {
            rawValues[i] = rawData[i];
        }
    }

    public void run()
    {
        runClock();
```

307

Table 11-21 Listing: *ReconPlotter.java (continued)*

```
        }
    public void runClock()
    {
        DecimalFormat dfmt = new DecimalFormat("0.00");
        keepRunning = true;
        long nextSleepTime = normalSleepTime;
        int counter = 0;
        long startTime = System.currentTimeMillis();
        try {
            Thread.sleep( nextSleepTime );
        }
        catch ( InterruptedException iex )
        {
         System.err.println( " *** Thread Interrupted: " + iex + " ***");
        }
        counter++;
        double counterSeconds = counter / 10.0;
        double elapsedSeconds = ( System.currentTimeMillis() - startTime
) / 1000.0;
        double diffSeconds = counterSeconds - elapsedSeconds;
        nextSleepTime = normalSleepTime + ( (long) (diffSeconds * 1000.0)
);
        if ( nextSleepTime < 0 )
        {
            nextSleepTime = 0;
        }
        timeMsg = dfmt.format(counterSeconds) + " - " +
                    dfmt.format(elapsedSeconds) + " = " +
                    dfmt.format(diffSeconds);
        repaint();
    } // end runClock()

    public void updatePlot( int reconDataCount, double [] reconData )
    {
        rawValueCount = reconDataCount;
        for ( int i = 0; i < rawValueCount; i++ )
        {
            rawValues[i] = reconData[i];
        }
        repaint();
    }

    public void stopClock()
    {
        keepRunning = false;
    }

    public void paint( Graphics g )
    {
        Graphics2D g2d = (Graphics2D)g;
        AffineTransform originalTransform = g2d.getTransform();

        // Find maximum plotting value

        double max = 0;
        for ( int i = 0; i < rawValueCount; i++ )
            if ( rawValues[i] > max ) max = rawValues[i];
        if ( ((int) max) > plotHeight ) plotHeight = (int) max;

        // We are constrained to a rectangle plotWidth x plotHeight in
area.
        // Let's first rotate the area and then begin plotting.

        g2d.setColor( Color.black );
        g2d.fillRect(0,0,plotWidth,plotHeight);
```

Table 11-21 Listing: *ReconPlotter.java (continued)*

```
        g2d.setColor( Color.green );
        for ( int i = 0; i < rawValueCount-1; i++ )
        {
            int x0 = (int) ((i+0) * plotWidth/rawValueCount);
            int x1 = (int) ((i+1) * plotWidth/rawValueCount);
            int y0 = plotHeight - (int) (rawValues[i] * 1/plotHeight );
            int y1 = plotHeight - (int) (rawValues[i+1] * plotHeight/max );
            g2d.drawLine( x0, y0, x1, y1 );
        }
    } // end paint
}
```

11.7 User Interface Program

In Chapter 8, a sample user interface is provided for which the source code is now listed. The user interface shown in Chapter 8 is constructed using several programs that are listed here. Note that the user interface created using the following programs is a close approximation to those depicted in Chapter 8. Nevertheless, the interested reader will be able to gain a fair understanding of function from the programs that follow. The first program creates a data feed that is used by the user interface program. The data feed program, UI_SendMain, reads a Microsoft Access database, uiDesign, and transmits these data to the plotting program, UI_PlotMain, which reads them through a socket connection and plots them. These methods were architected to simulate the near-real-time receipt of data from a source (i.e., through a live feed) which would then be plotted as they are received. The sending and plotting programs are compiled with the aid of batch files. These are defined as follows:

UISenderCompile.bat:

```
javac UI_SendMain.java UI_Send.java
```

UIPlotterCompile.bat:

```
javac UI_PlotMain.java UI_Plotter.java
    -Xlint:deprecation
```

UISenderRun.bat:

```
java UI_SendMain
```

UIPlotterRun.bat:

```
java UI_PlotMain
```

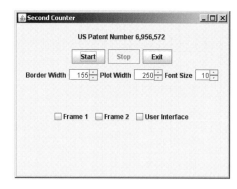

Figure 11-4
UIPlotter master user
interface window

Both programs must be executed concurrently within command shells, with UIPlotterRun.bat being launched first, followed by launching UISenderRun.bat. Select the user interface check box in UIPlotter along with Frame 1 (or Frame 2). This selection window is shown in Figure 11-4. Press the Start button. Next, select the parameters to be transmitted from the user interface window in UISender. Failure to execute in this order may result in a socket connection error between UISender and UIPlotter. Should this occur, simply press the stop buttons in both user interface windows and start the UIPlotter followed by UISender. If this still does not solve the problem, restart both and press the start buttons in the order instructed above.

UI_SendMain retrieves data from an MS Access database. The database table listing together with a sampling of the table content is shown in Figure 11-5. Data are read from this table and transmitted to

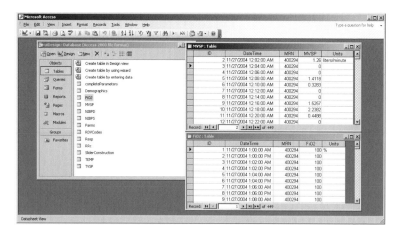

Figure 11-5 uiDesign.mdb database view

UI_PlotMain, listed in Table 11-22, where they are displayed in the user interface. Communication from the sender to plotter is via a TCP/IP port. Table 11-23 is a listing of UI_Plotter.java. Table 11-24 lists UI_SendMain.java (the main program), and Table 11-25 lists UI_Send.java.

Table 11-22 Listing: *UIPlotMain.java*

```java
import javax.comm.*;
import javax.imageio.ImageIO;
import javax.swing.*;
import javax.swing.AbstractButton;
import javax.swing.border.*;
import javax.swing.ButtonModel;
import javax.swing.JCheckBox;
import javax.swing.JFrame;
import javax.swing.event.*;
import javax.swing.event.ChangeEvent;
import javax.swing.event.ChangeListener;
import javax.swing.plaf.*;
import javax.swing.text.NumberFormatter;
import javax.swing.Timer;

import java.sql.*;
import java.sql.Connection;
import java.sql.DriverManager;
import java.sql.SQLException;

import java.applet.*;
import java.awt.*;
import java.awt.BorderLayout;
import java.awt.Color;
import java.awt.Container;
import java.awt.event.*;
import java.awt.event.ActionEvent;
import java.awt.event.ActionListener;
import java.awt.event.ItemEvent;
import java.awt.event.ItemListener;
import java.awt.event.KeyEvent;
import java.awt.Graphics;
import java.awt.Image;
import java.awt.List;
import java.awt.Scrollbar;
import java.awt.Toolkit;
import java.io.*;
import java.io.BufferedInputStream;
import java.lang.*;
import java.lang.Math;
import java.lang.Thread;
import java.net.*;
import java.net.URL;
import java.text.*;
import java.text.DecimalFormat;
import java.util.Date;
import java.util.GregorianCalendar;
import java.util.Properties;
import java.util.Vector;

import javax.swing.border.*;
import javax.swing.event.*;
import javax.swing.JInternalFrame;
import javax.swing.JDesktopPane;
import javax.swing.JMenu;
import javax.swing.JMenuItem;
```

Table 11-22 Listing: *UIPlotMain.java (continued)*

```
import javax.swing.JMenuBar;
import javax.swing.JFrame;
import javax.swing.KeyStroke;

import java.util.Hashtable;

public class UI_PlotMain extends JPanel
{
    static int MaxParameters = 10;
    JSlider threshold1;
    JSlider threshold2;
    JSlider threshold3;
    JSlider threshold4;
    JSlider threshold5;
    JSlider threshold6;
    JSlider threshold7;
    JSlider threshold8;
    JCheckBox checkbox1;
    JCheckBox checkbox2;
    JCheckBox showuiCheckbox;
    JPanel sliderPanel1;
    JPanel sliderPanel2;
    String [] sliderType = new String[MaxParameters];
    String [] sliderCaption = new String[MaxParameters];
    int [] minSliderValue = new int[MaxParameters];
    int [] maxSliderValue = new int[MaxParameters];
    int [] initSliderValue = new int[MaxParameters];
    JDesktopPane desktop;
    public UI_Plotter uip;
    private JButton startB;
    private JButton stopB;
    private JButton exitB;

    /* MS Access SQL Connection */

    public boolean respiratory = false;
    public boolean temperature = false;

    Connection conn;
    Statement st;
    ResultSetMetaData rsmd;
    ResultSet rec;
    String dbURL = "jdbc:odbc:uiDesign";
    String uname = "";
    String pword = "";
    int nCols = 0;

    /* Width of the window */

    public static int MasterWindowWidth = 400;
    public static int MasterWindowHeight = 300;
    public static int UIWindowWidth = 465;
    public static int UIWindowHeight = 465;
    public static int Frame1Width = 400;
    public static int Frame1Height = 300;
    public static int Frame2Width = 400;
    public static int Frame2Height = 300;

    /* Window location */

    public static int MasterWindowLocation_x = 20;
    public static int MasterWindowLocation_y = 0;
    public static int UIWindowLocation_x = 420;
    public static int UIWindowLocation_y = 0;
    public static int Frame1Location_x = 20;
    public static int Frame1Location_y = 300;
```

Table 11-22 Listing: *UIPlotMain.java (continued)*

```java
public static int Frame2Location_x = 20;
public static int Frame2Location_y = 320;

/* Set plot width */

public int minplotwidth = 150;
public int maxplotwidth = 350;
public int plotstep = 5;
public int initplotvalue = 250;

SpinnerModel pmodel = new SpinnerNumberModel( initplotvalue,
                                              minplotwidth,
                                              maxplotwidth,
                                              plotstep );
JSpinner plotWidth = new JSpinner( pmodel );

/* Set plot border */

public int minborderwidth = 50;
public int maxborderwidth = maxplotwidth/2;
public int borderstep = plotstep;
public int initbordervalue = 155;

SpinnerModel bmodel = new SpinnerNumberModel( initbordervalue,
                                              minborderwidth,
                                              maxborderwidth,
                                              borderstep );
JSpinner borderWidth = new JSpinner( bmodel );

/* Set font size */

public int minfontsize = 8;
public int maxfontsize = 14;
public int fontstep = 1;
public int initfontvalue = 10;

SpinnerModel fmodel = new SpinnerNumberModel( initfontvalue,
                                              minfontsize,
                                              maxfontsize,
                                              fontstep );
JSpinner fontSize = new JSpinner( fmodel );

//----------------------------------------------------------------
// Constructor
//----------------------------------------------------------------
public UI_PlotMain()
{
    uip = new UI_Plotter( initplotvalue, initbordervalue );
    startB = new JButton("Start");
    stopB = new JButton("Stop");
    exitB = new JButton("Exit");
    stopB.setEnabled(false); // begin with this disabled
    exitB.setEnabled(true); // begin with this enabled
    startB.addActionListener( new ActionListener() {
      public void actionPerformed(ActionEvent e ) {
      // disable to stop more "start" requests
      startB.setEnabled( false );
      // thread to run the counter
      Thread counterThread = new Thread( uip, "UI_Plotter");
      counterThread.start();
      stopB.setEnabled( true );
      stopB.requestFocus();
    }
    });
    stopB.addActionListener( new ActionListener() {
      public void actionPerformed(ActionEvent e ) {
```

313

Table 11-22 Listing: *UIPlotMain.java (continued)*

```java
                    stopB.setEnabled( false );
                    uip.stopClock();
                    startB.setEnabled( true );
                    startB.requestFocus();
                }
            });
            exitB.addActionListener( new ActionListener() {
                public void actionPerformed(ActionEvent e ) {
                    exitB.setEnabled( false );
                    uip.stopClock();
                    System.exit( 0 );
                }
            });
            borderWidth.addChangeListener( new ChangeListener() {
                public void stateChanged( ChangeEvent evt ) {
                    JSpinner spinner = (JSpinner)evt.getSource();
                    // get the new value
                    Object value = spinner.getValue();
                    uip.updateBorder( value );
                }
            });
            plotWidth.addChangeListener( new ChangeListener() {
                public void stateChanged(ChangeEvent evt ) {
                    JSpinner spinner = (JSpinner)evt.getSource();
                    // get the new value
                    Object value = spinner.getValue();
                    uip.updatePlotWidth( value );
                }
            });
            fontSize.addChangeListener( new ChangeListener() {
                public void stateChanged(ChangeEvent evt ) {
                    JSpinner spinner = (JSpinner)evt.getSource();
                    // get the new value
                    Object value = spinner.getValue();
                    uip.updateFontSize( value );
                }
            });

            /* Sliders : Retreive relevant information from tables */

            mdbConn();
            int nSliders = qryGen( "SliderConstruction" );
            clsConn();

            JLabel [] sliderLabel = new JLabel[MaxParameters];

            /* Update the slider values in the plotter */

                uip.updateSlider( sliderType[0], sliderCaption[0], initSlider-
            Value[0], 0, 8 );
                uip.updateSlider( sliderType[1], sliderCaption[1], initSlider-
            Value[1], 1, 8 );
                uip.updateSlider( sliderType[2], sliderCaption[2], initSlider-
            Value[2], 2, 8 );
                uip.updateSlider( sliderType[3], sliderCaption[3], initSlider-
            Value[3], 3, 8 );
                uip.updateSlider( sliderType[4], sliderCaption[4], initSlider-
            Value[4], 4, 8 );
                uip.updateSlider( sliderType[5], sliderCaption[5], initSlider-
            Value[5], 5, 8 );
                uip.updateSlider( sliderType[6], sliderCaption[6], initSlider-
            Value[6], 6, 8 );
                uip.updateSlider( sliderType[7], sliderCaption[7], initSlider-
            Value[7], 7, 8 );

            /************************/
```

Table 11-22 Listing: *UIPlotMain.java (continued)*

```
/* JSlider constructor */
/***********************/

System.out.println( " slider1: " +
                     minSliderValue[0] +
                     " " +
                     maxSliderValue[0] +
                     " " +
                     initSliderValue[0] );

threshold1 = new JSlider( JSlider.HORIZONTAL,
                          minSliderValue[0],
                          maxSliderValue[0],
                          initSliderValue[0] );

sliderLabel[0] = new JLabel( sliderCaption[0],
                             JLabel.CENTER);

sliderLabel[0].setAlignmentX(Component.CENTER_ALIGNMENT);

threshold1.setMajorTickSpacing( maxSliderValue[0]/5 );
threshold1.setMinorTickSpacing( maxSliderValue[0]/10 );
threshold1.setPaintTicks( true );
threshold1.setPaintLabels( true );
threshold1.setSnapToTicks(true);
threshold1.setBorder(BorderFactory.createEmptyBorder(0,0,10,0));
threshold1.setBorder(BorderFactory.createEmptyBorder(0,0,10,0));

/***********************/
/* JSlider constructor */
/***********************/

System.out.println( " slider2: " +
                     minSliderValue[1] +
                     " " +
                     maxSliderValue[1] +
                     " " +
                     initSliderValue[1] );

threshold2 = new JSlider( JSlider.HORIZONTAL,
                          minSliderValue[1],
                          maxSliderValue[1],
                          initSliderValue[1] );

sliderLabel[1] = new JLabel( sliderCaption[1],
                             JLabel.CENTER);

sliderLabel[1].setAlignmentX(Component.CENTER_ALIGNMENT);

threshold2.setMajorTickSpacing( maxSliderValue[1]/5 );
threshold2.setMinorTickSpacing( maxSliderValue[1]/10 );
threshold2.setPaintTicks( true );
threshold2.setPaintLabels( true );
threshold2.setSnapToTicks(true);
threshold2.setBorder(BorderFactory.createEmptyBorder(0,0,10,0));
threshold2.setBorder(BorderFactory.createEmptyBorder(0,0,10,0));

/***********************/
/* JSlider constructor */
/***********************/

System.out.println( " slider3: " +
                     minSliderValue[2] +
                     " " +
                     maxSliderValue[2] +
                     " " +
```

315

Table 11-22 Listing: *UIPlotMain.java (continued)*

```
                                initSliderValue[2] );

   threshold3 = new JSlider( JSlider.HORIZONTAL,
                             minSliderValue[2],
                             maxSliderValue[2],
                             initSliderValue[2] );

   sliderLabel[2] = new JLabel( sliderCaption[2],
                               JLabel.CENTER);

   sliderLabel[2].setAlignmentX(Component.CENTER_ALIGNMENT);

   threshold3.setMajorTickSpacing( maxSliderValue[2]/5 );
   threshold3.setMinorTickSpacing( maxSliderValue[2]/10 );
   threshold3.setPaintTicks( true );
   threshold3.setPaintLabels( true );
   threshold3.setSnapToTicks(true);
threshold3.setBorder(BorderFactory.createEmptyBorder(0,0,10,0));
threshold3.setBorder(BorderFactory.createEmptyBorder(0,0,10,0));

   /***********************/
   /* JSlider constructor */
   /***********************/

   System.out.println( " slider4: " +
                       minSliderValue[3] +
                       " " +
                       maxSliderValue[3] +
                       " " +
                       initSliderValue[3] );

   threshold4 = new JSlider( JSlider.HORIZONTAL,
                             minSliderValue[3],
                             maxSliderValue[3],
                             initSliderValue[3] );
   sliderLabel[3] = new JLabel( sliderCaption[3], JLabel.CENTER);
   sliderLabel[3].setAlignmentX(Component.CENTER_ALIGNMENT);

   threshold4.setMajorTickSpacing( maxSliderValue[3]/5 );
   threshold4.setMinorTickSpacing( maxSliderValue[3]/10 );
   threshold4.setPaintTicks( true );
   threshold4.setPaintLabels( true );
   threshold4.setSnapToTicks(true);
threshold4.setBorder(BorderFactory.createEmptyBorder(0,0,10,0));
threshold4.setBorder(BorderFactory.createEmptyBorder(0,0,10,0));

   /***********************/
   /* JSlider constructor */
   /***********************/

   System.out.println( " slider5: " +
                       minSliderValue[4] +
                       " " +
                       maxSliderValue[4] +
                       " " +
                       initSliderValue[4] );

   threshold5 = new JSlider( JSlider.HORIZONTAL,
                             minSliderValue[4],
                             maxSliderValue[4],
                             initSliderValue[4] );
   sliderLabel[4] = new JLabel( sliderCaption[4],
                               JLabel.CENTER);
   sliderLabel[4].setAlignmentX(Component.CENTER_ALIGNMENT);

   threshold5.setMajorTickSpacing( maxSliderValue[4]/5 );
```

Table 11-22 Listing: *UIPlotMain.java (continued)*

```
threshold5.setMinorTickSpacing( maxSliderValue[4]/10 );
threshold5.setPaintTicks( true );
threshold5.setPaintLabels( true );
threshold5.setSnapToTicks(true);
threshold5.setBorder(BorderFactory.createEmptyBorder(0,0,10,0));
threshold5.setBorder(BorderFactory.createEmptyBorder(0,0,10,0));

/***********************/
/* JSlider constructor */
/***********************/

System.out.println( " slider6: " +
                    minSliderValue[5] +
                    " " +
                    maxSliderValue[5] +
                    " " +
                    initSliderValue[5] );

threshold6 = new JSlider( JSlider.HORIZONTAL,
                          minSliderValue[5],
        maxSliderValue[5],
        initSliderValue[5] );
        sliderLabel[5] = new JLabel(sliderCaption[5],
        JLabel.CENTER);
sliderLabel[5].setAlignmentX(Component.CENTER_ALIGNMENT);

threshold6.setMajorTickSpacing( maxSliderValue[5]/5 );
threshold6.setMinorTickSpacing( maxSliderValue[5]/10 );
threshold6.setPaintTicks( true );
threshold6.setPaintLabels( true );
threshold6.setSnapToTicks(true);
threshold6.setBorder(BorderFactory.createEmptyBorder(0,0,10,0));
threshold6.setBorder(BorderFactory.createEmptyBorder(0,0,10,0));

/***********************/
/* JSlider constructor */
/***********************/

System.out.println( " slider7: " +
                    minSliderValue[6] +
                    " " +
                    maxSliderValue[6] +
                    " " +
                    initSliderValue[6] );

threshold7 = new JSlider( JSlider.HORIZONTAL,
                          minSliderValue[6],
                          maxSliderValue[6],
                          initSliderValue[6] );
        sliderLabel[6] = new JLabel( sliderCaption[6],
                          JLabel.CENTER);
sliderLabel[6].setAlignmentX(Component.CENTER_ALIGNMENT);

threshold7.setMajorTickSpacing( maxSliderValue[6]/5 );
threshold7.setMinorTickSpacing( maxSliderValue[6]/10 );
threshold7.setPaintTicks( true );
threshold7.setPaintLabels( true );
threshold7.setSnapToTicks(true);
threshold7.setBorder(BorderFactory.createEmptyBorder(0,0,10,0));
threshold7.setBorder(BorderFactory.createEmptyBorder(0,0,10,0));

/***********************/
/* JSlider constructor */
/***********************/

System.out.println( " slider8: " +
```

Table 11-22 Listing: *UIPlotMain.java (continued)*

```
                            minSliderValue[7] +
                            " " +
                            maxSliderValue[7] +
                            " " +
                            initSliderValue[7] );

     threshold8 = new JSlider( JSlider.HORIZONTAL,
                               minSliderValue[7],
                               maxSliderValue[7],
                               initSliderValue[7] );
     sliderLabel[7] = new JLabel( sliderCaption[7],
                                  JLabel.CENTER );
     sliderLabel[7].setAlignmentX(Component.CENTER_ALIGNMENT);

     threshold8.setMajorTickSpacing( 2 );
     threshold8.setMinorTickSpacing( 1 );
     threshold8.setPaintTicks( true );
     threshold8.setPaintLabels( true );
     threshold8.setSnapToTicks(true);
threshold8.setBorder(BorderFactory.createEmptyBorder(0,0,10,0));
threshold8.setBorder(BorderFactory.createEmptyBorder(0,0,10,0));

     /***********************************/
     /* Add Action Listeners to JSliders */
     /***********************************/

     threshold1.addChangeListener( new ChangeListener() {
         public void stateChanged( ChangeEvent evt ) {
             JSlider source = (JSlider)evt.getSource();
             int minValue = (int)source.getValue();
             if ( !source.getValueIsAdjusting()) {
                 uip.updateSlider( sliderType[0],
                                   sliderCaption[0],
                                   minValue, 0, 8 );
             } else { // value is adjusting; just set the text
                 uip.updateSlider( sliderType[0],
                                   sliderCaption[0],
                                   minValue, 0, 8 );
             }
         }
     });
     threshold2.addChangeListener( new ChangeListener() {
         public void stateChanged( ChangeEvent evt ) {
             JSlider source = (JSlider)evt.getSource();
             int minValue = (int)source.getValue();
             if ( !source.getValueIsAdjusting()) {
                 uip.updateSlider( sliderType[1],
                                   sliderCaption[1],
                                   minValue, 1, 8 );
             } else { // value is adjusting; just set the text
                 uip.updateSlider( sliderType[1],
                                   sliderCaption[1],
                                   minValue, 1, 8 );
             }
         }
     });
     threshold3.addChangeListener( new ChangeListener() {
         public void stateChanged( ChangeEvent evt ) {
             JSlider source = (JSlider)evt.getSource();
             int minValue = (int)source.getValue();
             if ( !source.getValueIsAdjusting()) {
                 uip.updateSlider( sliderType[2],
                                   sliderCaption[2],
                                   minValue, 2, 8 );
             } else { // value is adjusting; just set the text
                 uip.updateSlider( sliderType[2],
```

Table 11-22 Listing: *UIPlotMain.java (continued)*

```
                                sliderCaption[2],
                                minValue, 2, 8 );
            }
        }
    });
    threshold4.addChangeListener( new ChangeListener() {
        public void stateChanged( ChangeEvent evt ) {
            JSlider source = (JSlider)evt.getSource();
            int minValue = (int)source.getValue();
            if ( !source.getValueIsAdjusting()) {
                uip.updateSlider( sliderType[3],
                                sliderCaption[3],
                                minValue, 3, 8 );
            } else { // value is adjusting; just set the text
                uip.updateSlider( sliderType[3],
                                sliderCaption[3],
                                minValue, 3, 8 );
            }
        }
    });
    threshold5.addChangeListener( new ChangeListener() {
        public void stateChanged( ChangeEvent evt ) {
            JSlider source = (JSlider)evt.getSource();
            int minValue = (int)source.getValue();
            if ( !source.getValueIsAdjusting()) {
                uip.updateSlider( sliderType[4],
                                sliderCaption[4],
                                minValue, 4, 8 );
            } else { // value is adjusting; just set the text
                uip.updateSlider( sliderType[4],
                                sliderCaption[4],
                                minValue, 4, 8 );
            }
        }
    });
    threshold6.addChangeListener( new ChangeListener() {
        public void stateChanged( ChangeEvent evt ) {
            JSlider source = (JSlider)evt.getSource();
            int minValue = (int)source.getValue();
            if ( !source.getValueIsAdjusting()) {
                uip.updateSlider( sliderType[5],
                                sliderCaption[5],
                                minValue, 5, 8 );
            } else { // value is adjusting; just set the text
                uip.updateSlider( sliderType[5],
                                sliderCaption[5],
                                minValue, 5, 8 );
            }
        }
    });
    threshold7.addChangeListener( new ChangeListener() {
        public void stateChanged( ChangeEvent evt ) {
            JSlider source = (JSlider)evt.getSource();
            int minValue = (int)source.getValue();
            if ( !source.getValueIsAdjusting()) {
                uip.updateSlider( sliderType[6],
                                sliderCaption[6],
                                minValue, 6, 8 );
            } else { // value is adjusting; just set the text
                uip.updateSlider( sliderType[6],
                                sliderCaption[6],
                                minValue, 6, 8 );
            }
        }
    });
    threshold8.addChangeListener( new ChangeListener() {
```

Table 11-22 Listing: *UIPlotMain.java (continued)*

```
            public void stateChanged( ChangeEvent evt ) {
                JSlider source = (JSlider)evt.getSource();
                int minValue = (int)source.getValue();
                if ( !source.getValueIsAdjusting()) {
                    uip.updateSlider( sliderType[7],
                                      sliderCaption[7],
                         minValue, 7, 8 );
            }      else { // value is adjusting; just set the text
                    uip.updateSlider( sliderType[7],
                                      sliderCaption[7],
                                      minValue, 7, 8 );
                }
            }
        });

        /********************/
        /* All Other Labels */
        /********************/

        JLabel patentLabel =
        new JLabel("<html><font = arial color = blue size = 3>US Patent
Number 6,956,572</font></html>",
        JLabel.CENTER);
        patentLabel.setAlignmentX(Component.CENTER_ALIGNMENT);
        JLabel fontLabel =
        new JLabel("<html><font = arial color = blue size = 3>Font Size</
font></html>",
        JLabel.CENTER);
        fontLabel.setAlignmentX(Component.CENTER_ALIGNMENT);
        JLabel plotLabel =
        new JLabel("<html><font = arial color = blue size = 3>Plot Width</
font></html>",
        JLabel.CENTER);
        plotLabel.setAlignmentX(Component.CENTER_ALIGNMENT);
        JLabel borderLabel =
        new JLabel("<html><font = arial color = blue size = 3>Border
Width</font></html>",
        JLabel.CENTER);
        borderLabel.setAlignmentX(Component.CENTER_ALIGNMENT);

        /***********************************/
        /* Slider panels and their labels */
        /***********************************/

        JPanel borderWidthPanel = new JPanel( new BorderLayout() );
        borderWidthPanel.add( borderWidth, BorderLayout.WEST );
        JPanel plotWidthPanel = new JPanel( new BorderLayout() );
        plotWidthPanel.add( plotWidth, BorderLayout.WEST );
        JPanel fontSizePanel = new JPanel( new BorderLayout() );
        fontSizePanel.add( fontSize, BorderLayout.WEST );

        JPanel sseButtonPanel = new JPanel();
        sseButtonPanel.setLayout( new FlowLayout( FlowLayout.CENTER ) );
        sseButtonPanel.add(startB);
        sseButtonPanel.add(stopB);
        sseButtonPanel.add(exitB);

        JPanel masterPanel = new JPanel();
        masterPanel.setLayout( new GridLayout( 2, 2  ) );
        JPanel controlPanel = new JPanel();
        controlPanel.setLayout( new FlowLayout() );

        sliderPanel1 = new JPanel();
        sliderPanel1.setLayout( new GridLayout( 4, 2  ) );
        sliderPanel2 = new JPanel();
```

Table 11-22 Listing: *UIPlotMain.java (continued)*

```
        sliderPanel2.setLayout( new GridLayout( 4 /* rows */, 2 /* cols
*/, 5 /* hgap */, 4 /* vgap */ ) );

        masterPanel.add( patentLabel ); masterPanel.add( sseButtonPanel
);
        controlPanel.add( borderLabel ); controlPanel.add( borderWidth-
Panel );
        controlPanel.add( plotLabel ); controlPanel.add( plotWidthPanel
);
        controlPanel.add( fontLabel ); controlPanel.add( fontSizePanel );

        sliderPanel1.add( sliderLabel[0] ); sliderPanel1.add( threshold1
);
        sliderPanel1.add( sliderLabel[1] ); sliderPanel1.add( threshold2
);
        sliderPanel1.add( sliderLabel[2] ); sliderPanel1.add( threshold3
);
        sliderPanel1.add( sliderLabel[3] ); sliderPanel1.add( threshold4
);

        sliderPanel2.add( sliderLabel[4] ); sliderPanel2.add( threshold5
);
        sliderPanel2.add( sliderLabel[5] ); sliderPanel2.add( threshold6
);
        sliderPanel2.add( sliderLabel[6] ); sliderPanel2.add( threshold7
);
        sliderPanel2.add( sliderLabel[7] ); sliderPanel2.add( threshold8
);

        /**********************************************/
        /* Checkbox panel                             */
        /**********************************************/

        checkbox1 = new JCheckBox("Frame 1");
        checkbox1.setSelected( false );
        checkbox2 = new JCheckBox("Frame 2");
        checkbox2.setSelected( false );
        showuiCheckbox = new JCheckBox("User Interface");
        showuiCheckbox.setSelected( false );

        JPanel checkboxPanel = new JPanel();
        checkboxPanel.setLayout( new FlowLayout() );
        checkboxPanel.add(checkbox1);
        checkboxPanel.add(checkbox2);
        checkboxPanel.add(showuiCheckbox);

JPanel mainPanel = new JPanel();
        mainPanel.setLayout( new GridLayout(3,1) );
        mainPanel.add( masterPanel );
        mainPanel.add( controlPanel );
        mainPanel.add( checkboxPanel );

        this.setLayout( new FlowLayout() );
        this.add( mainPanel );

        /**********************************/
        /* JCheckbox ItemListeners        */
        /**********************************/

        final JFrame myFrame1 = new JFrame("Frame 1");
        final JFrame myFrame2 = new JFrame("Frame 2");
        final JFrame uiFrame  = new JFrame("Interface");

        showuiCheckbox.addItemListener( new ItemListener() {
            public void itemStateChanged( ItemEvent evt1)
            {
```

Table 11-22 Listing: *UIPlotMain.java (continued)*

```
                uiFrame.setSize( UIWindowHeight, UIWindowWidth );
             uiFrame.setLocation( UIWindowLocation_x, UIWindowLocation_y
);
                uiFrame.add( uip );
                uiFrame.setVisible( true );
                if ( evt1.getStateChange() == 1 ) uiFrame.setVisible(
true );
                if ( evt1.getStateChange() == 2 ) uiFrame.setVisible(
false );
           }
        });
        checkbox1.addItemListener( new ItemListener() {
           public void itemStateChanged( ItemEvent evt1)
           {
              myFrame1.setSize( Frame1Width, Frame1Height );
           myFrame1.setLocation( Frame1Location_x, Frame1Location_y );
              myFrame1.add( sliderPanel1 );
              uiFrame.setVisible( true );
              if ( evt1.getStateChange() == 1 ) myFrame1.setVisible(
true );
              if ( evt1.getStateChange() == 2 ) myFrame1.setVisible(
false );
           }
        });
        checkbox2.addItemListener( new ItemListener() {
           public void itemStateChanged( ItemEvent evt2)
           {
              myFrame2.setSize( Frame2Width, Frame2Height );
           myFrame2.setLocation( Frame2Location_x, Frame2Location_y );
              myFrame2.add( sliderPanel2 );
              if ( evt2.getStateChange() == 1 ) myFrame2.setVisible(
true );
              if ( evt2.getStateChange() == 2 ) myFrame2.setVisible(
false );
           }
        });
    }

    //-------------------------------------------------------------------
    // Make database connection.
    //-------------------------------------------------------------------
    public void mdbConn()
    {
        try
        {
            //::::
            //:::: JDBC Driver
            //::::

            Class.forName("sun.jdbc.odbc.JdbcOdbcDriver");

            //::::
            //:::: JDBC url link to USER DSN object in Settings->
            //:::: Control Panel->Administrative Tools->ODBC
            //::::

            String url = "jdbc:odbc:uiDesign";

            //::::
            //:::: User, Pword set to nothing
            //::::

            String user = "";
            String password = "";

            //::::
```

Table 11-22 Listing: *UIPlotMain.java (continued)*

```
                //:::: Connect to database
                //::::

                conn = DriverManager.getConnection(url,user,password);

                //::::
                //:::: Create a statement object instance
                //::::

                st = conn.createStatement();
        }
        catch(Exception e)
        {
            System.out.println("Error - "+e.toString());
        }
    }

//--------------------------------------------------------------------
// Query database with WHERE clause.
//--------------------------------------------------------------------
public int qryGen( String tableName )
{
    int nRows = 0;
    try {
        //::::
      //:::: Query the database for data objects. Select two objects.
        //::::

            String queryString = "SELECT * FROM " + tableName;
            System.out.println( " queryString......" + queryString );
            rec = st.executeQuery( queryString );

            //::::
            //:::: Get some data about the data.
            //::::

            rsmd = rec.getMetaData();
            int nCols = rsmd.getColumnCount();

            //::::
            //:::: Print all instances of these objects out
            //::::

            while(rec.next() && nRows < MaxParameters )
            {
                sliderType[nRows] = rec.getString(2);
                sliderCaption[nRows] = rec.getString(3);
                minSliderValue[nRows] = rec.getInt(4);
                maxSliderValue[nRows] = rec.getInt(5);
                initSliderValue[nRows] = rec.getInt(6);

                System.out.println( "/// " +
                                        sliderType[nRows] +
                                        " " +
                                        sliderCaption[nRows] +
                                        " " +
                                        minSliderValue[nRows] +
                                        " " +
                                        maxSliderValue[nRows] +
                                        " " +
                                        initSliderValue[nRows] );
                nRows++;
            } // end while
    }
    catch(Exception e)
    {
```

Table 11-22 Listing: *UIPlotMain.java (continued)*

```
            System.out.println("Error - "+e.toString());
      }
      return nRows;
}

//-------------------------------------------------------------------
// Close database connection.
//-------------------------------------------------------------------
public void clsConn()
{
    try {
        conn.close();
        st.close();
    }
    catch ( Exception e )
    {
        System.err.println( " Cannot close database " + e );
    }
}

//-------------------------------------------------------------------
// Main
//-------------------------------------------------------------------
public static void main(String[] args)
{
    UI_PlotMain uipm = new UI_PlotMain();
    JFrame jf = new JFrame("Second Counter");
    jf.setContentPane( uipm );
    jf.setSize( MasterWindowWidth, MasterWindowHeight );
    jf.setVisible( true );
  jf.setLocation( MasterWindowLocation_x, MasterWindowLocation_y );
    jf.addWindowListener( new WindowAdapter() {
        public void windowClosing(WindowEvent e ) {
            System.exit( 0 );
        }
    });
} // end main
} // end UI_PlotMain
```

Table 11-23 Listing: UI_Plotter.java

```
import javax.comm.*;
import javax.imageio.ImageIO;
import javax.swing.*;
import javax.swing.AbstractButton;
import javax.swing.border.*;
import javax.swing.ButtonModel;
import javax.swing.JCheckBox;
import javax.swing.JFrame;
import javax.swing.event.*;
import javax.swing.event.ChangeEvent;
import javax.swing.event.ChangeListener;
import javax.swing.plaf.*;
import javax.swing.SwingUtilities;
import javax.swing.text.NumberFormatter;
import javax.swing.Timer;

import java.applet.*;
import java.awt.*;
import java.awt.BorderLayout;
import java.awt.Color;
import java.awt.Container;
import java.awt.event.*;
import java.awt.event.ActionEvent;
```

Table 11-23 Listing: UI_Plotter.java *(continued)*

```java
import java.awt.event.ActionListener;
import java.awt.event.ItemEvent;
import java.awt.event.ItemListener;
import java.awt.event.KeyEvent;
import java.awt.Graphics;
import java.awt.Graphics2D;
import java.awt.color.ColorSpace;
import java.awt.geom.AffineTransform;
import java.awt.image.AffineTransformOp;
import java.awt.image.BufferedImage;
import java.awt.image.BufferedImageOp;
import java.awt.image.ByteLookupTable;
import java.awt.image.ColorConvertOp;
import java.awt.image.ConvolveOp;
import java.awt.image.Kernel;
import java.awt.image.LookupOp;
import java.awt.image.RescaleOp;

import java.awt.Image;
import java.awt.image.*;

import java.awt.List;
import java.awt.Scrollbar;
import java.awt.Toolkit;
import java.io.*;
import java.io.BufferedInputStream;
import java.lang.*;
import java.lang.Math;
import java.lang.Thread;
import java.net.*;
import java.net.URL;
import java.text.*;
import java.text.DecimalFormat;
import java.util.Date;
import java.util.GregorianCalendar;
import java.util.Properties;
import java.util.Vector;

import javax.swing.border.*;
import javax.swing.event.*;
import javax.swing.JInternalFrame;
import javax.swing.JDesktopPane;
import javax.swing.JMenu;
import javax.swing.JMenuItem;
import javax.swing.JMenuBar;
import javax.swing.JFrame;
import javax.swing.KeyStroke;
import java.util.Random;

// **************************************************
//
// UI_Plotter.java
//
// Called by UI_PlotMain.java to plot data from
// UI_Send.java
//
// Author: J. Zaleski
//
// **************************************************
public class UI_Plotter extends JComponent implements Runnable
{
    static int MaxParameters = 10;
    static int MaxValues = 2000;
    public boolean debug = true;
    long normalSleepTime = 100; // ms
```

Table 11-23 Listing: UI_Plotter.java *(continued)*

```
// Processing thread controls

private volatile boolean suspended;
private volatile boolean keepRunning;
private Font labelFont;
private Font patentFont;
private Font textFont;
private Font smalltextFont;
private volatile String timeMsg;
private volatile int arcLen;
private volatile int rotAngle = 0;
private volatile String[] parms = new String[MaxParameters];
public int outsideBorder = 0;
public int plotDiameter = 0;
public int fontSize = 10;

double angle = 45.0;

public int NumParameters = 0;
public String [] sType = new String[MaxParameters];
public String [] sCapt = new String[MaxParameters];
public int [] sThreshold = new int[MaxParameters];

// Arrays to hold parameter values

protected String [] paramName = new String[MaxParameters];
protected static int nsp = 0;
protected double [] paramValue = new double[MaxParameters];
protected double [] lastparamValue = new double[MaxParameters];
protected double []paramMax = new double[MaxParameters];
protected double []paramMean = new double[MaxParameters];
protected double [] paramSqrd = new double[MaxParameters];
protected String [] paramDT = new String[MaxParameters];
protected String [] paramTM = new String[MaxParameters];
protected int [] paramCount = new int[MaxParameters];
protected int [] previousTM = new int[MaxParameters];
protected int [] deltaTM = new int[MaxParameters];
protected int [] meanLoc = new int[MaxParameters];
protected int [] sdevLoc = new int[MaxParameters];
protected int [] instLoc = new int[MaxParameters]; // mean tick
location

//----------------------------------------------------------------
// UI_Plotter -- Constructor
//----------------------------------------------------------------
public UI_Plotter( int initplotvalue, int initbordervalue )
{
    super();
    plotDiameter = initplotvalue;
    outsideBorder = initbordervalue;
    labelFont = new Font("Monaco", Font.BOLD, 14 );
    patentFont = new Font("Tahoma", Font.BOLD,9 );
    textFont = new Font("Monaco", Font.BOLD, 10 );
    smalltextFont = new Font("Monaco", Font.BOLD, 9 );
  for ( int k = 0; k < MaxParameters; k++ ) paramName[k] = "empty";
    for ( int j = 0; j < MaxParameters; j++ ) paramMax[j] = 0.0;
    timeMsg = "Not Started";
    arcLen = 0;
    for ( int m = 0; m < MaxParameters; m++ )
    {
        previousTM[m] = 0;
        lastparamValue[m] = 0.0;
        paramMean[m] = 0.0;
        paramCount[m]= 0;
        paramSqrd[m] = 0.0;
    }
```

Table 11-23 Listing: UI_Plotter.java *(continued)*

```java
}
//---------------------------------------------------------------
// run method
//---------------------------------------------------------------
public void run()
{
    runClock();
}

//---------------------------------------------------------------
// runClock method -- receives data from sender method
//---------------------------------------------------------------
public void runClock()
{
    DecimalFormat dfmt = new DecimalFormat("0.00");
    long nextSleepTime = normalSleepTime;
    int counter = 0;
    long startTime = System.currentTimeMillis();
    keepRunning = true;
    try {
        ServerSocket srvr = new ServerSocket(1234);
        Socket skt = srvr.accept();
        BufferedReader in = new BufferedReader(new
                        InputStreamReader(skt.getInputStream()));

        while ( keepRunning )
        {
            // Read in the data one record at a time

            String inputData = in.readLine();

            // extract names and numbers

            parseData( inputData,
                        paramName,
                        paramValue,
                        lastparamValue,
                        paramMax,
                        paramDT,
                        paramTM,
                        previousTM,
                        deltaTM);

            // get number of parameters

            for( int m = 0; m < paramName.length; m++ )
            {
                if ( !paramName[m].equals("empty") )
                {
                    nsp=m+1;
                }
            }

            // sleep

            try
            {
                Thread.sleep( nextSleepTime );
            }
            catch ( InterruptedException x )
            {
                System.err.println( "Thread Interrupted: " + x);
            }

            counter++;
```

327

Table 11-23 Listing: UI_Plotter.java *(continued)*

```
                double counterSecs = counter / 10.0;
                double elapsedSecs =
                    ( System.currentTimeMillis() - startTime ) / 1000.0;
                double diffSecs = counterSecs - elapsedSecs;

                nextSleepTime = normalSleepTime +
                    ( (long) ( diffSecs * 1000.0 ) );

                if ( nextSleepTime < 0 )
                {
                    nextSleepTime = 0;
                }

                timeMsg = dfmt.format(counterSecs) + " - " +
                          dfmt.format(elapsedSecs) + " = " +
                          dfmt.format(diffSecs);

                // paint anew

                repaint();

            } // end while
            in.close();
        }
        catch(Exception e) {
            System.out.print("Lost Connection\n");
        }
    }

//----------------------------------------------------------------
// stopClock method
//----------------------------------------------------------------
public void stopClock()
{
    keepRunning = false;
}

//----------------------------------------------------------------
// paint method
//----------------------------------------------------------------
public void paint ( Graphics g )
{
    // Define geometry drawing parameters

    int xPos = 100;
    int yPos = 100;

    // Set the plot width, subject to constraints

    int xDiam = 0;
    if ( plotDiameter > xDiam ) xDiam = plotDiameter;

    // Set the border around the plot, subject to constraints

    int border = 0;
        border = outsideBorder;
    int yDiam = xDiam;
    int textOffset = 0;
    int zeroOffset = 10; // pixels
    int lineLen = xDiam/2 - zeroOffset; // Draws the axis line
    int xCentroid = xDiam/2 + xPos; // Locate center of circle
    int yCentroid = yDiam/2 + yPos; // Locate center of circle
    int boxWidth = 6; // pixels
    int boxHeight = 14; // pixels
    int startAngle = 0;
```

Table 11-23 Listing: UI_Plotter.java *(continued)*

```java
// angle axes about the circle

int nAxes = nsp;
int drotAngle = 0;

if ( nAxes == 0 ) drotAngle = 360;
if ( nAxes > 0  ) drotAngle = 360/nAxes;

// Write some parameter information for diagnostics

g.setFont( textFont );

// Define decimal place limits for drawing values on axes

DecimalFormat dfmt = new DecimalFormat("0.00");
String valueMsg = "";
String deltaMsg = "";
String meanValueMsg = "";
String lastvalueMsg = "";

//
// Draw the basic circle and prepare to place the axes for each
// data point
//
// Valid Colors:
//
// black, blue, cyan, darkGray, gray, green, lightGray,
//             // magenta, orange, pink, red, white, yellow
//

g.setColor( Color.darkGray );
g.fillOval( xPos-border/2,
            yPos-border/2,
            xDiam+border,
            yDiam+border );

g.setColor( Color.black );
g.fillOval(xPos, yPos, xDiam, yDiam ); // fill with black
g.setColor( Color.blue ); // blue for text drawn on circle portion

// Define the 2d graphics environment

Graphics2D g2d = (Graphics2D)g;

// Draw each axis and the data box at the
// location of the data point.

for ( int iAxes = 0; iAxes < nAxes; iAxes++ )
{
    // Define the rotation angle

    angle = (double) (1.0 * iAxes * drotAngle);

    //
    // increase the text offset so that parameters and values
    // do not overlap into plot area as they are located around
    // the circumference of the UI
    //
    // y = A * x^4 + B * x^3 + C*x^2 + D*x + E
    //

    double A =  1.0e-8;
    double B = -8.0e-6;
    double C =  0.0014;
    double D =  0.054;
    double E =  30.0;
```

Table 11-23 Listing: UI_Plotter.java *(continued)*

```
                   double x = angle;

                   textOffset = (int) (A*x*x*x*x +
                                       B*x*x*x +
                                       C*x*x +
                                       D*x +
                                       E );

               // Plot the location of the "value box"

               instLoc[iAxes] = iScale( paramValue[iAxes],
                                        lineLen, paramMax[iAxes] );

               // Compute the mean of each parameter

               paramMean[iAxes] += paramValue[iAxes];
               paramSqrd[iAxes] += paramValue[iAxes]*paramValue[iAxes];
               paramCount[iAxes] += 1;
               double meanValue = paramMean[iAxes] / paramCount[iAxes];
               double sumXSquared = paramSqrd[iAxes];
               double sumX = paramMean[iAxes];
               int N = paramCount[iAxes];
               double sdevValue = Math.sqrt((sumXSquared - (sumX*sumX/N))/
(N-1));
        meanLoc[iAxes] = iScale( meanValue, lineLen, paramMax[iAxes] );
        sdevLoc[iAxes] = iScale( sdevValue, lineLen, paramMax[iAxes] );

               // write the parameter value at the location of the mean,
               // above the parameter.

               meanValueMsg = dfmt.format( meanValue );
               valueMsg = dfmt.format(paramValue[iAxes]);
               deltaMsg = ""+paramTM[iAxes]; // deltaTM[iAxes] + "sec";
               lastvalueMsg = dfmt.format(lastparamValue[iAxes]);

               // get original transform

               AffineTransform originalTransform = g2d.getTransform();

               // Plot parameter names, values along the circumferential
               // ring of the UI

               int xBorderPosition =
               (int) ((lineLen + zeroOffset) *
               Math.cos( Math.toRadians( angle ) ) );
               int yBorderPosition =
               (int) ((lineLen + zeroOffset) *
               Math.sin( Math.toRadians( angle ) ) );

               int xLabelPosition =
               (int) ((lineLen + zeroOffset + textOffset) *
               Math.cos( Math.toRadians( angle ) ) );
               int yLabelPosition =
               (int) ((lineLen + zeroOffset + textOffset) *
               Math.sin( Math.toRadians( angle ) ) );

               int xValuePosition =
               (int) ((instLoc[iAxes]) * Math.cos( Math.toRadians( angle )
  ) );
               int yValuePosition =
               (int) ((instLoc[iAxes]) * Math.sin( Math.toRadians( angle )
  ) );

               int xMeanValuePosition =
               (int) ((meanLoc[iAxes]) * Math.cos( Math.toRadians( angle )
  ) );
```

Table 11-23 Listing: UI_Plotter.java *(continued)*

```
                  int yMeanValuePosition =
                  (int) ((meanLoc[iAxes]) * Math.sin( Math.toRadians( angle )
  ) );

                  // Draw axes

                  g2d.setColor( Color.gray );
                  g2d.drawLine(xCentroid + xBorderPosition,
                               yCentroid + yBorderPosition,
                               xCentroid + xLabelPosition,
                               yCentroid + yLabelPosition );

                  // Write parameter labels

                  g2d.setFont( labelFont );
                  g2d.setColor( Color.yellow );
                  g2d.drawString( paramName[iAxes],
                                  xCentroid + xLabelPosition,
                                  yCentroid + yLabelPosition );

                  FontMetrics fm = g2d.getFontMetrics();
                  int valueWidth = fm.stringWidth( valueMsg );
                  int valueHeight = fm.getHeight();
                  int deltaWidth = fm.stringWidth( deltaMsg );
                  int deltaHeight = fm.getHeight();
                  int lastvalueWidth = fm.stringWidth( lastvalueMsg );
                  int lastvalueHeight = fm.getHeight();
                  int meanvalueWidth = fm.stringWidth( meanValueMsg );

                  if ( angle < 90 || angle > 270 )
                  {
                      // Text transform

                      g2d.transform(
                  AffineTransform.getRotateInstance(Math.toRadians(angle),
                                  xCentroid,
                                  yCentroid));

                      // Draw zero point

                      g2d.setColor( Color.green );
                      g2d.drawLine( xCentroid + zeroOffset,
                                    yCentroid + 3,
                                    xCentroid + zeroOffset,
                                    yCentroid - 3 );

                      // Draw axis line

                      g2d.setColor( Color.blue );
                      g2d.drawLine( xCentroid + zeroOffset,
                                    yCentroid,
                                    xCentroid + zeroOffset + lineLen,
                                    yCentroid );

                      // Draw line at the mean location

                      g2d.setColor( Color.yellow );
                      g2d.drawLine( xCentroid + zeroOffset + meanLoc[iAxes],
                                    yCentroid + 5,
                                    xCentroid + zeroOffset + meanLoc[iAxes],
                                    yCentroid - 5 );

                      // Write mean value

                      g2d.setFont( textFont );
                      g2d.setColor( Color.yellow );
```

Table 11-23 Listing: UI_Plotter.java *(continued)*

```
                    g2d.drawString( meanValueMsg,
                    xCentroid + zeroOffset + meanLoc[iAxes] - meanvalueWidth/
2,
                                 yCentroid - valueHeight/2);

            // Draw line at +/-1 standard deviation of mean
            // location

                    g2d.setColor( Color.blue );
                    g2d.drawLine(
            xCentroid + zeroOffset + meanLoc[iAxes] + sdevLoc[iAxes],
                    yCentroid + 3,
            xCentroid + zeroOffset + meanLoc[iAxes] + sdevLoc[iAxes],
                            yCentroid - 3 );
                    g2d.drawLine(
            xCentroid + zeroOffset + meanLoc[iAxes] - sdevLoc[iAxes],
                    yCentroid + 3,
            xCentroid + zeroOffset + meanLoc[iAxes] - sdevLoc[iAxes],
                            yCentroid - 3 );

            // Select color for parameter rectangle based upon
            // value with respect to selected threshold.

            for ( int k = 0; k < NumParameters; k++ )
            {
                if ( sType[k].equals(paramName[iAxes]) )
                {
                    if ( paramValue[iAxes] < sThreshold[k] )
                        g2d.setColor( Color.red );
                    if ( paramValue[iAxes] > sThreshold[k] )
                        g2d.setColor( Color.green );
                    if ( paramValue[iAxes] ==sThreshold[k] )
                        g2d.setColor( Color.yellow );
                }
            }

            // Draw rectangle

                    g2d.fillRect( xCentroid + zeroOffset + instLoc[iAxes] -
boxWidth/2,
                                yCentroid - boxHeight/2,
                                boxWidth,
                                boxHeight );

            // Write instantaneous value

                    g2d.setFont( textFont );
                    g2d.setColor( Color.cyan );
                    g2d.drawString( valueMsg,
                            xCentroid + zeroOffset + instLoc[iAxes] -
valueWidth/2,
                            yCentroid + valueHeight + 4) ;

                    g2d.setColor( Color.gray );

            // Write time between last and current measurement

                    g.setFont( smalltextFont );
                    g2d.drawString( deltaMsg,
                            xCentroid + zeroOffset + instLoc[iAxes] + 4,
                            yCentroid + valueHeight + deltaHeight );

                    g2d.drawString( lastvalueMsg,
                            xCentroid + zeroOffset + instLoc[iAxes] -
lastvalueWidth,
                            yCentroid + valueHeight + lastvalueHeight );
```

Table 11-23 Listing: UI_Plotter.java *(continued)*

```
                // Transform back

                g2d.setTransform( originalTransform );
            }

            if ( angle >= 90 && angle <= 270 )
            {
                // Text Transform

                g2d.transform( AffineTransform.getRotateInstance(
                            Math.toRadians(angle-180),
                            xCentroid,
                            yCentroid));

                // Draw zero point

                g2d.setColor( Color.green );
                g2d.drawLine( xCentroid - zeroOffset,
                            yCentroid + 3,
                            xCentroid - zeroOffset,
                            yCentroid - 3 );

                // Draw axis line

                g2d.setColor( Color.blue );
                g2d.drawLine( xCentroid - zeroOffset,
                            yCentroid,
                            xCentroid - zeroOffset - lineLen,
                            yCentroid );

                // Draw line at the mean location

                g2d.setColor( Color.yellow );
                g2d.drawLine( xCentroid - zeroOffset - meanLoc[iAxes],
                            yCentroid + 5,
                            xCentroid - zeroOffset - meanLoc[iAxes],
                            yCentroid - 5 );

                g2d.setFont( textFont );
                g2d.setColor( Color.yellow );
                g2d.drawString( meanValueMsg,
                xCentroid - zeroOffset - meanLoc[iAxes] - meanvalueWidth/
2,
                        yCentroid - valueHeight/2 );

                // Draw line at +/-1 standard deviation of mean location

                g2d.setColor( Color.blue );
                g2d.drawLine(
                    xCentroid - zeroOffset - meanLoc[iAxes] -
sdevLoc[iAxes],
                    yCentroid + 3,
                    xCentroid - zeroOffset - meanLoc[iAxes] -
sdevLoc[iAxes],
                    yCentroid - 3 );
                g2d.drawLine(
                    xCentroid - zeroOffset - meanLoc[iAxes] +
sdevLoc[iAxes],
                    yCentroid + 3,
                    xCentroid - zeroOffset - meanLoc[iAxes] +
sdevLoc[iAxes],
                    yCentroid - 3 );

                // Select color for parameter rectangle based upon
                // value with respect to selected threshold.
```

Table 11-23 Listing: UI_Plotter.java *(continued)*

```
                for( int k = 0; k < NumParameters; k++ )
                {
                    if ( sType[k].equals(paramName[iAxes] ))
                    {
                        if ( paramValue[iAxes] < sThreshold[k] )
                            g2d.setColor( Color.red );
                        if ( paramValue[iAxes] > sThreshold[k] )
                            g2d.setColor( Color.green );
                        if ( paramValue[iAxes] ==sThreshold[k] )
                            g2d.setColor( Color.yellow );
                    }
                }

                // Draw rectangle

                g2d.fillRect(
                    xCentroid - zeroOffset - instLoc[iAxes] - boxWidth/2,
                        yCentroid - boxHeight/2,
                        boxWidth,
                        boxHeight );

                g2d.setFont( textFont );
                g2d.setColor( Color.cyan );
                g2d.drawString( valueMsg,
                        xCentroid - zeroOffset - instLoc[iAxes] -
valueWidth/2,
                        yCentroid + valueHeight + 4);

                // Write time between last and current measurement

                g.setFont( smalltextFont );
                g2d.setColor( Color.gray );
                g2d.drawString( deltaMsg,
                        xCentroid - zeroOffset - instLoc[iAxes] + 4,
                            yCentroid + valueHeight + deltaHeight );

                g2d.drawString( lastvalueMsg,
                        xCentroid - zeroOffset - instLoc[iAxes] -
lastvalueWidth,
                        yCentroid + valueHeight + lastvalueHeight );

                // Transform back

                g2d.setTransform( originalTransform );
            }
        } // end for
    } // end paint()

    //----------------------------------------------------------------
    // Find the sine of the passed angle
    //----------------------------------------------------------------
    public double sin( int rotAngle )
    {
        double value = 0.0;
        double s = 0.0;
        value = rotAngle * Math.PI / 180.0;
        s = Math.sin(value);
        return s;
    }

    //----------------------------------------------------------------
    // Find the cosine of the passed angle
    //----------------------------------------------------------------
    public double cos( int rotAngle )
    {
```

Table 11-23 Listing: UI_Plotter.java *(continued)*

```java
            double value = 0.0;
            double c = 0.0;
            value = rotAngle * Math.PI / 180.0;
            c = Math.cos(value);
            return c;
        }

        //----------------------------------------------------------------
        // parse the input data
        //----------------------------------------------------------------
        public void parseData( String  id,
                               String [] pn,
                               double [] pv,
                               double [] lpv,
                               double [] pm,
                               String [] pdt,
                               String [] ptm,
                               int    [] otm,
                               int    [] dtm)
        {
            double d = -1;
            int spaceLocation1= id.indexOf(" ");
            int spaceLocation2= id.indexOf(" ", spaceLocation1+1 );
            int spaceLocation3= id.indexOf(" ", spaceLocation2+1 );
            String parmName = id.substring(0,spaceLocation1);
        String parmValue = id.substring(spaceLocation1+1,spaceLocation2);
          String parmDate = id.substring(spaceLocation2+1, spaceLocation3
);
            String parmTime = id.substring(spaceLocation3+1, id.length() );
            int colonLocation1 = parmTime.indexOf(":");
            int colonLocation2 = parmTime.indexOf(":", colonLocation1+1 );
            int spaceLocation = parmTime.indexOf(" ", colonLocation2+1 );
            String shour = parmTime.substring( 0, colonLocation1 );
            String sminute = parmTime.substring( colonLocation1+1,
                                                 colonLocation2 );
            String ssecond = parmTime.substring( colonLocation2+1, spaceLo-
cation );
            System.out.println( " ....HOUR: " + shour );
            System.out.println( " ....MINUTE: " + sminute );
            System.out.println( " ....SECOND: " + ssecond );
            int hour = Integer.parseInt( shour );
            int minute = Integer.parseInt( sminute );
            int second = Integer.parseInt( ssecond );
            int ctime = hour * 3600 + minute * 60 + second;

            try {
                d = Double.valueOf( parmValue.trim() ).doubleValue();
            } catch ( NumberFormatException nfe ) {
                System.err.println( " *** Number format error: " + nfe + "
*** " );
            }

            boolean inArray = false;
            int insertLocation = -1;

            for ( int i = 0; i < pn.length; i++ )
            {
                if ( parmName.equals( pn[i] ) ) insertLocation = i;
            }

            if ( insertLocation == -1 )
            {
                int k = 0;
                do {
                    if ( pn[k].equals("empty") )
                    {
```

335

Table 11-23 Listing: UI_Plotter.java *(continued)*

```
                     pn[k] = parmName;
                     pdt[k] = parmDate;
                     ptm[k] = parmTime;
                     dtm[k] = ctime - otm[k];
                     otm[k] = ctime;
                     insertLocation = k;
                }
                k++;
            } while ( insertLocation == -1 );
        }

        // copy new value

        for ( int m = 0; m < pn.length; m++ )
        {
            lpv[m] = pv[m];
            if ( parmName.equals( pn[m] ) )
            {
                pv[m] = d;
                pdt[m] = parmDate;
                ptm[m] = parmTime;
                dtm[m] = ctime - otm[m];
                otm[m] = ctime;
                if ( d > pm[m] ) pm[m] = d;
            }
        }
    } // end parseData

    //----------------------------------------------------------------
    // scale the raw input data point to the circular axis radius
    //----------------------------------------------------------------
    public int iScale( double d, int l, double dm )
    {
        int x = 0;
        if ( dm > 0.0 )
        {
            x = (int) (l * d / dm);
        }
        return x;
    }

    //----------------------------------------------------------------
    // update the Border
    //----------------------------------------------------------------
    public void updateBorder( Object b )
    {
        String d = "";
        d = b.toString();
        outsideBorder = Integer.parseInt( d );
        repaint();
    }

    //----------------------------------------------------------------
    // update the Plot Width
    //----------------------------------------------------------------
    public void updatePlotWidth( Object w )
    {
        String d = "";
        d = w.toString();
        plotDiameter = Integer.parseInt( d );
        repaint();
    }

    //----------------------------------------------------------------
    // update the Font Size
    //----------------------------------------------------------------
```

Table 11-23 Listing: UI_Plotter.java *(continued)*

```java
    public void updateFontSize( Object w )
    {
        String d = "";
        d = w.toString();
        fontSize = Integer.parseInt( d );
        textFont = new Font("Monaco", Font.BOLD, fontSize );
        repaint();
    }

    //--------------------------------------------------------------
    // update the slider
    //--------------------------------------------------------------
    public void updateSlider( String sliderType,
                              String sliderCaption,
                              int value,
                              int index,
                              int n )
    {
        sType[index] = sliderType;
        sCapt[index] = sliderCaption;
        sThreshold[index] = value;
        NumParameters = n;
        repaint();
    }
} // end UI_Plotter
```

Table 11-24 Listing: UI_SendMain.java

```java
import javax.comm.*;
import javax.imageio.ImageIO;
import javax.swing.*;
import javax.swing.AbstractButton;
import javax.swing.border.*;
import javax.swing.ButtonModel;
import javax.swing.JCheckBox;
import javax.swing.JFrame;
import javax.swing.event.*;
import javax.swing.event.ChangeEvent;
import javax.swing.event.ChangeListener;
import javax.swing.plaf.*;
import javax.swing.text.NumberFormatter;
import javax.swing.Timer;

import java.sql.*;
import java.sql.Connection;
import java.sql.DriverManager;
import java.sql.SQLException;


import java.applet.*;
import java.awt.*;
import java.awt.BorderLayout;
import java.awt.Color;
import java.awt.Container;
import java.awt.event.*;
import java.awt.event.ActionEvent;
import java.awt.event.ActionListener;
import java.awt.event.ItemEvent;
import java.awt.event.ItemListener;
import java.awt.event.KeyEvent;
import java.awt.Graphics;
import java.awt.Image;
import java.awt.List;
import java.awt.Scrollbar;
```

Table 11-24 Listing: UI_SendMain.java *(continued)*

```java
import java.awt.Toolkit;
import java.io.*;
import java.io.BufferedInputStream;
import java.lang.*;
import java.lang.Math;
import java.lang.Thread;
import java.net.*;
import java.net.URL;
import java.text.*;
import java.text.DecimalFormat;
import java.util.Date;
import java.util.GregorianCalendar;
import java.util.Properties;
import java.util.Vector;

import javax.swing.border.*;
import javax.swing.event.*;
import javax.swing.JInternalFrame;
import javax.swing.JDesktopPane;
import javax.swing.JMenu;
import javax.swing.JMenuItem;
import javax.swing.JMenuBar;
import javax.swing.JFrame;
import javax.swing.KeyStroke;


// ************************************************************
//
// UI_SendMain.java
//
// Transmits vitals parameters to UI_PlotMain.java
//
// Author: J. Zaleski
//
// ************************************************************

public class UI_SendMain extends JPanel
{
    JDesktopPane desktop;
    public UI_Send ui_send;
    private JButton startB;
    private JButton stopB;
    private JButton exitB;
    public static int  maxWidth = 400;
    public static int  maxHeight = 300;

    //-----------------------------------------------------------
    // Constructor
    //-----------------------------------------------------------
    public UI_SendMain ()
    {
        ui_send = new UI_Send();
        startB = new JButton("Start");
stopB = new JButton("Stop");
exitB = new JButton("Exit");
stopB.setEnabled(false); // begin with this disabled
exitB.setEnabled(true);
startB.addActionListener( new ActionListener() {
            public void actionPerformed(ActionEvent e1 ) {

                // disable to stop more "start" requests

                startB.setEnabled( false );

                // thread to run the counter
```

Table 11-24 Listing: UI_SendMain.java *(continued)*

```
            Thread counterThread =
                new Thread( ui_send, "UI ui_send" );
            counterThread.start();
            stopB.setEnabled( true );
            stopB.requestFocus();
        }
    });

    stopB.addActionListener( new ActionListener() {
        public void actionPerformed(ActionEvent e3 ) {
            stopB.setEnabled( false );
            ui_send.stopClock();
            startB.setEnabled( true );
            startB.requestFocus();
        }
    });

    exitB.addActionListener( new ActionListener() {
        public void actionPerformed(ActionEvent e4 ) {
            ui_send.stopClock();
            System.exit(0);
        }
    });

    JPanel innerButtonP = new JPanel();
    innerButtonP.setLayout( new GridLayout(0, 1, 0, 3 ) );
    innerButtonP.add(startB);
    innerButtonP.add(stopB);
    innerButtonP.add(exitB);

    JPanel buttonP = new JPanel();
    buttonP.setLayout(new BorderLayout());
    buttonP.add(innerButtonP, BorderLayout.NORTH);

    JPanel listPanel = new JPanel();
    listPanel.add( ui_send.scrollingList1 );
    listPanel.add( ui_send.scrollingList2 );

    this.setLayout( new BorderLayout(10, 10) );
    this.setBorder(new EmptyBorder(20,20,20,20));
    this.add(buttonP, BorderLayout.WEST);
    this.add(ui_send, BorderLayout.CENTER);
    this.add(listPanel, BorderLayout.EAST );
}

//------------------------------------------------------------
// Main
//------------------------------------------------------------
public static void main( String[] args )
{
    UI_SendMain uis = new UI_SendMain();
    JFrame jf = new JFrame("Second Counter");
    jf.setContentPane( uis );
    jf.setSize( maxWidth, maxHeight );
    jf.setVisible( true );
    jf.setLocation( 100,100);
    jf.addWindowListener( new WindowAdapter() {
        public void windowClosing(WindowEvent e ) {
            System.exit( 0 );
        }
    });
} // end Main
} // end UI_SendMain
```

Table 11-25 Listing: UI_Send.java

```
import javax.comm.*;
import javax.imageio.ImageIO;
import javax.swing.*;
import javax.swing.AbstractButton;
import javax.swing.border.*;
import javax.swing.ButtonModel;
import javax.swing.JCheckBox;
import javax.swing.JFrame;
import javax.swing.event.*;
import javax.swing.event.ChangeEvent;
import javax.swing.event.ChangeListener;
import javax.swing.plaf.*;
import javax.swing.text.NumberFormatter;
import javax.swing.Timer;

import java.sql.*;
import java.sql.Connection;
import java.sql.DriverManager;
import java.sql.SQLException;

import java.applet.*;
import java.awt.*;
import java.awt.BorderLayout;
import java.awt.Color;
import java.awt.Container;
import java.awt.event.*;
import java.awt.event.ActionEvent;
import java.awt.event.ActionListener;
import java.awt.event.ItemEvent;
import java.awt.event.ItemListener;
import java.awt.event.KeyEvent;
import java.awt.Graphics;
import java.awt.Image;
import java.awt.List;
import java.awt.Scrollbar;
import java.awt.Toolkit;
import java.io.*;
import java.io.BufferedInputStream;
import java.lang.*;
import java.lang.Math;
import java.lang.Thread;
import java.net.*;
import java.net.URL;
import java.text.*;
import java.text.DecimalFormat;
import java.util.Date;
import java.util.GregorianCalendar;
import java.util.Properties;
import java.util.Vector;

import javax.swing.border.*;
import javax.swing.event.*;
import javax.swing.JInternalFrame;
import javax.swing.JDesktopPane;
import javax.swing.JMenu;
import javax.swing.JMenuItem;
import javax.swing.JMenuBar;
import javax.swing.JFrame;
import javax.swing.KeyStroke;
import java.util.Random;

// ******************************************
//
// UI_Send.java
//
// Called by UI_SendMain.java
```

Table 11-25 Listing: UI_Send.java *(continued)*

```
//
// Author: J. Zaleski
//
// *******************************************
public class UI_Send extends JComponent
                    implements Runnable, ListSelectionListener
{
    static int MaxParameters = 10;
    static int MaxValues = 300;
    public boolean debug = true;
    public int sleepDelay = 1500; // 1.5 seconds
    private volatile boolean suspended;
    private volatile boolean keepRunning;
    private Font paintFont;

    String[] data = new String[40];
    String[] returnValues = new String[MaxValues];
    String[] returnDTs= new String[MaxValues];
    String[][] matrix = new String[MaxParameters][MaxValues];
    Socket clientConnection = null;
    Socket inbound = null;
    ServerSocket welcomeSocket = null;

    /* MS Access SQL Connection */

    Connection conn;
    Statement st;
    ResultSetMetaData rsmd;
    ResultSet rec;
    String dbURL = "jdbc:odbc:uiDesign";
    String uname = "";
    String pword = "";
    int nCols = 0;

    /* Lists for scrollpanes */

    DefaultListModel model1 = new DefaultListModel();
    DefaultListModel model2 = new DefaultListModel();
    JList List1 = new JList( model1 );
    JList List2 = new JList( model2 );
    int visible = 7;
    staticint TotalListItems = 0;
    JScrollPane scrollingList1;
    JScrollPane scrollingList2;

    /* Arrays to hold parameter values */

    protected String  [] paramName = new String[MaxParameters];
    protected int  [] selectedParamNum = new int[MaxParameters];
    protected static intnumberSelectedParams = 0;

    //-----------------------------------------------------------
    // Constructor
    //-----------------------------------------------------------
    public UI_Send()
    {
        getParameterList();
    }

    //-----------------------------------------------------------
    // Get parameter list
    //-----------------------------------------------------------
    public void getParameterList()
    {
        scrollingList1 = new JScrollPane( List1 );
        scrollingList2 = new JScrollPane( List2 );
```

341

Table 11-25 Listing: UI_Send.java *(continued)*

```
    // List panels

    List1.setFont( new Font( "mono", Font.BOLD, 12 ) );
    List1.setForeground( Color.yellow );
    List1.setBackground( Color.black );
    List1.setEnabled( true );
    List1.setPrototypeCellValue("My Sample Item");
    List1.addListSelectionListener( this );
    List2.setFont( new Font( "mono", Font.BOLD, 12 ) );
    List2.setForeground( Color.red );
    List2.setBackground( Color.black );
    List2.setEnabled( true );
    List2.setPrototypeCellValue("My Sample Item");
    List2.addListSelectionListener( this );

    String dataObjects = "";

    mdbConn();
    int nCols = qryConnGen( "Parms", "parmName", paramName );
    clsConn();

    // Add items to List1

    for ( int i = 0; i < paramName.length; i++ )
    {
        model1.add(i, paramName[i]);
    }

    // Listen for multiple clicks on a single item

    List1.addMouseListener( new MouseAdapter() {
        public void mouseClicked( MouseEvent evt ) {
            JList list = (JList)evt.getSource();
            if ( evt.getClickCount() == 2 ) { // Double-click
                // Get item index
                int index = list.locationToIndex(evt.getPoint());
            } else if ( evt.getClickCount() == 3 ) { // Triple-click
                // Get item index
                int index = list.locationToIndex(evt.getPoint());
                // Note that this list will receive a double-click
                // event before this triple-click event.
            }
        }
    });

} // end getParameterList()

//-----------------------------------------------------------
// valueChanged -- list listeners
//-----------------------------------------------------------
public void valueChanged(ListSelectionEvent e) {
    if ( e.getValueIsAdjusting() == false ) {
        if ( List1.getSelectedIndex() == -1 ) {
                /* Do nothing if list is empty */
        }
        else {
            // Get the selected item from List1

            String name = List1.getSelectedValue().toString();

            // Check to see whether item is in List2 already

            int size2 = List2.getModel().getSize();

            // If something in List2, find out what it is and add
```

Table 11-25 Listing: UI_Send.java *(continued)*

```
                  // to List2 only if does not exist

                  boolean inList2 = false;
                  int pos = -1;
                  for ( int i = 0; i < size2; i++ )
                  {
                      String item2 = List2.getModel().getElemen-
tAt(i).toString();
                      if ( item2.equals( name ) ) {
                          inList2 = true;
                          pos = i;
                      }
                  }
                  if ( !inList2 ) {
                      model2.addElement(name);
                      size2 = List2.getModel().getSize();
                      numberSelectedParams = size2;
                      for ( int j = 0; j < MaxParameters; j++ )
                          paramName[j] = "";
                      for ( int k = 0; k < size2; k++ )
                      {
                          paramName[k] =
                          List2.getModel().getElementAt(k).toString();;
                      }
                  }
                  if ( inList2 ) {
                      model2.remove(pos);
                      size2 = List2.getModel().getSize();
                      numberSelectedParams = size2;
                      for ( int j = 0; j < MaxParameters; j++ )
                          paramName[j] = "";
                      for ( int k = 0; k < size2; k++ )
                      {
                          paramName[k] =
                          List2.getModel().getElementAt(k).toString();;
                      }
                  }
                  numberSelectedParams = size2;
                  retrieveData( paramName, size2);
              }
          }
      }

      //-----------------------------------------------------------
      // run()
      //-----------------------------------------------------------
      public void run()
      {
          runClock();
      }

      //-----------------------------------------------------------
      // runClock -- Executes thread
      //-----------------------------------------------------------
      public void runClock()
      {
          keepRunning = true;
          try {
              Socket skt = new Socket("localhost", 1234);
              PrintWriter out = new PrintWriter(skt.getOutputStream(),
true);
              System.out.println( " keepRunning = " + keepRunning );
              while ( keepRunning ) {
                  if ( keepRunning = false ) break;
                  for ( int m = 0; m < MaxValues; m++ ) {
                      for (int k = 0; k < numberSelectedParams; k++ ) {
```

Table 11-25 Listing: UI_Send.java *(continued)*

```
                        System.out.print("Sending string: '" +
                                    matrix[k][m] + "'\n");
                        out.println( matrix[k][m] );
                        Thread.sleep( sleepDelay );
                    } // for k
                } // for m
            } // end while
        } catch ( Exception e ) {
            System.out.println( "Attempting TCP binding " + e );
        } // try
    } // run

    //---------------------------------------------------------
    // Retrieve data from database
    //---------------------------------------------------------
    public void retrieveData( String [] pn, int n )
    {
        int Rows = 0;
        int Rows1= 0;

        // Open database connection

        mdbConn();

        // Retrieve data and copy to matrix

        for( int i = 0; i < n; i++ ) {
            System.out.println( " pn = " + pn[i] );
            Rows = qryConnGen( pn[i], pn[i], returnValues );
            Rows1= qryConnGen( pn[i], "DateTime", returnDTs );
            if ( Rows > MaxValues ) Rows = MaxValues;
            for( int j = 0; j < Rows; j++ ) {
                matrix[i][j] = pn[i] + " " + returnValues[j] + " " +
                                returnDTs[j];
            }
        }
        clsConn();
    }

    //---------------------------------------------------------
    // mdbConn -- Make database connection.
    //---------------------------------------------------------
    public void mdbConn()
    {
        try
        {
// JDBC Driver

            Class.forName("sun.jdbc.odbc.JdbcOdbcDriver");

            // JDBC url link to USER DSN object in
            // Settings->Control Panel->Administrative Tools->ODBC

            String url = "jdbc:odbc:uiDesign";

            // User, Pword set to nothing

            String user = "";
            String password = "";

            // Connect to database

            conn = DriverManager.getConnection(url,user,password);

            // Create a statement object instance
```

Table 11-25 Listing: UI_Send.java *(continued)*

```java
        st = conn.createStatement();

        // System.out.println( " Connected to database");
    }
    catch(Exception e)
    {
        System.out.println("Error  mdbConn()- "+e.toString());
    }
}


//----------------------------------------------------------
// qryConn -- Query database with WHERE clause.
//----------------------------------------------------------
public String qryConn( String tableName,
                       String queryItem,
                       String parameterValue,
                       String whereClauseItem )
{
    String columnValue = null;
    try {
        // Query the database for data objects.
        // Select two objects.

        String queryString = "SELECT " + queryItem +
                             " FROM " + tableName +
                             " WHERE " + whereClauseItem +
                             " = '" + parameterValue +
                             "'";
        rec = st.executeQuery( queryString );

        // Get some data about the data.

        rsmd = rec.getMetaData();
        int nCols = rsmd.getColumnCount();

        // Print all instances of these objects out

        while(rec.next())
        {
            for (int i = 1; i <= nCols; i++)
            {
                columnValue = rec.getString(i);
            }
        } // end while
    }
    catch(Exception e)
    {
        System.out.println("Error in qryConn - "+e.toString());
    }
    return columnValue;
}

//----------------------------------------------------------
// clsConn -- Close database connection.
//----------------------------------------------------------
public void clsConn()
{
    try {
        conn.close();
        st.close();
    }
    catch ( Exception e )
    {
        System.err.println( " Cannot close database " + e );
    }
}
```

Table 11-25 Listing: UI_Send.java *(continued)*

```
//------------------------------------------------------------
// qryConnGen -- Query database - NO WHERE clause.
//------------------------------------------------------------
public int qryConnGen( String tableName,
                       String queryItem,
                       String[] returnValues )
{
    String columnValue = null;
    int nRows = 0;
    try {
        // Query the database for data objects.
        // Select two objects.

        String queryString = "SELECT " + queryItem +
                             " FROM " + tableName;

        rec = st.executeQuery( queryString );

        // Get some data about the data.

        rsmd = rec.getMetaData();
        nCols = rsmd.getColumnCount();

        // Print all instances of these objects out

        while(rec.next() && nRows < MaxValues )
        {
            for (int i = 1; i <= nCols; i++)
            {
                columnValue = rec.getString(i);
                returnValues[nRows] = columnValue;
                nRows++;
                System.out.println( " columnValue......" + columnValue
);
            }
        } // end while
    }
    catch(Exception e)
    {
        System.out.println("Error qryConnGen() - "+e.toString());
    }
    return nRows;
}


//------------------------------------------------------------
// qryConnGen2 -- Query database - NO WHERE clause.
//------------------------------------------------------------
public int qryConnGen2( String tableName,
                        String queryItem,
                        int q,
                        String[][] returnValues )
{
    String columnValue = null;
    int nRows = 0;
    try {
        // Query the database for data objects.
        // Select two objects.

        String queryString = "SELECT " + queryItem +
                             " FROM " + tableName;

        rec = st.executeQuery( queryString );

        // Get some data about the data.
```

Table 11-25 Listing: UI_Send.java *(continued)*

```java
            rsmd = rec.getMetaData();
            nCols = rsmd.getColumnCount();

            // Print all instances of these objects out

            while(rec.next())
            {
                for (int i = 1; i <= nCols; i++)
                {
                    columnValue = rec.getString(i);
                    returnValues[q][nRows] = columnValue;
                    nRows++;
                }
            } // end while
        }
        catch(Exception e)
        {
            System.out.println("Error qryConnGen2() - "+e.toString());
        }
        return nRows;
    }

    //-----------------------------------------------------------
    // stopClock -- Stop the clock
    //-----------------------------------------------------------
    public void stopClock()
    {
        keepRunning = false;
    }
} // UI_Send
```

List of Abbreviations

AAMI	Association for the Advancement of Medical Instrumentation
ABG	Arterial Blood Gas
ABP	Arterial Blood Pressure
ACC	American College of Cardiology
ACCE	American College of Clinical Engineers
ACS	Automatic Control System
ADT	Admission, Transfer, and Discharge
AFEHCT	Association for Electronic Health Care Transactions
ANSI	American National Standards Institute
API	Application Programming Interface
APOC	Architecture for Medical Device Communication at-Point-of-Care
ASCII	American Standard Code for Information Interchange
ASTM	American Society for Testing and Materials
BP	Blood Pressure
CABG	Coronary Artery Bypass Grafting
CCR	Continuity of Care Record
CDRH	Centers for Devices and Radiological Health
CDS	Clinical Decision Support
CFR	Code of Federal Regulations
CHR	Computerized Health Record
CIE	Computer Interface Emulator
CIMIT	Center for Integration of Medicine & Innovative Technology
CMR	Computerized Medical Record
COPD	Chronic Obstructive Pulmonary Disease
CPAP	Continuous Positive Airway Pressure
CPOE	Computerized Physician Order Entry
CPR	Computer-based Patient Record
CPRI	Computer-based Patient Record Institute
CRC	Cyclic Redundancy Check
CT	Computed Tomography
CVR	Coded Value Response
DARPA	Defense Advanced Research Projects Agency
DCI	Digital Communications Interface
.dll	Dynamic Link Libraries
DP	Data Processing Manager
DWT	Discrete Wavelet Transform
EAP	Extensible Application Protocol

ECG, EKG	Electrocardiogram
EHR	Electronic Health Record
EMR	Electronic Medical Record
EPR	Electronic Patient Record
ETT	Endotracheal Tube
FDA	Food and Drug Administration
FV	Finding Value
GMP	Good Manufacturing Practice
HFMA	Healthcare Financial Management Association
HHS	Department of Health and Human Services
HIMSS	Health Information Management Systems Society
HIS	Health Information System
HL7	Health Level Seven
HR	Pulse or Heart Rate
HTML	Hyper-Text Markup Language
I & O	Intake & Output
ICU	Intensive Care Unit
IEEE	Institute of Electrical and Electronics Engineers
IHE	Integrating the Health Enterprise
IMV	Intermittent Mandatory Ventilation
IOM	Institute of Medicine
IP	Internet Protocol
IR	Infrared
IRB	Institutional Review Board
IrDA	Infrared Device Association
ISO	International Standards Organization
ISP	Internet Service Provider
LAN	Local Area Network
LIS	Laboratory Information Systems
LOINC	Logical Observation Identifiers Names and Codes
LVAD	Left Ventricular Assist Device(s)
MAC	Media Access Control
MD PnP	Medical Device "Plug-and-Play"
MDDL	Medical Device Data Language
MDDS	Medical Device Data System(s)
MDER	Medical Device Encoding Rule(s)
MDG	Medical Device Gateway
MIB	Medical Information Bus
MPEG	Moving Picture Experts Group
MRI	Magnetic Resonance Imaging
MRN	Medical Record Number
MSH	Message Header
MV	Minute Ventilation
NIC	Network Interface Card
NIST	National Institute for Standards and Technology

NIBP	Non-invasive Blood Pressure
NM	Numeric Value
OBR	Observation Request Segment
OBX	Observation Record or Result
ORU	(HL7) Observation Report—Unsolicited (also ORU^R01)
PAN	Patient Account Number
PDA	Personal Digital Assistant
PHR	Personal Health Record
PID	Patient Identification
PII	Patient Identifying Information (or Personal Identifying Information)
PMA	Pre-Market Approval
PMN	Pre-Market Notification
PSRS	Pennsylvania Safety Reporting System
PTN	Patient Number
QoS	Quality of Service
QSR	Quality System Regulation(s)
RFID	Radio Frequency Identification
RIM	Reference Information Model
RSBI	Rapid-Shallow Breathing Index
RR	Respiratory Rate
RSNA	Radiological Society of North America
RSS	Root-Sum-Square
RTSP	Real-Time Streaming Protocol
SDK	Software Development Kit
SDO	Standards Development Organization(s)
SEDES	Standard for Electronic Data Exchange specification
SICU	Surgical Intensive Care Unit
SPD	Send Patient Data
SPP	Serial Port Profile
SQL	Structured Query Language
SSE	Sum-of-Squares Error
SSID	Service Set Identifier
TCP/IP	Transmission Control Protocol / Internet Protocol
TV	Tidal Volume
UDP	User (or Universal) Datagram Protocol
UI	User Interface
UPC	Universal Product Code
USB	Universal Serial Bus
WAN	Wide Area Network
WEDI	Workgroup on Electronic Data Interchange
WEP	Wireless Equivalency Protocol
WLAN	Wireless Local Area Network
WPA	Wi-Fi-Protected Access

Index

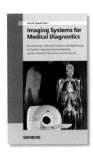

Arnulf Oppelt (Editor)

Imaging Systems for Medical Diagnostics

Fundamentals, technical solutions and applications for systems applying ionization radiation, nuclear magnetic resonance and ultrasound

2nd revised and enlarged edition, 2005,
996 pages, 692 illustrations, 23 tables, hardcover
ISBN 978-3-89578-226-8
€ 119.00 / sFr 188.00

The book provides a comprehensive compilation of fundamentals, technical solutions and applications for medical imaging systems. It is intended as a handbook for students in biomedical engineering, for medical physicists, and for engineers working on medical technologies, as well as for lecturers at universities and engineering schools. For qualified personnel at hospitals, and physicians working with these instruments it serves as a basic source of information. This also applies for service engineers and marketing specialists.

The book starts with the representation of the physical basics of image processing, implying some knowledge of Fourier transforms. After that, experienced authors describe technical solutions and applications for imaging systems in medical diagnostics. The applications comprise the fields of X-ray diagnostics, computed tomography, nuclear medical diagnostics, magnetic resonance imaging, sonography, molecular imaging and hybrid systems. Considering the increasing importance of software based solutions, emphasis is also laid on the imaging software platform and hospital information systems.

Contents

Physiology of vision · Subjective assessment of image quality · Image rendering · Image fusion · Navigation · X-ray and gamma-radiation · Concepts in magnetic resonance imaging · Physical principles of medical ultrasound · System theory · Principles of image reconstruction · Image displays · X-ray systems · Computed X-ray tomography · Nuclear medicine · Magnetic resonance imaging · Ultrasound imaging systems · Special and hybrid systems · Molecular imaging · Software platform for medical imaging · Computer-aided detection and diagnosis (CAD) · Hospital information systems.

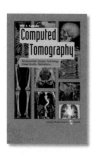

Willi A. Kalender

Computed Tomography

Fundamentals, System Technology,
Image Quality, Applications

2nd revised and enlarged edition, 2005,
306 pages, 130 illustrations, 18 tables, hardcover
ISBN 978-3-89578-216-9
€ 49.90 / sFr 80.00

The book offers a comprehensive and user-oriented description of the theoretical and technical system fundamentals of computed tomography (CT) for a wide readership, from conventional single-slice acquisitions to volume acquisition with multi-slice and cone-beam spiral CT. It covers in detail all characteristic parameters relevant for image quality and all performance features significant for clinical application. Readers will thus be informed how to use a CT system to an optimum depending on the different diagnostic requirements. This includes a detailed discussion about the dose required and about dose measurements as well as how to reduce dose in CT. All considerations pay special attention to spiral CT and to new developments towards advanced multi-slice and cone-beam CT.

For the 2nd edition many sections of this book have been updated. In particular, material on new x-ray technology, on 64-slice spiral and cone-beam CT scanning have been added.

The enclosed CD-ROM offers attractive case studies, including many examples from the most recent 64-slice acquisitions, and interactive exercises for image viewing and manipulation.

This book is intended for all those who work daily, regularly or even only occasionally with CT: physicians, radiographers, engineers, technicians and physicists. A glossary describes all the important technical terms in alphabetical order.

Contents

System concepts · System components · Image reconstruction · Spiral CT · Multi-slice spiral CT · Dynamic CT · Quantitative CT · Image quality · Spatial resolution · Contrast · Pixel noise · Homogeneity · Routine and special applications · 3D displays · Post-processing · Quality assurance

www.publicis.de/books